高等学校
"十四五"医学规划新形态教材

 浙江省普通本科高校
"十四五"重点教材

（供卫生检验与检疫、医学检验技术、预防医学等专业用）

卫生检验与检疫专业英语

English for Health Inspection and Quarantine

U0304964

主　编　李　敏　楼永良

副主编　徐向东　黄东萍　李迎丽

编　者　（按姓氏汉语拼音排序）

安　康（山东第一医科大学）　　　柏琴琴（南华大学）

陈　阳（福建医科大学）　　　　　关万春（温州医科大学）

黄东萍（广西医科大学）　　　　　黄　颖（安徽医科大学）

李　敏（温州医科大学）　　　　　李　琴（首都医科大学）

李淑荣（包头医学院）　　　　　　李　祥（温州医科大学）

李雪霞（海南医学院）　　　　　　李迎丽（重庆医科大学）

楼永良（温州医科大学）　　　　　王　涛（武汉科技大学）

吴淑春（杭州医学院）　　　　　　徐向东（河北医科大学）

杨红茹（河北大学）　　　　　　　张定梅（中山大学）

中国教育出版传媒集团

高等教育出版社·北京

内容简介

本书共 24 章，主要介绍分析化学、仪器分析、微生物学检验、理化检验、流行病学、实验室安全等领域的专业基础知识与技术。教材第一模块为绪论，第二模块为专业词汇特征与结构分析，第三与第四模块介绍了微生物与理化检验知识，第五与第六模块讨论了检疫与实验室安全等内容。本书的特色在于围绕专业与人才培养理念和需求，从英语听、说、读、写结合的角度，分专题详细介绍专业领域方面的应用。

本书结构新颖、逻辑清晰，启发性与引导性较强，可供卫生检验与检疫、医学检验技术、预防医学等专业教师与学生使用，也可作为相关专业研究人员的参考书。

图书在版编目（CIP）数据

卫生检验与检疫专业英语 / 李敏，楼永良主编. --
北京：高等教育出版社，2023.11
供卫生检验与检疫、医学检验技术、预防医学等专业
用
ISBN 978-7-04-060529-7

Ⅰ. ①卫… Ⅱ. ①李… ②楼… Ⅲ. ①卫生检验 – 英
语 – 教材②卫生检疫 – 英语 – 教材 Ⅳ. ①R115②R185

中国国家版本馆 CIP 数据核字（2023）第 089395 号

Weisheng Jianyan Yu Jianyi Zhuanye Yingyu

策划编辑 张映桥 责任编辑 张映桥 封面设计 王 洋 责任印制 朱 琦

出版发行	高等教育出版社	网 址	http://www.hep.edu.cn
社 址	北京市西城区德外大街4号		http://www.hep.com.cn
邮政编码	100120	网上订购	http://www.hepmall.com.cn
印 刷	北京宏伟双华印刷有限公司		http://www.hepmall.com
开 本	787mm×1092mm 1/16		http://www.hepmall.cn
印 张	19.75		
字 数	468 千字	版 次	2023 年 11 月第 1 版
购书热线	010-58581118	印 次	2023 年 11 月第 1 次印刷
咨询电话	400-810-0598	定 价	49.80元

本书如有缺页、倒页、脱页等质量问题，请到所购图书销售部门联系调换
版权所有 侵权必究
物 料 号 60529-00

新形态教材·数字课程（基础版）

卫生检验与
检疫专业英语

主编　李敏　楼永良

登录方法：

1. 电脑访问 http://abooks.hep.com.cn/60529，或微信扫描下方二维码，打开新形态教材小程序。

2. 注册并登录，进入"个人中心"。

3. 刮开封底数字课程账号涂层，手动输入 20 位密码或通过小程序扫描二维码，完成防伪码绑定。

4. 绑定成功后，即可开始本数字课程的学习。

绑定后一年为数字课程使用有效期。如有使用问题，请点击页面下方的"答疑"按钮。

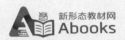
新形态教材网 Abooks

关于我们 ｜ 联系我们　　登录/注册

卫生检验与检疫专业英语

李敏　楼永良

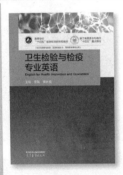

开始学习　　收藏

　　卫生检验与检疫专业英语数字课程与纸质教材一体化设计，紧密配合。数字课程涵盖教学课件、自测题等资源，充分运用多种形式的媒体资源，与纸质教材相互配合，丰富了知识呈现形式。在提升课程教学效果的同时，为学习者提供更多思考与探索的空间。

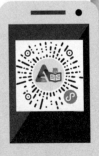

http://abooks.hep.com.cn/60529

前　言

随着健康中国战略持续推进，卫生检验与检疫专业人才在卫生健康服务领域的地位和重要性日益凸显。随着世界范围内知识与信息技术交流的增强，卫生检验领域岗位工作任务的更迭及新技术、新业态和新需求的不断涌现，对高素质、高技能卫生检验与检疫复合型人才的培养提出了更高的要求。

卫生检验与检疫专业英语是面向高年级本科生开设的课程，旨在培养学生阅读和理解外文专业文献的能力、以英语进行学术交流和书面科学阐述的意识与能力，并为英文专业写作打下基础，从而提升学生在专业领域内的英语综合运用能力与国际化视野，使卫生检验与检疫专业教学与人才培养更上一个台阶。

本教材根据专业人才培养目标和要求，遵循"三基、五性、三特定"的原则，构建了内容多样和方式灵活的综合学习体系，结合技术赋能的高效教学，达到学科交叉、分模块进行能力培养的目标，从而培养学生语言应用与思维能力。

全书共24章，均为经过精心选择且贴近专业培养与工作岗位实际，又适合在校大学生学习的内容。每章围绕卫生检验与检疫某特定主题开展，附有相应的词汇表、练习题和参考答案，内容相对独立，有利于教师在教学过程中自主选择教学内容和学生的课后知识巩固。在纸质教材的基础上，本教材还为读者提供了网络数字资源，更有利于个性化自主学习。

本教材编写团队由来自全国15所高等院校长期在教学一线工作的专家组成。高等教育出版社为本书出版做了大量的工作，温州医科大学为本书的编写提供了诸多支持与帮助，本书的编写也得到全体编者工作单位与领导的大力支持，在此一并表示衷心感谢。

限于编写团队的学识水平，书中难免存在不足之处，敬请广大同仁与读者批评指正。

李　敏　楼永良

2023 年 5 月

Contents

PART I Introduction

PART II Terminology

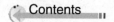

PART III   Microbiology

PART IV   Physicochemical Analysis

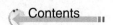

PART V Sanitary Quarantine

PART VI Lab Management

PART I
Introduction

Chapter 1
Overview of Health Inspection and Quarantine

Learning objectives:

- Understand the concept of HIQ.
- Understand the significance of HIQ.
- Be familiar with the development history of HIQ .
- Gain awareness of the HIQ-related laws.

1.1 Concept and Significance of HIQ

Public health is the science and art of preventing disease, prolonging life, and promoting the health of all people through the organized efforts and informed choices of society, organizations, public and private, communities, and individuals. One of the core and foundational parts of public health is Health Inspection and Quarantine (hereinafter referred to as HIQ). HIQ is the science and technology focused on disease surveillance, environment surveillance, and pathogenic microorganisms diagnostic testing for public health; it also offers measures to prevent the spread of communicable diseases, pests, and other harmful agents domestic and abroad.

HIQ plays a crucial role in protecting public health, promoting international trade, and safeguarding ecosystems and the environment. The importance of HIQ is reflected in the following four aspects. Firstly, it plays an essential role in ensuring the safety of both living and working environments, as well as food safety. Scientists of HIQ test water, soil, air, food, manufactured products, and specimens from people (such as blood, stool, sputum, and urine) that could harm humans, animals, or the environment. They also identify harmful chemicals in people's bodies, such as lead and pesticides. Secondly, HIQ provides infectious diseases monitoring. It includes carrying out identification of the pathogen, confirming the nature of the epidemic situation, tracking the source of infectious diseases, and finding out the potential source of infection. Scientists of HIQ conduct monitoring to detect new or re-emerging diseases, such as COVID-19, Ebola virus disease, Zika virus disease, and influenza, to provide early warning for public health. Thirdly, HIQ promotes international trade. It involves inspecting and monitoring people, animals, plants, and goods entering or leaving a country or region to ensure they meet certain health and safety standards. Its measures are necessary to protect against the introduction of pests and diseases from foreign countries, and they facilitate the movement of goods across borders by ensuring compliance with international regulations and standards. Fourthly, knowledge gained from HIQ can also be applied in the field of clinical medicine. It can aid in the development of improved diagnostic tests, new drugs, vaccines, and other medical technologies to enhance clinical outcomes for patients. It also can provide valuable information on the epidemiology and pathogenesis of infectious diseases.

HIQ major is becoming increasingly important with the improvement of health awareness and living standards. The goal of this major is to educate students with a broad understanding and expertise in public health, especially in health inspection and quarantine. Students of HIQ need to learn courses such as epidemiology, biostatistics, environmental health, physical and chemical analysis, microbiological testing, etc. These courses aim to help students in building the preliminary ability to deal with public health emergencies along with developing critical thinking and innovative ideas. A student of HIQ can work for public health laboratories in disease control and prevention institutions, customs, hospitals, and related institutions or companies. One question that is frequently asked is: What are the differences between public health laboratories and clinical laboratories? The answer is: public health laboratories focus on safeguarding the health of the general population, while hospital and commercial clinical laboratories primarily provide support for the diagnosis and treatment of individual patients. For a laboratory scientist working in HIQ, dealing with non-routine situations is commonplace. They are heroes who work behind-the-scenes. For instance, after conducting a *Salmonella* investigation on Monday, they may have to deal with a chemical contamination incident on Tuesday. There are many career opportunities for students and young professionals who want to challenge themselves.

1.2   Brief History of HIQ

The primal health inspection and quarantine has been mentioned since biblical times. In the Biblical book of Leviticus, written in the 7th century BC or perhaps earlier, it described the procedure for separating out people infected with the skin disease Tzaraath. The word "quarantine" is believed to be derived from the Venetian language, specifically from the Italian words "quaranta giorni", which mean "forty days". In the 14th century, ships arriving in Venice from overseas were required to anchor offshore for 40 days before landing as a preventive measure against the spread of plague. The practice was based on the belief that the incubation period for the disease was 40 days. So, if a ship waited offshore for this period and nobody fell ill, it was considered safe to enter the port. The consciousness of HIQ is ubiquitous in different cultures and countries. China's history of HIQ can be traced back to ancient times. As early as the Han Dynasty, there were records of adopting isolation measures to prevent the spread of diseases. During the Ming and Qing Dynasties in China, the isolation and quarantine system for epidemics was further developed through a series of measures. One of the most significant developments was the establishment of designated quarantine stations at key ports of entry throughout the country, where incoming travelers and cargo would be examined and isolated if necessary. For example, in 1873, a cholera epidemic broke out in Siam (now Thailand) and various areas of the Malay Archipelago. The customs offices in Shanghai and Xiamen established and implemented China's earliest quarantine regulations. According to the regulations, if a ship came from an epidemic area, it was ordered to raise a yellow flag on the foremast and undergo inspection by medical officers.

The education on HIQ in China can be traced back to late Qing Dynasty. In 1902, the "Beiyang Military Medical School" was founded in Tianjin and was then renamed as "Army Military Medical School" in 1906. Dr. Wu Lien Teh, plague fighter and father of the Chinese public health system, was once vice-president of this school. In 1910, a deadly epidemic broke out in Northeast China. Dr. Wu discovered *Yersinia Pestis* in the body tissues and concluded that the epidemic was pneumonic plague, which could be transmitted by human breath or sputum. On the advice of Dr. Wu, corpses and coffins of plague victims were gathered and cremated to cut off the transmission of the disease. It turned out to be the turning point of the epidemic.

Pioneers of HIQ education in China include scholars such as Gongji Lin and Yingchuan Li. In 1934 and 1936, Gongji Lin published *the Water Inspection Law* and *Sanitary Chemistry*, which are considered as groundbreaking works in the field of HIQ education. Yingchuan Li, on the other hand, made significant contributions to the development of HIQ education through his research and teaching in the 1950s and 60s. In 1946, Yingchuan Li, who worked in Shanghai Commodity Inspection Bureau, compiled and published the *Food Inspection and Analysis Method*. In the preface, the author said that the book was modified according to the *Food Inspection and Analysis* document written by the US scholar Leach, while it also complied with the methods actually applied by China's commodity inspection bureaus. This book is appointed as the textbook for undergraduates majoring in agriculture or chemistry.

After the founding of the People's Republic of China, China's medical education entered a period of rapid development. The first and second national health work conferences were held in 1950 and 1952, respectively. The health work policy was formally established and summarized as "to serve workers, peasants, and soldiers; to focus on the prevention of diseases; to combine traditional Chinese medicine and Western medicine; to embed health work in mass movement" . This indicated that the national health and epidemic prevention system entered a period of comprehensive construction. The health and epidemic prevention stations were generally established in 1953 in all the provinces, autonomous regions, and municipalities, as well as prefectures (cities) and counties (banners and districts). In 1954, the Ministry of Health issued *the Interim Measures and Regulations on the Organization & Personnel Establishment for Health & Epidemic Prevention Stations at All Levels*, which is considered as an important document in the construction of China's health and epidemic prevention system. This document defined the business scope and specific responsibilities of the stations, including environmental health, labor health, food hygiene, school health supervision, prevention of infectious and parasitic diseases, and health publicity and education. In 1957, Wuhan Medical College held a special course for health laboratory doctors, while the Sichuan Medical College (West China School of Medicine of Sichuan University) in 1958 started a three-year specialized course in health inspection. In 1974, the Health Department of Sichuan Medical College established a three-year health inspection major. After the resumption of the college entrance examination in 1977, the Health Department of Sichuan Medical College recruited undergraduates for a four-year health inspection major. This indicated a development in the training of college students from vocational training to senior professional training in China.

In 1981, Health Inspection was officially included in *the Catalogue of Undergraduate Majors in Ordinary Colleges & Universities in China (the Catalogue)*. In 1982, it was changed to a five-year education major and was awarded as "the Bachelor of Medicine". In *the Revised Catalogue* (1998), Health Inspection was incorporated into the preventive medicine major. The separate enrollment for health inspection major was stopped. In 1999, West China Medical University invited many domestic colleges and universities to conduct a demonstration meeting on health inspection major. There was a consensus among the participating schools on pleading with the Ministry of Education to restore the health inspection major. In 2003, a public health emergency known as SARS raised a deep awareness of the importance of health inspection in far-sighted people. After the appeal of Sichuan and other universities, the Ministry of Education in 2004 provided the approval to pilot Health Inspection major (Major Code: 100204S, Science, 4-Year Education). Henceforth, between 1999 and 2012, groups of health inspection professionals were trained by 19 universities, including Sichuan University, Guangdong Pharmaceutical University, Anhui Medical University, Nanjing Medical University, *etc.*

In 2012, the Ministry of Education issued *The Newly Edited Catalogue*, in which "Health Inspection and Quarantine (Major Code: 101007)" was adopted. HIQ was included in the formal professional directory under the category of "Medical Technology". It was clarified that HIQ major mainly included the detection of health risk factors and inspection of quarantine. Moreover, it was deemed as crucial technical assistance for the top-tier academic program in Public Health and Preventive Medicine. Since then, there has been a rapid increase in the number of colleges and universities offering this major. Overall, the colleges and universities have enrolled a total of 3,300 undergraduates every year. As of December 2022, more than 60 colleges and universities in China have set up HIQ major.

With the rapid development of international trade, a number of laws related to HIQ have been established in China since the founding of the People's Republic of China. The following are some of the HIQ-related laws: the Quarantine Law of the People's Republic of China on Entry and Exit Animals and Plants; the Frontier Health and Quarantine Law of the People's Republic of China; the Food Safety Law of the People's Republic of China; the Law of the People's Republic of China on Prevention and Treatment of Infectious Diseases; the Law of the People's Republic of China on Import and Export Commodity Inspection. By preventing the spread of diseases and pests across borders, protecting domestic agriculture and food safety, and promoting safe and sustainable development, these laws fulfill a crucial role in safeguarding public health, ecological balance, and economic growth.

1.3 Prospect of HIQ in China

HIQ is changing with the reforms of the public health system in the new era. After the SARS incident in 2003, the Chinese government has adopted a series of measures, which greatly promoted the construction of public health inspection laboratories at all levels along with the development of education in HIQ field. In response to the outbreak of COVID-19, China called for efforts to develop a strong public health system to safeguard people's health. Only by developing a strong public health system, improving the early warning and response mechanisms, comprehensively enhancing the capacity for prevention, control and treatment, weaving a tight prevention and control network, and consolidating the wall of quarantine, can we provide a strong guarantee for safeguarding the people's health. The pressing need for boosting the early-stage epidemic monitoring and warning capacity to improve the public health system was emphasized, including efforts for a better monitoring system for epidemics and public health emergencies, and a better monitoring mechanism for diseases of unknown causes and abnormal health incidents. A consensus was reached that science and technology are sharp weapons in human's battle against diseases, and human cannot defeat a major disaster or epidemic without scientific development and technological innovation. National Health Commission have called for increasing scientific and technological inputs in the health sector and attracting more talent for scientific research.

Nowadays, China has established a complete infectious disease prevention, control, and biosafety system which effectively reduces the prevalence of infectious diseases. With the development of the economy, the living environment and the spectrum of human diseases have also changed in recent years. Malignant tumors and chronic diseases have become major public health problems globally, with new infectious diseases and zoonoses emerging constantly. Today, humans are facing many new challenges, but one of the most pressing is how to improve healthcare and well-being through more effective health inspection and quarantine measures. It is a question that demands our careful consideration and reflection.

Glossary

quarantine *n.* 检疫 a state, period, or place of isolation in which people or animals that may have been exposed to infectious disease are placed; *v.* place (a person or animal) in quarantine in order to prevent the spread of an infectious disease

disease surveillance 疾病监测 an information-based epidemiological practice by which the spread of disease is monitored in order to establish patterns of progression

COVID-19 2019 新型冠状病毒感染 Corona Virus Disease 2019

Ebola virus disease 埃博拉病毒病 a deadly viral infection caused by the Ebola virus, that leads to profuse internal and external bleeding and eventually leading to organ failure

Zika virus disease 寨卡病毒病 a viral infection transmitted by the Aedes aegypti mosquito

foodborne illness 食源性疾病 an illness acquired by consuming foods or beverages that have been contaminated by pathogens

sanitary chemistry 卫生化学 a component of environmental chemistry, based on the issues of general, organic and instrumental chemistry

Yersinia pestis 鼠疫耶尔森菌 a short gram-negative rod that causes plague

Salmonella *n.* 沙门菌 a group of bacteria that can cause gastrointestinal illness and fever called salmonellosis

（徐向东）

新形态教材网·数字课程学习……

💻教学 PPT   📄自测题   💬推荐阅读

Chapter 2
Health Management

Learning objectives:

- Know the importance of community health management and school health management.
- Understand the basic contents of health management.
- Be familiar with the basic strategies of health management.
- Master the basic process of health management.

Health is not everything, but without health, you can lose everything, including your dream, life, and so on. People are paying more and more attention to health,with the development of economy.However, there are still many people who do not know how to keep healthy in their daily life. Nowadays, the wrong way of life such as overeating, staying up late, drinking alcohol is more and more common in modern people's life. As a result, the death spectrum has changed and the prevalence of chronic diseases has gradually increased. Therefore, health management, including personal health management and population health management, is very necessary. Health management needs multidisciplinary support, and health inspection and quarantine can provide necessary data for health management.

2.1 Overview of Health Management

2.1.1 Definition of Health Management

At present, there is no perfect and universally recognized definition of health management. Health management is interpreted as a combination of the words "health" and "management". Throughout history, the concept of health has been constantly improved. The history of mankind is the history of the theory and practice of health management. The early understanding of health was that it is a general condition of body and mind. It is a healthy state of well-being free from disease. Now the health is defined by the World Health Organization (WHO) as a state of complete physical, mental and social well-being, and not merely the absence of disease or infirmity. There are three levels of health. The first level is physical health, that is, the structure of the body is intact, functioning properly and in relative balance with the environment. The second level is mental health, also known as referring to people's psychological state in good condition, including correct understanding of oneself, correct understanding of the environment, timely adaptation to the environment. The third level is good social adaptability, which refers to the ability of individuals to fully play their roles in the social system. Individuals can effectively play the role corresponding to their identity, and their behaviors are consistent with social norms and harmoniously integrated. The definition of health reflects the positive multidimensional view of health and is the highest goal of health. It not only fully explains the relationship between biological factors and health, but also emphasizes the influence of psychological factors and social factors on health. That's the three dimensional view of health. In 1986, the WHO defined health as a resource for everyday life rather than a purpose for life. Health is a resource for society and the individual, a reflection of the individual's capabilities. Good health is a major resource for socio-economic and personal development, and health is an important aspect of quality of life. This definition enriches the connotation of health and emphasizes the importance of health. Since health is a resource, health needs to be managed because all resources are finite. Only through effective management can resources be fully utilized.

Management is an ancient discipline, which is an act of managing something. Management is to optimize the allocation and use of resources through planning, organizing, directing, coordinating and controlling. The goal is to use the most suitable things in the most suitable place at the most appropriate time and play the most appropriate role, so as to achieve the goal. Therefore, management is a method that people adopt in order to achieve certain goals. Putting health and management two words together, is health management. Health management is a process of planning, organizing, directing, coordinating and controlling health resources to achieve maximum health effects according to health needs. Protecting health resources, saving health resources, maximizing rational use of health resources and making the best use of it is health management.

Health management service is becoming a significant supplement to the medical service system. Now, health management has evolved into a distinct profession in China. Health management is defined as the use of modern biomedical and information management technology to conduct comprehensive monitoring, analysis and health assessment, health management, health consultation, whole process intervention and risk factor analysis of individual or group health status, lifestyle and social environment from social factors, psychological factors and biological factors. The purpose of health management is to mobilize the enthusiasm of individuals, groups and even the whole society, and effectively use limited resources to achieve the maximum health effect. The specific approach of health management is to provide individuals, groups and governments with targeted scientific health information and create conditions for action to improve health.

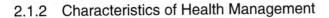

2.1.2　Characteristics of Health Management

Health management is targeted at individuals as well as populations. The main reasons for the increased demand for health management are the rising of medical costs, the aging population, the significant increase in the incidence of chronic diseases, and the decline in productivity due to the poor health of employees. The need for health is not only about adequate medical resources, but also includes managing health risk factors such as overweight, obesity, hypertension and dyslipidemia. The means of health management can be the analysis of health risk factors, the quantitative assessment of health risks, or the supervision and guidance of the intervention process. But health management generally does not involve the diagnosis and treatment of disease. Diagnosing and treating disease is the job of a clinician, instead of a health manager.

The characteristics of health management service are standardization, quantification, individualization and systematization. The service items and working process of health management must ensure their scientific nature. These efforts are determined and implemented in accordance with evidence-based medicine, hygienic standards and guidelines that have been accepted by the academic community. Health management services should be repeatable and effective, and be able to produce optimal results through the cooperation of multiple organizations.

The process of health management, also known as the health management cycle, begins with the examination of health risk factors (detection of health problems), continues with the evaluation of health risk factors (recognition of health problems, guiding intervention), and ends with the intervention of health risk factors (solving health problems). The health management process cannot be completed by a cycle, but should run several cycles over and over again. Each cycle of the health management addresses some health hazards. Through the continuous running of the health management cycle, the health problems of managed objects are constantly solved and the health level of managed objects is constantly improved.

2.1.3　Public Health

Public health is the science and art of preventing disease, prolonging life and promoting health through the organized efforts and informed choices of society, organizations, public and private organizations, communities and individuals. Instead of focusing on treatment of the individual ailment, public health addresses the health of the population as a whole. It focuses on threats to health based on population health analysis. Public health includes the prevention, monitoring and treatment of serious diseases, especially infectious diseases, food supervision and control, drugs and public environmental health, as well as related publicity, health education and immunization. There is a difference between public health and medical services. Medical services are mostly for individuals, but public health works for the population. Public health service is a kind of service with low cost and good effect, but it is also a kind of service with relatively long period of social benefit return. Governments play an important role in public health services, and government intervention is irreplaceable in public health work. In many countries, the responsibilities of governments at all levels in public health are clearly defined in order to make better use of the role of governments at all levels and to facilitate monitoring and evaluation.

The emphasis on public health has led to a gradual separation between clinical medicine and public health. After the separation of clinical medicine from public health, excessive resources were invested in the technical development, education and practice of clinical medicine. While clinical medicine had immediate benefits in terms of effectiveness in the early years, the benefits of public health were gradually found to be undeniable. Clinical medicine and public health are inextricably linked. The integration of clinical medicine and public health is the general trend. It is recognized that, in addition to material factors, social factors also play an important role in influencing health, but the health sector alone cannot fulfill this task.

Health management is an important service of public health. China's national basic public health services include health management for children, the elderly, pregnant and lying-in women. The health management of some patients with chronic diseases is also included in the basic national public health services, such as the hypertensive, the diabetic, the lunger and the severe mentally disturbed.

The COVID-19 outbreak has raised public awareness about public health and encouraged countries to increase public health spending.In the fight against COVID-19, it has been recognized that individual health behavior management (wearing masks, washing hands frequently, etc.) plays an important role in preventing respiratory infections. Good health management helps to achieve public health goals, which benefits all.

The health inspection and quarantine profession has shown an irreplaceable role in the prevention and control of COVID-19, especially in the detection of viral nucleic acid in samples such as throat swabs and cold chain food. Based on the work of health inspection and quarantine, the virus carriers can be found as early as possible, so that isolation measures and other effective methods can be taken in time. Health inspection and quarantine professionals are called detectives in the field of public health and health management. Achieving health for all requires the combined efforts of clinicians, public health physicians, laboratory technicians, scientists, health managers and everyone.

2.2　Basic Strategy of Health Management

The basic strategy of health management is to control health risks and improve health through health information collection, health risk assessment and health intervention. Forms of health management, including life-style management, health demand management, disease management, management of catastrophic injuries, disability management and population health management.

2.2.1　Lifestyle Management

The lifestyle is a manner of living that reflects the person's values and attitudes, including dietary structure, work, sleep, sports, cultural entertainment, social communication and many other aspects. It is economy-based and culture-oriented. The key element of lifestyle is living habit, which is greatly influenced by humanistic values, ethics and other factors, and is closely related to health. Now people also recognized excessive mental pressure and unhealthy lifestyles are bad factors of human health.

Human health consists of four parts: reasonable diet, proper exercise, moderately positive attitude and adequate health care knowledge. Lifestyle management can tell people what a healthy lifestyle is, such as exercising, eating reasonably, quitting smoking, etc. There are many ways and channels to help people make choices and provide conditions for them to experience a healthy lifestyle and to guide them to master the skills to change their lifestyle. But none of them is a substitute for individuals to make decisions about how to live their lives. The core of lifestyle management is to guide or help people correct bad lifestyle through scientific methods. Therefore, the effectiveness of lifestyle management depends on how behavior intervention skills are used to motivate individuals and the public to form health behaviors. The lifestyle management can also be a fundamental component of other health management.

Scientific lifestyle health management is inseparable from the participation of multiple professionals, and a lot of health guidance comes from other related professionals. Test results from health inspection and quarantine can be used to guide lifestyle health management. For example, the results of food physical and chemical test can be used for dietary guidance, and the data of air inspection can be used to judge whether the outdoor environment is suitable for physical exercise.

2.2.2　Health Demand Management

In the realm of management, demand management is a planning methodology used to manage and forecast the demand for products and services. The health demand management is a population-based approach to control health consumption expenditure and improve the utilization of health care services by helping healthy consumers to maintain health and seek appropriate medical care methods. Health demand management seeks to reduce the use of expensive, clinically unnecessary health care services that are thought to be necessary. Health demand management, through telephone, internet and other remote patient management methods to guide individuals to correctly use a variety of medical care services to meet their health needs.

2.2.3　Disease Management

Disease management is defined as "a system of coordinated health-care interventions and communications for populations with conditions in which patient self-care efforts are significant". The cost of the prevention of disease is lower than the cost of treating them. This concept has been widely recognized. Disease management is a comprehensive and integrated health care and cost management system based on the natural process of disease development. The purpose of disease management is to improve the disease recovery rate, the quality of life of the target population and the satisfaction of health care services through the collaboration of organizations and sectors of the health industry chain to provide continuous quality health care services, improve the cost effectiveness. The characteristics of the disease management is based on people and to pay attention to the whole process of disease development, to provide a full range of disease diagnosis and treatment monitoring maintenance services, to help patients to control the happening of the disease development, to prevent the deterioration of the illness and the occurrence of complications, and to improve the quality of life of patients and family members. The disease management requires the cooperation of prevention medicine, rehabilitation medicine, clinical medicine, medical laboratory technology and other disciplines. Disease management emphasizes active individual involvement and self-management. The disease management advocates early use of resources to reduce medical costs after the occurrence of diseases and improve the efficiency of health resources and funds.

Disease management is the provision of health care services that are needed by people with a particular disease. It is mainly the coordination of medical resources for patients throughout the health service system. Disease management emphasizes the importance of patient's self-care, which is essentially patient's self-management. Patients must monitor the progress of their disease and improve their behavior in various areas, such as medication adherence, dietary adjustments and symptom monitoring. Patients must communicate their illness status regularly with health care professionals. Through the long-term development of disease management, the method and strategy have been standardized. But the disease management techniques are still evolving. The target population of disease management mainly focuses on the disease, but in order to achieve the health goal of the whole population, disease management needs to shift from personal health management to population-based health management.

2.2.4 Management of Catastrophic Injuries

Management of catastrophic injuries is a special type of disease management, which provides various medical care services for patients and their families. The catastrophic injuries are the injuries caused by a major disease, such as tumors, organ failure, or severe injuries. The medical expenditure of the disease is huge and has a "catastrophic" impact on the patient's family. The huge medical expenditure is also called catastrophic health expenditures (CHE). Standardized care in times of disaster is called crisis standards of care (CSC). In the face of disaster rescue and management, the CSC is mainly implemented by five systems, including hospital emergency rescue, public health service, out-of-hospital service system, pre-hospital and emergency medicine service, emergency management and public security.

2.2.5　Disability Management

Disability management was first used to prevent disability, control costs, improve the level of security and improve services as an important management means. In recent years, disability management strategies have evolved from simple case management to comprehensive management strategies consisting of quality case management, cycle management, vocational rehabilitation and re-employment support. At present, disability management is increasingly handled from the perspective of the employer according to the degree of disability, with the aim of minimizing the loss of working and living capacity and reducing costs caused by disability. The purpose of disability management is to reduce the frequency and cost of disability accidents. Many factors can influence the onset and duration of disability, such as the severity of the disease or injury, treatment options, rehabilitation process, age, complications, side effect of drug, etc. Quality case management and cycle management strategies constitute the gatekeeper of industrial injury insurance, which is conducive to improving the efficiency of fund use.

2.2.6　Population Health Management

Population health management is to provide more comprehensive health and welfare management for both groups and individuals by coordinating different health management strategies. On the basis of analyzing the health management needs of a certain group, it provides effective management objects, management objectives and management paths for health management implementors, and formulates scientific and reasonable health management programs, so as to improve the effect, utility and benefit of health management as a whole. The population health management can adopt three-grade prevention. Primary prevention is preventing diseases before they occur. Primary prevention should be made top priority. Secondary prevention is the early diagnosis and monitoring of diseases before they develop. Tertiary prevention aims to prevent the development and spread of a disease once it has occurred, in order to reduce pain and disability, etc. With the development of society, economy and medicine, population health management has received more and more attention and will play an increasingly important role in the field of public health services.

2.3　Basic Process of Health Management

Basic process of health management includes health information collection and management, physical examination, health risk assessment, health intervention program formulation, and effective evaluation of health management.

2.3.1　Health Information Collection and Management

Health information is an important information produced in the course of health service, including total population, electronic health records, electronic medical records, population health statistics, etc. Health information mainly comes from health service records. When some special problems need to be solved, it is necessary to obtain information through special investigation, including questionnaire survey, interview, direct observation and so on. Health information entry should follow the principle of easy entry, easy verification and easy analysis. Attention should be paid to follow the principles of medical ethics to ensure information security and protect personal privacy. The utilization principles of health information include classified utilization, authorized utilization, and individuals' utilization of their own population health information to ensure that personal information is not disclosed without authorization.

Health record is a record of every person's changes in all vital signs, from birth to death, and of all health-related actions and events undertaken by himself. It mainly includes: each person's habits, past history, diagnosis and treatment, family history, all previous physical findings, and the occurrence of diseases, development, treatment and outcome of the process, etc. It is a continuous and comprehensive recording process. Health records include personal health records, family health records and community health records. The electronic health record research is a hot concern both in China and abroad. Health records can be collected by means of household investigation, disease screening, physical examination, etc., and health records can be set up by grass-roots health service personnel for residents. Health records can also be set up by medical personnel when residents receive services at grass-roots health service departments. The establishment of health records should follow the combination of voluntary and guidance, and mainly protect the privacy of service objects. In principle, the health records are kept and coded uniformly by the basic health service departments in charge of residential districts. China proposes to gradually establish a unified health record for residents throughout the country and implement standardized management.

2.3.2　Physical Examination

The primary objective of physical examination is to find diseases. Previously, the medical examination was to understand the physical condition of the examinee and determine whether the examinee was suitable for a job or activity. In the past, the traditional physical examination was mainly carried out in the outpatient department of the hospital, and only a few physical examinations were carried out in special physical examination centers. Since the 21st century, third-party medical detection institutions have sprung up rapidly in China. Physical examination is important in the health management. Physical examination is the main way to collect health information and the basis of health assessment. It is the period when the examinee pays the most attention to their own health, and it is the best time for health education. It is also the best time to promote the marketization of health management. Nowadays, a physical examination includes many tests. It is necessary to formulate a health examination plan scientifically and rationally according to the specific situation of the patient.

2.3.3 Health Risk Assessment

Health risk factor refers to various inducing factors existing in the internal and external environment of the body that are related to the occurrence, development and prognosis of diseases, including biological, psychological, behavioral, economic and social factors. Health risk factors are characterized by long incubation period, weak specificity, combined effect and widespread presence. Health risk assessment is based on the health risk factors and health status of individuals or groups to predict the life span of individuals and the incidence of chronic and common diseases or mortality. In general, the steps of health risk assessment include gathering information, risk calculations, and assessment reports. Now there are many kinds of risk calculation methods and models that can be used, which should be reasonably selected according to the actual situation.

2.3.4 Health Intervention Program Formulation

In the field of management, the planning is an act of formulating a program for a definite course of action. There are six basic procedures for health intervention plan design. The first step is the assessment of the health intervention needs. Analysis of health problems objectively identifies the main health problems of the target population and ultimately identifies the health problems for priority intervention. The analysis of influencing factors for health problems is designed to make health intervention program easily accepted by the intervention population. Prioritizing health interventions takes into account the severity of the threat to the health of the population. The second step is to identify intervention targets. The requirements can be summarized as "SMART" (S: special; M: measurable; A: achievable; R: reliable; T: time-bound). Specific targets can be classified into health targets, behavioral targets, educational targets, and so on. The third step is to develop intervention strategies and activities. The fourth step is to formulate the plan evaluation program. The fifth step is to make a plan to implement the plan. The sixth step is to prepare a budget for health interventions. A complete health intervention program should include the health intervention plan design, implementation and evaluation of three stages. These three stages are a continuous process, and they affect each other.

2.3.5 Effect Evaluation of Health Management

Effect evaluation of health management includes behavioral factors evaluation, behavioral lifestyle evaluation, health risk evaluation, health status evaluation, quality of life evaluation, social and economic evaluation, etc. Sometimes there are some interference factors that affect the accuracy of effect evaluation of health management, such as time, testing or observation error, choice factor, loss of follow-up, etc. Common health intervention effect evaluation schemes include before-after test without control group and nonequivalent control group design.

2.4   Community Health Management

Community is a group of people having ethnic or cultural or religious characteristics in common, living in a particular local area. Communities are usually made up of several families. It has many functions such as politics, economy, culture, education and health service. Community health service is an important content in the work, of providing the most effective coherent community health care services, including the management of high-risk population and the health education of whole community members. Good standardized community health management can reduce the incidence of chronic diseases and improve the health level of community members.

Resident health records are the basis of community health management, including personal basic information, physical examination, health management records of key groups and other medical and health service records. It is established when residents receive services in township health centers, village clinics and community health service centers, or through household services, disease screening, health check-ups and other ways. When medical institutions provide medical and health services, they should update and supplement health records in time. All service records are consolidated and filed in time by responsible medical personnel or file management personnel. Institutions that have established electronic health record information systems should update their electronic health records at the same time.

Community health education is one of the important contents of community health management. Community health education aims to help residents establish health awareness, improve health literacy, change unhealthy life-style, prevent diseases and promote health. Community health education can be carried out in various ways, including providing health education materials, setting up health education propaganda column, carrying out public health consultation activities, holding health knowledge lectures and so on.

The key groups of community health management are children, the elderly, pregnant women, patients with chronic disease, etc.The health management of children aged between 0 and 6 can be divided into three stages: neonatal period, infancy and preschool period. For these children, township health centers and community health service centers should provide corresponding health services. Women from the beginning of pregnancy to postpartum 42d can be divided into four stages of health management according to the first trimester, second trimester, third trimester and postpartum. Township health centers and community health service centers should provide appropriate health testing and health guidance for pregnant women. Community health management provides services once a year for residents aged 65 and above, including lifestyle and health status assessment, physical examination, auxiliary examination and health guidance. Community health management provides services for patients with essential hypertension and type 2 diabetes among permanent residents aged 35 and above within the jurisdiction, including at least 4 face-to-face follow-up visits and health intervention guidance every year. The program of national basic public health services have clear provisions on community health management.

2.5　School Health Management

As a special group, students learn and live together in school. They are in the critical period of growth and development, their bodies and brains are not fully developed, easy to be affected by the external environment. Due to the aggregation of population public health emergencies such as infectious disease outbreaks, foodborne disease outbreaks and other student health risk incidents are easy to occur in schools. School health management is an important part of health management, aiming at protecting and enhancing the physical and mental health of young children. School health management is related to the health of teachers and students, the happiness of millions of families, social harmony and stability and the future health quality of the whole nation.

In recent 30 years, China's school health management has been mainly invested in the following aspects, such as school food hygiene and safety, school disease prevention and control, school health education, school health facilities construction, student nutrition improvement, school health institutions and personnel management, and a series of school health system construction. The health of Chinese children has improved across the board, and the mortality rate of school-age children related to tuberculosis, the leading cause of death among young people, has been declining. But serious problems still exist. The physical quality of Chinese adolescents has been continuously declining, the detection rate of poor vision remains high, and the poor vision continues to appear at younger age. The detection rate of overweight, obesity and high blood pressure continues to increase. Recently, chronic non-communicable diseases such as juvenile diabetes and metabolic syndrome have been increasing year by year, and the health status of adolescents is not optimistic.

School health management needs to enhance the awareness of the health of the students, on a regular basis to collect information about student health information and related risk factors, establish an effective and sustainable health records. Growth and development status detection includes height, weight morphological indicators, vital capacity, blood pressure and pulse and other functional indicators, reflecting speed, muscle strength and other physical indicators, as well as understanding personality, interpersonal communication, social adaptation and other mental health status. To investigate diseases or abnormalities such as myopia, amblyopia, dental caries, malnutrition, obesity, spinal curvature and neurosis. Investigate absences from school due to illness. Study the occurrence and fluctuation of various acute and chronic infectious diseases and collective food poisoning. Prevent and monitor of health risk behaviors such as smoking, alcohol and drug abuse, accidents, violent injuries, suicide, unhealthy lifestyle, internet addiction and unhealthy behaviors. Carry out early prevention of obesity, hypertension, diabetes, hyperlipidemia and other adult diseases. Take practical preventive measures, including establishing emergency response mechanisms, preventing sources of infection, cutting off transmission routes and protecting vulnerable groups.

The evaluation of school health management is an important part of the overall plan of school health promotion, which runs through the whole process of the plan. It is an important index to measure the school health management, and provides objective feedback information for managers, teachers, students and parents.

Glossary

health management 健康管理 a process of planning, organizing, directing, coordinating and controlling health resources to achieve maximum health effects according to health needs

public health 公共卫生 the science and art of preventing disease, prolonging life and promoting health through the organized efforts and informed choices of society, organizations, public and private, communities and individuals

strategy *n.* 策略 an elaborate and systematic plan of action

life-style *n.* 生活方式 a manner of living that reflects the person's values and attitudes, including dietary structure, work, sleep, sports, cultural entertainment, social communication and many other aspects

demand *n.* 需求 an urgent or peremptory request

disease management 疾病管理 a system of coordinated health-care interventions and communications for populations with conditions in which patient self-care efforts are significant

catastrophic *adj.* 灾难性的 extremely harmful, bringing physical or financial ruin

disability *n.* 失能、残疾 the condition of being unable to perform as a consequence of physical or mental unfitness

evaluation *n.* 评估 an appraisal of the value of something

diagnosis *n.* 诊断 identifying the nature or cause of some phenomenon

community *n.* 社区 a group of people having ethnic or cultural or religious characteristics in common, living in a particular local area

（安康）

新形态教材网·数字课程学习……

💻 教学 PPT   📝 自测题   💬 推荐阅读

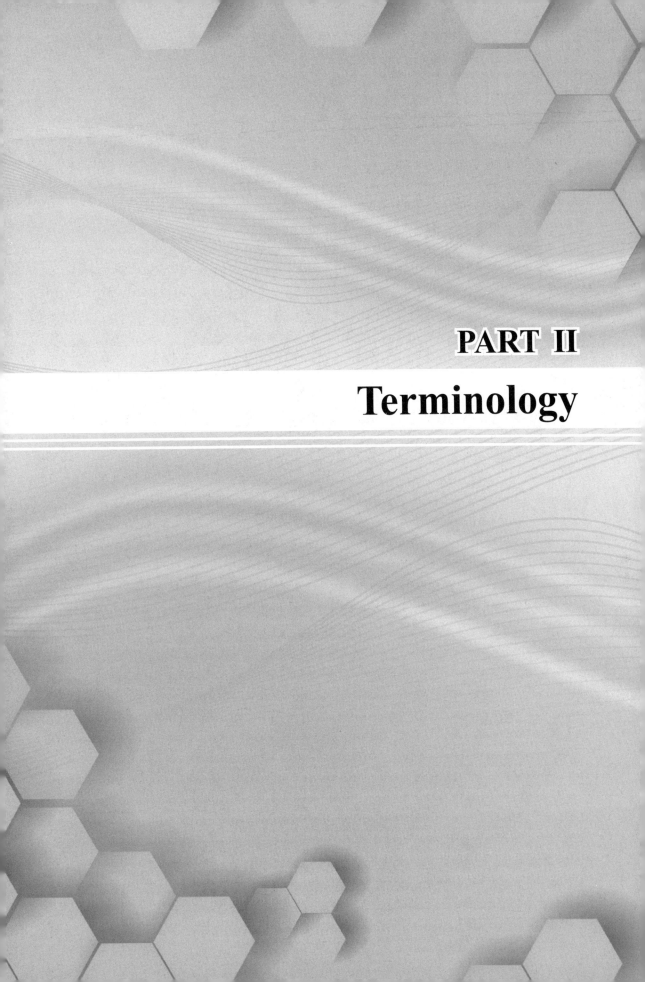

PART II
Terminology

Chapter 3
Medical Terminology

Learning objectives:
- Learn to break down and construct the medical words.
- Be familiar with medical terms and the use of prefixes, roots and suffixes.

3.1 Introduction to Medical Terminology

The formation of medical English words basically follows the rules of the structural characteristics of ordinary English words, which are often composed of prefixes, roots and suffixes. Due to the historical origin of medical profession, medical vocabulary mostly contains Greek and Latin components. The medical English vocabulary is the synthesis of English, Latin and Greek. Nevertheless, medical terms are mainly composed of nouns and adjectives, and the composition of medical English words has its own characteristics and rules. For example, the internal structure of medical English words is the same as that of ordinary English words, including morphemes, roots and affixes. Although the medical English vocabulary is huge, but as long as we find the similarities between them and master the most commonly used morphemes, the more words we can learn.

3.2 The Basic Elements and Composition of Medical Terms

The morpheme is a part of medical terms, which is the smallest combination of sound and meaning. Medical words may be composed of one morpheme or more morphemes. Semantically, there are two types of medical morphemes. One has a definite lexical meaning and expresses the main meaning of the word. These morphemes are called roots. For example, "orth (o) -" means "normal" , "reticul (o) -" means "reticular" . Another medical morpheme is affix.

Affixes can be divided into prefix and suffix according to their position in a word. Medical words can be broken down into parts. Just as in English words, there is always a root term. There also be a prefix, a suffix or both. The prefix will often appear in the beginning of the word, and the suffix at the end of the word. The prefix or suffix is a syllable or perhaps only a few letters, added to the root that will change its meaning. The roots are often connected to roots, or to suffixes, by combinational vowels.

Prefixes and suffixes are all morphemes, which were originally independent words or roots, but gradually become additional parts because they are often attached to other words or roots, auxiliary main meaning. The function of prefix and suffix are not exactly the same. Some common medical prefixes and suffixes are listed in Table 3-1 and Table 3-2, respectively. There are many other prefixes and suffixes, but the ones in these tables are those that will probably be encountered frequently in medical science. Note that prefixes are grouped with the term that gives a close meaning according to a practical root word. For example, the prefix "ab-" means "away from" and is grouped with the prefix "im-", which is indicated by "no". Also notice that there are several prefixes that have different meanings in the same group.

Table 3-1   Some common prefixes for medical terms

Prefix	Description	Example
无、抗、非（without, against, away from）		
a-	without, not	atypical 非典型的
an-	without, not	anemia 贫血
ab-	away from	abnormal 不正常的
anti-	against	antibody 抗体
de-	deactivate	deamination 脱氨作用
dis-	do the opposite of	disability 丧失劳动力
im-	not	imbalance 不平衡
in-	not	invalid 无效的
ir-	not, absence of	irreversible 不可逆的
non-	of little or no consequence	nonspecific 非特异的
un-	not	unusual 不寻常的
数量、量级、比重（quantity, magnitude, proportion）		
mono-	single, one	monoxide 一氧化碳
di-	double	diatomic 双原子的
tri-	three, the third	triphosphate 三磷酸盐
quadri-	four	quadrivalent 四价的
pent-	the fifth	pentose 戊糖
hex-	six, the sixth	hexose 己糖
hecto-	hundred	hectometer 百米
kilo-	thousand	kilometer 千米
deci-	a tenth	decimeter 分米

(*Continued*)

Table 3-1（*Continued*）

Prefix	Description	Example
centi-	one percent	centimeter 厘米
milli-	one thousandth	millimeter 毫米
micro-	small, tiny	microorganism 微生物
semi-	half	semitransparent 半透明的
mega-	huge, million	megaspore 大孢子
macro-	big, huge, much	macrophage 巨噬细胞
poly-	many, aggregate	polythene 聚乙烯
hyper-		hypertension 高血压
over-	over, too much	overexpression 过表达
super-		supernutrition 营养过剩
ultra-		ultrahigh 超高的
hypo-		hypoglycemia 低血糖症
oligo-	few, small, close to	oligopeptide 寡肽
sub-		subcellular 亚细胞的
方向、位置 (direction, position)		
pre-	before	precursor 前体
post-	after	postoperative 术后的
retro-	back	retropharyngeal 咽后的
centr-	middle	centrifuge 离心机
inter-	among	intermediate 中间物
endo-	inside	endocytosis 内吞作用
intra-	inside	intracellular 细胞内的
ec-		eccrine 外分泌的
exo-	outside	exosome 外泌体
extra-		extracellular 细胞外的
peri-	around	peripheral 外围的
epi-	upon	epithelium 上皮
异、同、新（different, same, new）		
co-	with, together	coagulation 凝结
iso-	equal	isopropanol 异丙醇 , isoenzyme 同工酶
neo-	young, fresh, new	neoplasm 新生物
homo-	some, similar, alike	homogeneity 同质性
hetero-	different, other	heterogeneity 异质性

（*Continued*）

Table 3-1 (*Continued*)

Prefix	Description	Example
不良、障碍、疾病（harmful, obstacle, disease）		
dys-	abnormal	dysfunction 功能障碍
auto-	self	autophagy 自噬
path-	disease	pathology 病理学
pedi-	children	pediatric 小儿科的
hemi-	half	hemiplegia 偏瘫
tachy-	fast	tachycardia 心动过速
brady-	slow	bradykinesia 运动迟缓
angi-	blood vessel	angiogenesis 血管再生术
颜色（color）		
leuk(o)-	white, colorless	leukemia 白血病
melano-	black	melanoderma 黑皮病
cyano-	blue	dithiocyano methane 二硫氰基甲烷
polio-	gray, grey	poliomyelitis 脊髓灰质炎
chlor-	green	chloroprene 氯丁二烯
porphyr(o)-	purple	porphyry spleen 斑岩脾
erythr(o)-, rhod(o)-	red	erythrocyte 红细胞
cirrh(o)-	red-yellow	cirrhosis 肝硬化
xanth(o)-	yellow	xanthomonas 黄单胞菌属

Table 3-2 Some common suffixes for medical terms

Suffix	Description	Example
-algia	pain	arthralgia 关节痛
-ase	enzyme	amylase 淀粉酶
-cyte	cell	erythrocyte 红细胞
-cele	hernia	bronchocele 支气管囊肿
-chrome	colored thing	cytochrome 细胞色素
-cide	act of killing	bactericide 杀菌剂
-emia	blood condition	hyperemia 充血
-ectomy	surgical removal	cholecystectomy 胆囊切除术
-gen	a combining form meaning "that which produces"	agglutinogen 凝集原
-genic	cause, origin	carcinogenic 致癌的
-gram	record of	cystogram 膀胱造影照片

(*Continued*)

Table 3–2（*Continued*）

Suffix	Description	Example
-graphy	way, method of recording	electrocardiography 心电图学
-ac/-al/-ar/-ary	pertaining to	cardiac 心脏的 , tonsillar 扁桃体的
-ism/-ia	condition of	alcoholism 酒精中毒 , anemia 贫血
-itis	inflammation	myocarditis 心肌炎
-ist	person who specializes	hematologist 血液学家
-logy	study of	microbiology 微生物学
-lysis	destruction or dissolution	hemolysis 溶血 , bacteriolysis 溶菌
-malacia	softening	osteomalacia 骨软化
-megaly	enlarge	cardiomegaly 心肥大
-meter	measure	barometer 气压计
-metry	process of measuring	chronometry 计时学
-oid	resembling	amoeboid 阿米巴样的
-oma	tumor	melanoma 黑色素瘤
-osis	state of, caused by	neurofibromatosis 神经纤维瘤病
-pathy	disease	neuropathy 神经病
-penia	deficiency	leukopenia 白细胞减少症
-phage, -phagia	eating of a (specified) type or substance	aerophagia 吞气症
-philia	tendency toward	hydrophilia 亲水性
-phobia	intolerance or aversion for	photophobia 恐光症
-plasia	growth	hypoplasia 发育不全
-plasty	repair	heteroplasty 异种移植
-poiesis	production, creation, formation	erythropoiesis 红细胞生成的
-rrhea	flow, discharge	diarrhea 腹泻
-scope	an instrument for viewing or observing	gastroscope 胃镜
-scopy	viewing, observation	microscopy 显微术
-stasis	slowing, stable state	homeostasis 稳态
-tomy	cutting, incision	lithotomy 取石术
-trophy	nutrition, nurture, growth	hypertrophy 肥大
-uria	presence in the urine	proteinuria 蛋白尿

Prefix only changes the meaning of the word, generally does not change the word property, while suffix not only changes the meaning of the word, but also changes the word property. Moreover, some suffixes themselves have specific meanings. For example, "-ate" means "hydrochloric acid" , "-ase" means "enzyme", "-ectomy" means "surgical removal". Words formed by prefixes are called "compound words" and words formed by suffixes are called "derivative words" . It is worth noting that the prefix is not necessarily in the front of the word, but must be before the root. For example, the prefixes of "en-" (inside) and "ex-" (outside) in "strephenopodia" and "strephexopodia" precede the root "pod-" (foot). The root does not have to be in the middle of a word, but can not be before the prefix. Some suffixes, especially compound suffixes or positional suffixes, often do not indicate the additional meaning of words, but tend to indicate the main meaning, as in the above word "-ia" (abnormal).

3.3 Construction of Medical Terms

Often someone may need to come up with the specific or medical terms for a short description of a condition. For example, you may need to know the term for a person who specializes in the diseases and conditions of the blood and hematological system. The root term pertaining to the blood is "hema-" ; the suffix for specialist is "-ist" . Therefore, a hematologist is a physician specializing in hematology.

If someone has been diagnosed with bacteria in the urine, the medical term would be derived from the term for bacteria and the suffix "-uria" , indicating the presence of some substances in the urine. Therefore, the word to describe the condition of bacteria in the urine is bacteriuria. However, if the bacteria were present in the blood, the term would be bacteremia. In this case, the suffix "-emia" refers to blood condition. There are also common root terms that describe diseases or conditions that can be applied to typical organs and body systems, see Table 3-3 for details.

Table 3–3 Some root terms for organs and body systems

Organs		Body systems	
Root	Description	Root	Description
osteo-	bone	hemat-	blood
encephalo-	brain	cardiovasculo-	heart and vessel
thoraco-	chest	entero-	intestine
oculo-	eye	arthro-	joint
genito-	genital	lympho-	lymphatic
cardio-	heart	meningo-	meninges
nephro-	kidney	myo-	muscle
hepato-	liver	neuro-	nerve
pneumo-, pulmono-	lung	dermato-	skin
oro-	mouth	dento-	teeth
naso-	nose	uro-	urinary
gastro-	stomach	vaso-	vessel

Most of medical words are made from combination of the four elements, including base, prefix, suffix, and vowel. The vowel is also called "combining vowel" , usually "o" or "i" and less frequently "e" , placed between two elements to constitute combining form of words. There are some situations related to the formation of medical English words.

3.3.1 Derivation Method

These words are formed by combining derived affixes with roots, or just combining adhesive roots. Words constructed in this way are called derivative words. The derivation method is the most common and also the most commonly used word formation method. Based on this method, a large number of derivation words can be formed. The root is the basis of derivative words, and different affixes can be added to the same root to indicate different meanings and different word class. Prefixes, roots and suffixes can form different medical words according to different combinations rules. Here are some examples.

(1) Prefix + Root

"an-" + "aerobic" ➜ anaerobic
（无）（需氧的）　厌氧的

(2) Prefix + Root + Suffix

"hyper-" + "glyco" + "-emia" ➜ hyperglycemia
（高）　（糖）　（血液中）　高血糖症

(3) Prefix + Root + Suffix + Suffix

"re-" + "gen" + "-er" + "-ate" ➜ regenerate
（再）（生产）　　　使再生

(4) Prefix + Prefix + Root

"re-" + "im-" + "port" ➜ reimport
（再）（进入）（输运）　再输入

(5) Root + Root + Suffix

"myo-" + "cardio-" + "-pathy" ➜ myocardiopathy
（肌肉）（心脏的）（疾病）　心肌病

(6) Root + Suffix

"hepato-" + "-itis" ➜ hepatitis
（肝）　（炎症）　肝炎

(7) Root + Suffix + Suffix

"onco-" + "gene" + "-tic" ➜ oncogenetic
（肿瘤）（发生）　（的）　肿瘤发生的

(8) Root + Root + Root

"stern" + "o" + "cleid" + "o" + "mastoid" ➜ sternocleidomastoid
（胸骨）　（锁骨）　（乳突的）　胸锁乳突肌

3.3.2 Composition Method

Under this way, two or more roots are combined to form a new word. Words constructed based on this method are called compound words. Some roots of these compound words are connected together, while another some roots are connected by a connection vowel, also some roots of the compound words are separated. It is worth noting that medical compound words have semantic integrity, which is different from the characteristics of phrase. The meaning of some compound words is not a simple addition of the meanings of two word formation elements. There are many kinds of medical compound words, but two kinds account for the largest number, including compound nouns and compound adjectives.

(1) The word formation methods of compound nouns are generally as follows.

noun + noun: For example, thermosphere（电离层）

noun + verb: For example, eyeshade（眼罩）

noun + gerund: For example, bottle feeding（人工喂养）

verb + noun: For example, playground（操场）

gerund + noun: For example, operating theatre（手术室）

adjective + noun: For example, greenhouse（温室）

preposition + noun: For example, overexpression（过表达）

(2) There are several commonly used word formation methods for compound adjectives.

noun + adjective: For example, label-free（无标记的）

noun + present participle: For example, peace-loving（爱好和平的）

noun + past participle: For example, man-made（人造的）

numeral + noun: For example, zero-gravity（零重力的）

numeral + noun + adjective: For example, ten-year-old（十岁的）

adjective + noun: For example, long-chain（长链的）

adjective + noun + ed: For example, far-sighted（远视的）

adjective + adjective: For example, deaf-mute（听障的）

adverb + adjective: For example, evergreen（常青的）

preposition + noun: For example, in-line（内嵌的）

（陈阳　王涛）

新形态教材网·数字课程学习……

🖥 教学 PPT　　　　📝 自测题　　　　💬 推荐阅读

Chapter 4
Technical Terminology

Learning objectives:

- Be familiar with the main terms in physicochemical and microbiological analysis.
- Master the common word stems, prefixes and suffixes.

4.1　Introduction to Terms of HIQ

Researches of health inspection and quarantine mainly involve environmental factors in the field of preventive medicine. The implementation sites are usually set up in central units for disease control and prevention, departments of clinical laboratory, and other inspection and quarantine units. Items of inspection and quarantine include, but are not limited to inspections and pathological tests for (1) large-scale epidemics such as COVID-19, (2) imported and exported animals and plants, (3) food, medicines, cosmetics, (4) microorganisms. All specimens involved must be carried out in professional units or qualified clinical laboratories. Terminologies related to health inspection and quarantine mainly come from two aspects, physical and chemical examination and microbiological inspection. Some common prefixes and suffixes are listed in Table 4-1 and Table 4-2, respectively. There are many other prefixes and suffixes, but the ones in these tables are those that will be encountered frequently in health inspection and quarantine.

Table 4–1　Some common prefixes for terms of HIQ

Prefix	Description	Prefix	Description
化学类（chemical category）			
aceto-	乙酰	hydroxy(l)-	羟基
acyl-	酰基	imino-	亚氨基
amidino-	脒基	iso-	同、等、异
amino-	氨基	keto-	酮基

（*Continued*）

31

Table 4-1 (*Continued*)

Prefix	Description	Prefix	Description
amylo-	淀粉的	mercapto-	巯基
bromo-	溴的	meth-, methyl-	甲基
carb(o)-	碳的	nitro-	硝基
carboxy(l)-	羧基	oxy-	氧
enol-	烯醇	thi(o)	二硫
formyl-	甲酰	phenyl-	苯基
ferri-	高铁	phosphor-	磷酸基
ferro-	亚铁	phosphoryl-	磷酰基

生物类（biological category）

Prefix	Description	Prefix	Description
aden(o)-	腺	uro-	尿
aer(o)-	空气的	lipo-	脂
agro-	土壤、农业	lympho-	淋巴
bio-	生物的	megal(o)-	巨大
carcin(o)-	癌	meso-	内消旋、中（间）
cardio-	心脏	myco-	真菌
chlor(o)-	绿	nucle(o)-	核
chrom(o)-, chromat (o)-	颜色	oligo-	寡
cyto-	细胞	onco-	肿瘤
deoxy-	脱氧	path(o)-	病
electr(o)-	电	peri-	周、周围
end(o)-	内	per-	过
enter(o)-	肠	rib(o)-	核糖
epi-	表、变化	plasm(o)-	原生质、血浆
erythr(o)-	红、赤	poly-	多、聚
eu-	真正	pro-	原、前
glyc(o)-	糖	pseud(o)-	假、拟
hem(o, a)-, haem(o, a)-, haemat(o)-	血的	pyro-	焦
hepat(o)-	肝的	quasi-	类似、准
hypo-	低、（过）少	radio-	辐射、放射
immuno-	免疫	thym(o)-	胸腺
kary(o)-	核、细胞核		

Table 4-2　Some common suffixes for terms of HIQ

Suffix	Description	Suffix	Description
化学类（chemical category）			
-aldehyde	醛	-ide	（构成名词）化合物
-amine	胺	-imine	亚胺
-ane	烷	-lactone	内酯
-ase	酶	-oid	类似物
-ate	盐、酯	-ol	醇
-ene	烯	-one	酮
生物类（biological category）			
-cide	杀、杀灭剂	-trophic	营养型
-cyte	细胞	-mycete	真菌
-gen, -genic, -genous	（形容词）原、产生	-mycin	霉素、菌素
-some	体	-sis	构成名词，表示作用
-itis	炎、发炎	-oma	瘤
-lysis	分解作用、过程	-ose	糖
-lytic	分解的	-oside	糖苷
-lyze, -lise	分解	-phoresis	移动
-lysate	分解液	-plasm	血浆、原生质
-troph	营养生物	-plast	体、粒、团

The main research objects of health inspection and quarantine are about the theory, methodology and technology related to the detection of chemical substances, poisonous and harmful organic matter, inorganic matter, and microorganisms in the environment (air, water, food, biomaterials) and other factors involved in human activities. According to the distribution of objects in health inspection and quarantine, the objects can be divided into the following five categories.

4.1.1　Air Quality

Air is essential for maintaining life. The body absorbs oxygen through the respiratory system, and produces carbon dioxide to be discharged from the body during the metabolic process. Presently, due to human industrial activities and unreasonable emissions, the normal components of the air have changed, causing adverse effects and harms to human health and the growth of animals and plants. Urban air, indoor air in daily life, and air quality in the work environment are all affected. Sources of man-made pollution can be divided into stationary pollution source (e.g., industrial enterprises, heating equipment and household stoves, etc.) and mobile pollution source (e.g., vehicles). There are thousands of pollutants emitted into the air. Common air pollutants mainly include dust of coal soot, sulfur dioxide, nitrogen dioxide, hydrocarbons (including polycyclic aromatic hydrocarbons), polychlorinated biphenyls, and pesticides. China has set series of limit on the concentration of 120 toxic and harmful pollutants in the production areas. These pollutants can be divided into primary pollutants and secondary pollutants according to different formation processes. The former includes sulfur dioxide, carbon monoxide, carbon dioxide, nitrogen oxides, hydrocarbons and other gases, vapors and particulate matter. The physical and chemical properties of these pollutants have not changed after they enter the atmosphere. The latter are new pollutants formed by primary pollutants under various physical, chemical conditions or biological effects. Such pollutants are often manifested as aerosols, with small particles ranging from 0.01 to 1.0 μm in size, and are generally more toxic than primary pollutants.

Air quality is the first priority for the quality of human life. The Chinese government has worked to change the situation of air pollution and established strict health standard of air quality. China has promulgated "Ambient Air Quality Standard (GB 3095-2012)", "Indoor Air Quality Standard (GB/T 18883-2002)", "Occupational Exposure Limits for Hazardous Factors in Industrial Sites (Part 1): Chemical Hazardous Factors (GBZ 2.1-2019)", and "Occupational Exposure Limits of Hazardous Factors in Industrial Sites (Part 2) (GBZ 2.2-2007)". These documents implement grading and layered management of ambient air quality, and the main indicators contain sulfur dioxide, nitrogen oxides, carbon monoxide, ozone, total organic carbon, dust, etc., as well as pollutant gases that may be generated or released during the production process. The terms related to air quality mainly cover the names and basic characteristics of air components, as well as some detection parameters and indicators related to air pollutants.

4.1.2 Water Quality

Due to human exploitation and endless waste, the world is seriously deficient in water resources, both in sources and water quality. China also faces water shortages. It is well known that 70% of the human body is made up of water, and his daily minimum water requirement is approximately 2.5 liter, mainly through drinking water and food intake. Various impurities can be brought to all kinds of water bodies after industrial and agricultural production, along with urban domestic water usage. One concern initiated by such impurities is the negative effects on water quality. Although various pollutants entering the water environment can be recovered through self-purification capacity, the self-purification capacity depends on the physical and chemical properties of pollutants and other environmental conditions, and its role is very limited. Water pollution not only causes human health problems, affects industrial and agricultural production, but also destroys ecological balance. Water pollution sources can be divided into natural pollution sources and man-made pollution sources. Most of the pollutants that pose hazard to human health are man-made pollution sources. Therefore, drinking water is the most important object of water quality inspection where the type and content of impurities determine the water quality.

Currently, more than 180 items of water quality sanitation inspection have been carried out, and the number is gradually increasing. Official documents promulgated in China have listed

42 conventional and 65 non-conventional inspection indicator, and more than 90 physical and chemical examination indicators according to "Standards for Drinking Water Quality (GB5749-2006)" . These conventional indicators cover wide range of factors such as sensory, chemical, toxicological, bacteriological and radioactive indicators. Actually, drinking water must convey a full inspection called general health project (e.g., temperature, pH, turbidity, conductivity, dissolved oxygen (DO), soluble solid, chemical oxygen demand (COD), biochemical oxygen demand (BOD), nitrite, nitrate, phosphate, oxide, total hardness). Besides, the drinking water inspection still needs additional project on harmful substances (e.g., phenol, mercury, arsenic, cyanide, and hexavalent chromium). The terms related to water quality mainly cover the traits and physical indicators of air components, also some pollution parameters and indicators related to water pollutants are included.

4.1.3   Food and Nutrition

There are many kinds of foods in daily life with wide sources and various forms. Some of them were shoddily produced or adulterated during production and selling process. In the case of alimentary toxicities, the poisoned substances should be identified through food inspection and used to provide circumstantial evidence for determining the legal responsibility of the perpetrator. The main testing objects of food inspection include two aspects, one is the detection of microorganisms and their metabolic products in food, which belongs to the food sanitary microbiology; the other one is the health inspection of chemical substances related to nutrition, which belongs to the physical and chemical examination. The harmful substances and nutrients in food are the main contents of food inspection.

The physical and chemical examination in health inspection of food is mainly based on the detection and analysis of the nutrients and harmful substances. The results will demonstrate the quality and content of nutrients in food, and thereafter conduct the health condition and quality surveillance for food production, processing, storage and sales. In addition, there are multiple sources of poisonous substance in food, (1) incorporation of natural poisonous plants and animals (e.g., fresh daylily, sprouted potatoes, animal thyroid, etc.); (2) concentration of industrial waste along food chain (e.g., waste water and gas, and waste residue concentrated in the ecosystem); (3) pesticide residues; (4) microorganisms (e.g., bacteria, mold and mycotoxin); (5) illegal food additives. Food inspection is an effective means for health management and meanwhile provides scientific basis for the formulation of relevant health standards, measures and policies. Currently, food inspection mainly includes sensory inspection, qualitative and quantitative examination by physical or chemical methods. The chemical methods are the most commonly used to identify nutrients and harmful substances, and the most popular methods include thin layer chromatography, UV-visible spectrophotometry, atomic absorption spectrometry, gas chromatography, high performance liquid chromatography, electrochemical analysis. Terms related to food and nutrition mainly include the names of nutrients, food additives and toxic and harmful substances, as well as the preservation and packaging of food.

4.1.4   Biomaterials

In the field of health laboratory science, biomaterials include tissues, organs and related metabolites from the body, as well as plants, animals and microorganisms related to the human health. The absorption, distribution, transformation and excretion of pollutants in organisms can be realized by monitoring the content and conformational forms of these pollutants in specimens like tissues, biofluids and other excretions from human body or animals. Mainly there are three ways for biological pollution, surface attachment, absorption and biological concentration. The theory and method for biomaterials test are basically consistent with those of air and water quality test. However, due to its complex conformation, the concentration and conformational form of pollutants show not only very significant temporal and temperature dependencies, but also individual variation. Currently, novel methods for biomaterials detection are still emerged in this field, and more sensitive and reliable indicators suitable for non-destructive monitoring are warranted.

4.1.5   Sanitary Microbiology

Sanitary microbiology refers to microorganisms in the environment related to human health. Sanitary microbiology is a science about the interaction between microorganisms and their environments, the impact on human health, and human strategies to deal with these microorganisms. Sanitary microbiology follows the idea of preventive medicine. From the perspectives of ecology, etiology and epidemiology, it formulates reasonable measures for people and the environment under the purpose of promoting benefits and avoiding harm. The research object of sanitary microbiology is the microorganisms in the environment and the environment in which they live, mainly including the non-biophysical environment such as atmosphere, soil, water, food, and drugs, as well as the biological environment inside and outside the organisms. It mainly studies the characteristics of physical factors (temperature, water, organic and inorganic substances, environmental pH, light, etc.) and biological factors (host and its state, bacterial colony), and their relationship with human health.

With the achievements of biomedical development, modern research methods and testing instruments and equipment will be more widely used in this field. Due to the accumulation of scientific achievements, the struggle between human intelligence and microbial infectious diseases will make people form a new understanding of infection and disease in health care. The terms related to sanitary microbiology are mainly composed of two aspects: one is the attributes and characteristics of bacteria and viruses; the second is the laboratory technology to measure these bacteria, viruses and other objects.

4.2　Common Terms in Health Physicochemical Analysis

4.2.1　Terms in Air Physicochemical Analysis

4.2.1.1　Atmosphere and air pollution

大气 atmosphere

对流层 troposphere

平流层 stratosphere

中间层 mesosphere

电离层 thermosphere

外层 exosphere

空气污染 air pollution

酸沉降 acid deposit

温室效应 greenhouse effect

温室气体 greenhouse gas

臭氧层耗损 ozone depletion

室内空气污染 indoor air pollution

气溶胶 aerosol

颗粒物 particulate matter, PM

一次污染物 primary pollutant

二次污染物 secondary pollutant

空气理化检验 physical and chemical examination for air

环境空气 ambient air

工业场所空气 workplace air

公共场所空气 public place air

室内空气 indoor air

室内空气质量 indoor air quality, IAQ

气象参数 meteorological parameter

气温 air temperature

气湿 air humidity

气流 air current

气压 atmosphere pressure

绝对湿度 absolute humidity

相对湿度 relative humidity, RH

最大湿度 maximum humidity

饱和差 saturated difference

生理饱和差 physiological saturated difference

风向 wind direction

风速 wind velocity

空气动力学直径 particle aerodynamic diameter, PAD

超细颗粒物和细颗粒物 ultrafine and fine particles

4.2.1.2　Sampling and testing

采样体积 sampling volume

质量浓度 mass concentration

体积分数 volume fraction

总悬浮颗粒物 total suspended substance, TSP

时间加权平均容许浓度 permissible concentration–time weighted average, PC–TWA

短时间接触容许浓度 permissible concentration–short time exposure limit, PC–STEL

最高容许浓度 maximum allowable concentration, MAC

空气样品 air sample

直接采样法 direct sampling method

注射器采样法 syringe sampling method

气袋采样法 sampling method using bag

采气管采样法 substitution sampling method

真空瓶采样法 vacuum sampling method

浓缩采样法 concentrated sampling method

溶液吸收法 solution absorption method

固体吸附剂采样法 solid adsorbent sampling method

冷阱法 cold trap method

静电沉降法 electrostatic sedimentation method

浸渍试剂滤料法 impregnated filter method

聚氨酯泡沫塑料 polyurethane foam plastic

多层滤料采样法 series filter method

扩散管和滤料联合采样法 denuder/filter pack sampling

被动式采样法 passive sampling

个体计量器 personal dosimeter

采样器 sampler

气泡吸收管 bubbling absorption tube

冲击式吸收管 impinger

多孔玻板吸收管 fritted glass bubbler

滤料采样夹 filter membrane sampler

填充式采样管 packed column sampler

气体流量计 gas flowmeter

皂膜流量计 soap bubble flowmeter

孔口流量计 orifice flowmeter

转子流量计 rotator flowmeter

采气动力 sampling power

最小采气量 minimum sampling volume

采样效率 sampling efficiency

采样点 sampled site

冷凝颗粒计数仪 condensation particle counter, CPC

粉尘分散度 distribution of particles

降尘 dustfall

二氧化硫 sulfur dioxide

氮氧化物 nitrogen oxides

一氧化碳 carbon monoxide

臭氧 ozone

零空气 zero air

氨 ammonia

甲醛 formaldehyde

苯 benzene

甲苯 toluene

二甲苯 xylene

汞 mercury

铅 lead

锰 manganese

快速测定 rapid analysis

检气管 detector tube

试纸法 test paper method

溶液法 solution method

空气质量自动监测系统 air quality monitoring system, AQMS

4.2.2   Terms in Water Physicochemical Analysis

4.2.2.1   Traits and physical indicators

水循环 water cycle

富营养化 eutrophication

水华 algal bloom

赤潮 red tide

浑浊度 turbidity

散射浊度单位 nephelometry turbidity unit, NTU

电导率 conductivity

4.2.2.2   Pollution parameters

溶解氧 dissolve oxygen, DO

化学需氧量 chemical oxygen demand, COD

生化需氧量 biochemical oxygen demand, BOD

总有机碳 total organic carbon, TOC

总碳 total carbon, TC

无机碳 inorganic carbon, IC

可吹扫有机碳 purgeable organic carbon, POC

不可吹扫有机碳 non-purgeable organic carbon, NPOC

石油 petroleum

氨氮 ammonia nitrogen

亚硝酸盐氮 nitrite nitrogen

硝酸盐氮 nitrate nitrogen

总硬度 total hardness

二苯碳酰二肼 diphenylcarbazide, DPC

4.2.3　Terms in Food Physicochemical Analysis

4.2.3.1　Nutrition

淀粉 starch

蛋白质 protein

粗蛋白 crude protein

脂肪 fat

粗脂肪 crude fat

总脂肪 total fat

粗纤维 crude fiber

膳食纤维 dietary fiber

维生素 vitamin

类胡萝卜素 carotenoids

硫胺素（维生素 B_1）thiamine

核黄素（维生素 B_2）riboflavin

抗坏血酸（维生素 C）ascorbic acid

钙 calcium

磷 phosphorus

铁 iron

锌 zinc

硒 selenium

碘 iodine

4.2.3.2　Food additives

食品添加剂 food additives

石膏 gypsum

防腐剂 preservative

苯甲酸 benzoic acid

山梨酸 sorbic acid

甘草 licorice root

糖精 saccharin

着色剂 coloring agent

胭脂红 carmine

苋菜红 amaranth

柠檬黄 tartrazine

靛蓝 indigo

日落黄 sunset yellow

赤藓红 erythrosine

亮蓝 brilliant blue

新红 new red

诱惑红 allura red

丁基羟基茴香醚 butylated hydroxyanisole, BHA

二丁基羟基甲苯 dibutyl hydroxy toluene, BHT

没食子酸丙酯 propyl gallate, PG

4.2.3.3　Toxic and harmful substances

六六六（六氯环己烷）hexachloroncy-clohexane, HCH

滴滴涕（二氯二苯三氯乙烷）dichlordiphenyl trichloroethane, DDT

敌敌畏 dichlorvos

甲拌磷 phorate

二嗪磷 diazinon

甲基对硫磷 methyl parathion

乙硫磷 ethion

稻丰散 phenthoate

乐果 dimethoate

对硫磷 parathion

黄曲霉毒素 aflatoxin, AFT

甲醇 methanol

杂醇油 fusel oil

醛类 aldehydes

氰化物 cyanide

亚硝酸盐 nitrite

亚硝酸钠 sodium nitrite

亚硝酸钾 potassium nitrite

巴比妥类 barbitones

巴比妥 barbital

苯巴比妥 phenobarbital

生物碱 alkaloids

雷因许法 Reinsch test

磷化锌 zinc phosphide

敌鼠 diphacinone

4.2.3.4 Other food (components)

马拉硫磷 malathion

氯化苦（三氯硝基甲烷）chloropicrin

酸败 rancidity

酸价 acid value

过氧化值 peroxide value

羰基价 carbonyl group value

棉酚 gossypol

酱油 soy sauce

食醋 vinegar

水产品 aquatic products

组胺 histamine

发酵酒 fermented wine

蒸馏酒 distilled wine

配制酒 mixed wine

4.2.3.5 Container and packaging

食品容器 food container

包装材料 packaging material

化学性食物中毒 chemical food poisoning

水浸法 soaking

4.2.3.6 Methodology

薄层色谱法 thin layer chromatography, TLC

4.3 Common Terms in Sanitary Microbiology

4.3.1 Objects in Sanitary Microbiology

报告基团 reporter, R

病毒 virus

病毒学 virology

大肠菌群 coliform

粪大肠菌群 faecal coliform, FC

禽流感 avian influenza

海水生境 marine habitat

呼肠病毒 reovirus

极端嗜热菌 *Extreme thermophile*

极端微生物 extremophiles

脊髓灰质炎病毒 poliovirus

兼性 facultative

嗜热菌 thermophile

嗜碱菌 alkaliphile

酵母菌 yeast

拮抗 amensalism

桔青霉素 citrinin

狂犬病 rabies

蓝绿藻 blue-green algae

冷休克蛋白 cold shock protein, CSP

裂谷热 rift valley fever

绿脓菌素 pyocin

霉菌 mould

耐冷微生物 crymophy lactic microorganism

耐热大肠菌群 thermo-tolerant coliform group

溶血素 hemolysin

耐受 tolerance

耐压菌 barotolerant

葡萄球菌素 staphylococcin

群落 community

人巨细胞病毒 human cytomegalovirus, HCMV

肉毒毒素 botulinum toxin

朊病毒 prion

生境 habitat

生态系统 ecosystem

平衡 balance

失调 disturbance

生物圈 biosphere

食品变败 food spoilage

食源性疾病 foodborne illness

适应性 adaptability

嗜冷菌 psychrophile

嗜酸菌 acidophile

嗜压菌 barophile

嗜盐菌 halophile

噬菌体 bacteriophage

丝状真菌 filamentous fungus

酸败 rancidity

突变体 mutant

外来微生物 foreign microorganism

土著微生物 autochthonous microbe

微环境 microenvironment

微生态学 microecology

微小生境 microhabitat

细胞器 organelle

细菌素 bacteriocin

细小病毒 parvovirus

腺病毒 adenovirus

驯化 domestication

烟曲霉震颤素 fumitremorgin

严重急性呼吸综合征 severe acute respiratory syndrome, SARS

原生动物 protozoa

藻类 algae

藻类学 algology

展青霉素 patulin

真菌 fungus

真菌毒素 mycotoxin

真菌毒素中毒症 mycotoxicosis

专性 obligate

4.3.2 Laboratory Technologies

半定量法 semi-quantitative method

变性 denaturation

变异 variation

变异性 variability

表型 phenotype

超高温瞬时杀菌技术 ultra-high temperature sterilization, UHT sterilization

超耐药 extensively drug resistance, XDR

超嗜热菌 hyper thermophile

存活时间 survival time, ST

消毒剂 disinfectant

碘酊 iodine tincture

碘附 iodophor

动物生物安全实验室 animal biosafety laboratory

多重耐药 multi-drug resistance, MDR

二相性 dimorphic

泛耐药 pan-drug resistance, PDR

防护实验室 containment laboratory

放线酮 actidione

分子信标 molecular beacon

伏马菌素 fumonisin

腐败 putrefaction

复苏 resuscitation

复性 renaturation

隔离 quarantine

共生 symbiosis

寡核苷酸微阵列 oligonucleotide array

关键控制点 critical control point, CCP

关键限值 critical limits

过氧化物 peroxides

杂交 hybridization

互惠共生 synergism

互利共生 mutualism

互生 alternation

基因型 genotype

基因组文库 metagenomic library

极端环境 extreme environment

寄生 parasitism

降解 degradation

交叉耐药 cross resistance

静水压 hydrostatic pressure

聚合酶链反应 polymerase chain reaction, PCR

菌落形成单位 colony forming unit, CFU

菌群失调 dysbacteriosis

氯己定 chlorhexidine

脉冲场凝胶电泳 pulsed field gel electrophoresis, PFGE

脉冲强光 intense pulsed light, IPL

脉动真空法 pulsing vacuum

米酵菌酸 bongkrekic acid

灭菌 sterilization

灭菌保证水平 sterility assurance level, SAL

偏利共生 commensalism

热原 pyrogen

人工选择 artificial selection

杀灭时间 killing time, KT

生物安全等级 biosafety level, BSL

生物安全柜 biological safety cabinet, BSC

生物被膜 biofilm, BF

衰减 decay

生物转化 bioconversion

退火 annealing

危险分析 hazard analysis

危害分析关键控制点 hazard analysis critical control point, HACCP

微波 microwave

微生物监测 microbial monitoring

卫生标准操作程序 sanitation standard operating procedure, SSOP

污水处理 sewage treatment

无菌保证水平 sterility assurance level, SAL

戊二醛 glutaraldehyde, GTA

眼点 eyespot

猝灭剂 quencher, Q

玉米赤霉烯酮 zearalenone

杂交 hybridization

最可能数 most probable number, MPN

最小抑菌浓度 minimum inhibitory concentration, MIC

（陈阳　王涛）

新形态教材网·数字课程学习……

💻 教学 PPT　　　📝 自测题　　　💬 推荐阅读

Chapter 5
Exercises in Terminology

Learning objectives:
- Know the application of terminology in practical cases.

In this section, the specific physicochemical and microbiological analyses are used to help demonstrate how terms of health inspection and quarantine describe conditions or procedures. These exercises will help to construct terms or determine the meaning.

For the following exercises, read the paragraph and find the terms that fit the given condition.

5.1   Terms Exercises in Medical Terminology

5.1.1   Terms Exercises in the Body as a Whole

The listed terms are parts of a cell. Match each term with its correct meaning.

cell membrane   chromosomes   cytoplasm   DNA   endoplasmic reticulum   genes
mitochondria   nucleus

(1) material of the cell located outside the nucleus and yet enclosed by the cell membrane

_____

(2) regions of DNA within each chromosome

_____

(3) small sausage-shaped structures that are the principal source of energy for the cell

_____

(4) network of canals within the cytoplasm; the site of protein synthesis _____

(5) structure that surrounds and protects the cell _____

(6) control center of the cell, containing chromosomes _____

(7) chemical found within each chromosome _____

(8) rod-shaped structures in the nucleus that contain regions called genes _____

5.1.2   Terms Exercises in the Body System

Match the term in Column Ⅰ with its definition or a term of similar meaning in Column Ⅱ. Write the correct letter in the spaces provided.

COLUMN Ⅰ

(1) voiding _____

(2) trigone _____

(3) renal cortex _____

(4) renal medulla _____

(5) urea _____

(6) erythropoietin _____

(7) renin _____

(8) electrolyte _____

(9) hilum _____

(10) calyx (calix) _____

COLUMN Ⅱ

A. hormone secreted by the kidney that stimulates formation of red blood cells

B. notch on the surface of the kidney where blood vessels and nerves enter

C. urination; micturition

D. nitrogenous waste

E. cup-like collecting region of the renal pelvis

F. small molecule that carries an electric charge in solution

G. inner region of the kidney

H. hormone made by the kidney; increases blood pressure

I. triangular area in the bladder

J. outer section of the kidney

5.1.3   Terms Exercises in the Blood Cells

A 6-year-old girl was taken to her pediatrician because she was tired all the time and bruised easily. The physician ordered a complete blood count (CBC) and the clinical laboratory technician performed a phlebotomy. Results of the CBC showed the presence of leukemia. Her leukocyte count was elevated and her erythrocyte count demonstrated anemia.

Find the word that means:

(1) A disease of the white cells:_____

(2) White blood cells:_____

(3) Red blood cells:_____

(4) A condition of too few red cells:_____

(5) Procedure to draw blood:_____

5.1.4   Terms Exercises in Diagnosis and Treatment

Match the following terms and write the appropriate letter to the left of each number.

(1) electrolyte (   )

(2) staging (   )

(3) symptom (   )

(4) syndrome (   )

(5) suture (   )

(6) cautery (   )

(7) scintiscan (   )

A. evidence of disease

B. classification of malignant tumors

C. substance that conducts electric current

D. to unite parts by stitching them together

E. a group of symptoms that characterizes a disease

F. removal of tissue for microscopic study

G. pain caused by cold

(8) cryalgesia (　　)　　　　　H. destruction of tissue with a damaging agent

(9) vasotripsy (　　)　　　　　I. image obtained with a radionuclide

(10) biopsy (　　)　　　　　　J. crushing of a vessel

(11) ergometer (　　)　　　　　K. instrument used to cut bone

(12) osteotome (　　)　　　　　L. organism that produces color

(13) acupuncture (　　)　　　　M. instrument to measure work output

(14) biofeedback (　　)　　　　N. method for controlling involuntary responses

(15) chromogen (　　)　　　　　O. treatment by insertion of thin needles

5.2　Terms Exercises in Health Physicochemical Analysis

5.2.1　Air Physicochemical Analysis

PM10 and PM2.5 are indicators that measure the hazards of suspended substance to the environment and human health, and are important indicators for indoor and outdoor air quality. Light scattering technique is an automatic method for detecting PM10 and PM2.5 based on the scattering effect of suspended particles on entrance light, and the intensity of scattered light is proportional to the concentration of particles. Briefly, PM10 and PM2.5 enter the darkroom for scattered light measurement, and interact with the optical source to generate scattered light. The scattered light signal is received by the photoelectric converter and converted into pulses per minute. The pulse count will be used to calibrate the mass concentration by standard criteria.

Now find the word that means:

Suspended substance in the air　　　　　　_____

Place for scattered light measurement　　　_____

5.2.2　Water Physicochemical Analysis

Organic pollutants in water have a broad source. They bring negative impact on human health and ecosystems in the way of inherent toxicity and reduction of dissolved oxygen (DO) in the water. The organic pollutants can be measured by comprehensive indicators. Commonly used comprehensive indicators are DO, chemical oxygen demand (COD) and biochemical oxygen demand (BOD), total organic carbon (TOC), volatile phenol and petroleum. For example, the TOC is a comprehensive indicator of carbon content that represents the total amount of organic matter in a water body, and it is also a direct indicator of the level of organic pollution in water quality. The TOC includes purgeable organic carbon (POC) and non-purgeable organic carbon (NPOC). The difference between these two is whether organic carbon can be purged from the water under specified conditions. Therefore, the inorganic carbon should be deducted when determining the TOC concentration of the water sample.

Construct the term that means:

Oxygen that dissolves in the water　　　　_____

Total amount of organic matter in a water body _____

Organic carbon can be purged from the water   _____

Organic carbon can't be purged from the water _____

5.2.3   Food Physicochemical Analysis

In order to prevent and control pests in warehouses, the grain is often stored by using fumigants in addition to hypoxia, radiation and low temperature storage. The main fumigants used are malathion, phosphide, cyanide, carbon disulfide and so on. Most fumigants can evaporate quickly after treatment, but some can remain in the grain even for a long time, and the large amount of residue is harmful to the human health. The limitation standards of fumigant residue are: malathion $\leqslant$ 3 mg/kg, phosphide $\leqslant$ 0.05 mg/kg, cyanide $\leqslant$ 5 mg/kg, carbon disulfide $\leqslant$ 10 mg/kg.

Now find the word that means:

Where to store the grain   _____

The main fumigants used   _____

5.3   Terms Exercises in Sanitary Microbiology

5.3.1   Plasmid Extraction and Electrophoresis Analysis

Since the characteristics of bacterial plasmids are stable, identification and typing of bacteria can be achieved according to the number and molecular weight of plasmids in different strains and the specific assignments in electrophoretic spectra of DNA fragments after digestion. Electrophoresis analysis of plasmid is deemed to determine the strain characteristics based on the plasmid DNA electrophoresis bands, including plasmid fingerprint maps and restriction maps. The difference between these electrophoresis methods is the processing after plasmid extraction. The former is to perform agarose gel electrophoresis on the extracted plasmid DNA and analyze the electrophoretic bands to determine the number and molecular weight. The latter is to use one or more restriction enzymes to digest the extracted plasmid DNA, and then subject to agarose gel electrophoresis. The different digestion sites of plasmid will decide the number of fragments and molecular weight are calculated, and the map also shows different band composition related to homology of plasmids.

Now, find the word that means:

Unique or distinctive pattern that presents specific person or substance   _____

Applied to sorting proteins according to their responses to an electric field   _____

Used in recombinant DNA procedures to transfer genetic material   _____

Capable of producing certain chemical changes by catalytic action   _____

5.3.2　Laboratory Biosafety

Laboratory biosafety containment needs to divide the hazard levels according to the risk of biotic factors. The biotic factors refer to all microorganisms and bioactive substances operated in the laboratory. According to the virulence, infectivity, as well as the risk to laboratory workers and the general population, the WHO has set up four hazard levels for biotic factors, namely, risk level 1, risk level 2, risk level 3, and risk level 4. The biosafety laboratory is accordingly divided into different biosafety levels (BSL), which corresponds to the risk level of biological factors. Risk level 1 is the lowest and denoted as BSL-1, while risk level 4 is the highest and denoted as BSL-4.

Now, find the word that means:

Maintenance of safe conditions in biological research　　＿＿＿＿＿＿＿＿＿＿

Any living thing that has an effect on an ecosystem　　＿＿＿＿＿＿＿＿＿＿

Having or producing an effect on living tissue　　＿＿＿＿＿＿＿＿＿＿

（陈阳　王涛）

新形态教材网·数字课程学习……

📺教学 PPT　　　📝自测题　　　💬推荐阅读

PART III
Microbiology

Chapter 6

Instruments for Microbiological Detection

Learning objectives

- Know applications of PCR and MALDI-TOF-MS.
- Be familiar with structures of PCR detection system and mass spectrometer.
- Master principles of PCR and MALDI-TOF-MS.

The microbiological examination by manual operation has been gradually replaced by the microbiology instruments with automatic operation and intelligent result interpretation. The automated instruments can perform the culture, identification, and antimicrobial susceptibility test of hundreds of suspected microorganisms, which mainly include automated blood culture system, automated microbial detection system and antibiotic sensitivity instrument. With the progress of microbial testing technology and related disciplines, the non-cultured microbial identification instruments are widely used in practice, due to its speed and simplicity. Here we focus on the rapid instruments, that is, polymerase chain reaction (PCR) instrument for detecting specific gene target sequences of microorganisms based on molecular biology technology; and mass spectrometer for detecting microbial components and metabolites based on matrix-assisted laser desorption/ionization time of flight mass spectrometry (MALDI-TOF MS).

6.1 Polymerase Chain Reaction

Polymerase chain reaction is a laboratory technique used to amplify target sequence of DNA to millions of copies in vitro. This technique was developed and described in 1983 by Kary Mullis, and the resulting manuscript was ultimately published in 1987.

6.1.1 Introduction of PCR

6.1.1.1 Principle of PCR

The essence of PCR technique is to amplify DNA fragments in vitro, so that the DNA template with low copies in the samples can be detected, and its specificity depends on the complementary oligonucleotide primers at both ends of the target sequences.

The reaction system of PCR includes DNA template, Taq DNA polymerase, oligonucleotide primers, four types of deoxyribonucleotide triphosphates (dNTP), appropriate buffer system, etc. A single target segment of DNA template is amplified into two pieces of double-stranded DNA by completing a cycle of high temperature denaturation, low temperature annealing and thermophilic extension. As the cycle repeats, a huge number of copies are produced.

6.1.1.2　Procedure of PCR

The process of PCR is carried out in small reaction tubes containing all the PCR components, which go through three main cycle steps, namely denaturation, annealing and extension.

Denaturation

In this step, the reaction mixture is heated to the denaturation temperature (about 94℃) for a certain time (15-30 seconds), and the hydrogen bonds between the double stranded DNA are broken and DNA templates are separated into two single strands.

Annealing

The temperature is descended to a certain degree (about 55°C). The two single stranded DNA as templates for PCR amplification can be combined with specific primers. The oligo-nucleotide primers complementarily attach to the single DNA strand to form hydrogen bonds with ends of target sequence.

Extension

In this step, Taq polymerase catalyzes the sequence starting from the 3' end of each primer and extending in the 5' to 3' direction at suitable temperature (about 72°C). The nucleotides added onto the primer are based on the principle that the A-T and C-G bases are complementary pairing.

The whole process takes place about 30-40 cycles and generates millions of copies of target sequence exponentially.

6.1.1.3　Types of PCR

At present, several specialized types of PCR have been developed based on the typical PCR procedures. The PCR techniques include reverse transcription PCR, real-time PCR, isothermal PCR, multiplex PCR, nested PCR, long-range PCR, single-cell PCR, hot start PCR, in situ PCR, digital PCR, etc. Some methods are introduced as follows:

Reverse Transcription PCR (RT-PCR)

Genetic material of some infectious agent like influenza virus is RNA. RNA is extracted and converted into complementary DNA (cDNA) by reverse transcriptase. The cDNA is then used as the template for the PCR reaction. The technique is called RT-PCR, which combines reverse transcription of RNA into DNA and amplification of target DNA sequence using PCR.

Real-time PCR

Real-time PCR, also quantitative real-time PCR, is a PCR technique that combines amplification of a target DNA sequence with real time detection of the DNA products in the reaction tube. DNA molecules are quantified using fluorescent dye or the fluorescent labelled oligonucleotides, which are used to monitor PCR products.

6.1.2   PCR Instrument

The earliest PCR instrument can be dated back to 1987. Cetus company and Perkin Elmer company (now ABI company) established Perkin Elmer Cetus instrument company, and began to develop nucleic acid amplification instrument based on PCR principle. The company launched the world's first PCR instrument "TC-1" at the end of that year. Higuchi reported the real-time fluorescence PCR technology in 1992. In 1996, ABI Company launched the first truly market-oriented real-time quantitative fluorescence PCR instrument–ABI 7700, which was introduced into China in 1997.

6.1.2.1   Structure of PCR Instrument

PCR instrument is a controllable fast temperature change device, which can complete three temperature cycles of denaturation, annealing and extension. Therefore, it is also called thermal cycler (thermocycler). The amplification instrument is usually composed of thermal cover parts, thermal cycling parts, transmission parts, control parts, and power supply parts (Figure 6-1). The PCR reaction tubes are placed into the instrument, and achieve the variation of required temperature controlled by the built-in program or computer software. The main ways of temperature change are heat block and air-driven circulation.

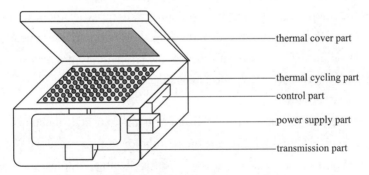

Figure 6–1   Structure of thermocycler

The PCR instrument with variable temperature heat block is to complete the alternating changes of three temperatures on the same heat block. The heat block is mainly made of aluminum or stainless steel, and has good thermal conductivity, making it more convenient to control the temperature than the water baths. There are different numbers or even different specifications of concave holes on it for placing PCR reaction tubes. The inner wall of the concave hole is processed accurately to ensure close contact with the sample tube to conduct heat. Two temperature modes of the instrument are controlled by the compressor and semiconductor. The former automatically controls the temperature rise and fall according to the set program, and semiconductor temperature controller is a current energy exchange device, which can not only cool, but also heat. By controlling the intensity and direction of input current, high-precision temperature control can be realized.

The temperature-adjustable PCR instrument can change the temperature of the tube via hot and cold air flow so that the three temperature cycles can be realized. It is heated by the metal coil, and cooled by the compressor. Air, as the medium, is in close contact with PCR tubes, with the good temperature uniformity and the fast temperature rise and fall speedily.

6.1.2.2　Types of PCR Instruments

PCR instruments are mainly divided into conventional PCR amplification instruments and fluorescence quantitative PCR amplification instruments. Compared with the later, conventional PCR instrument is usually called qualitative PCR instrument.

Conventional PCR Instruments

Conventional PCR instrument is equipped with temperature circulation which achieves a complete PCR experiment through cycles of temperature (the three steps of denaturation, annealing and extension), and the PCR products can be detected by agarose gel electrophoresis or fluorescence quantitative analysis, so that the unknown template can be detected.

Examples of other conventional PCR instruments are as follows:

Gradient PCR Instrument

PCR instrument with temperature gradient function is derived from conventional PCR instrument. The structure is basically the same as that of PCR instrument with variable temperature heat block, but the gradient function in the temperature control link is added. Gradient PCR instrument can be used to carry out gradient experiment on any of the three temperature cycles of high temperature denaturation, low temperature annealing and suitable temperature extension in PCR reaction. In practice, the temperature gradient of annealing step is commonly controlled in order to find the best annealing temperature.

In-situ PCR Instrument

In-situ PCR is the combination of hybridization in situ and PCR technique. The process of ·PCR is carried out in cells without destroying the morphology of tissues and cells. The instrument has several parallel aluminum grooves on the base for placing samples, and one slide can be placed vertically in each aluminum tank (cell suspension, tissue section, etc. are prefabricated on the slide). The surface of the slide is in close contact with the aluminum tank, with excellent temperature conduction and accurate temperature control.

6.1.2.3　Fluorescence Quantitative PCR Instrument

The fluorescence quantitative PCR instrument, combined with the PCR thermal cycler, fluorescence detection system and various application analysis software, can dynamically monitor the reaction process in real time and observe the gradual increase of PCR amplification products (fluorescence signal accumulation) in each reaction tube in each cycle of PCR. After the PCR process, quantitative results of the detected template can be obtained immediately with analyzing by standard curve. At the same time, PCR amplification efficiency and other information can be obtained.

The basic structure of fluorescence quantitative PCR instrument is composed of two main parts: PCR amplification system and fluorescence detection system. The PCR amplification system is similar to the conventional instrument. The fluorescence detection system mainly includes excitation light source and fluorescence detector. The excitation light source of fluorescence quantitative PCR instrument is mostly tungsten halogen lamp, equipped with 5-color filter, which can excite 96 samples at the same time. The detector is an ultra-low temperature charge coupled device (CCD) imaging system, which can detect multi-point and multi-color at the same time, and can effectively distinguish a variety of fluorescent dyes. Each type of fluorescence quantitative PCR instrument has real-time plate reading modes.

Digital PCR is a technique of detecting and absolutely quantifying nucleic acids. The quantitative process of digital PCR is divided into PCR amplification and fluorescence signal analysis. Firstly, the nucleic acid templates are diluted and distributed to tens of thousands of independent units, and theoretically there is only or less than a single template molecule in each reaction unit. Then the amplification reaction is carried out. Digital PCR instrument collects the fluorescence signal of each reaction unit after amplification. If the fluorescence signal can be detected, it is recorded as 1, otherwise 0. The reaction unit with fluorescence signal contains at least one copy of nucleic acid template. According to the total number of reaction units, the number of units with fluorescence signal and the dilution ratio of the sample, the initial copy number (concentration) of target molecules can be calculated using the Poisson statistics. According to the different ways of reaction unit formation, there are two mainstream digital PCR systems: microfluidic chip digital PCR systems and droplet digital PCR systems.

6.1.3　Common PCR Instruments

6.1.3.1　ABI PRISM 7000 Sequence Detection System

ABI PRISM 7000 Sequence Detection System (SDS) instrument is a quantitative and qualitative detector with fluorescent-based PCR chemistries. Quantitative detection employs real-time analysis, and qualitative detection uses end-point and dissociation-curve analysis. The instrument combines thermal cycling, fluorescence detection and analyzing software. It detects accumulated PCR products in real-time, thus obtaining detection results available immediately after completion of PCR, without further process analysis. At present, it is one of the mainstream PCR instruments used in domestic laboratories.

The instrument allows you to perform assays with 96-well plates or tubes. The assays can determine the quantity of a single nucleic acid specific sequence with a sample, including relative quantification and absolute quantification. And it can indicate the genotypes of samples and the presence or absence of a target sequence in a sample.

6.1.3.2　Roche LightCycler 96 System

LightCycler 96 system instrument is a real-time PCR system for absolute and relative quantification, melting curve analysis, and endpoint genotyping. It is also one of the mainstream PCR instruments used. The system consists of application software and amplification instrument.

The features of the instrument are plate-based system with 96-well block, standalone system, touchscreen with separate instrument software, and 4-plex multicolor. The detection performance of the system is dynamic range of 10 log, sensitivity of one copy, runtime of less than 1 hour.

6.1.3.3 Bio-Rad CFX96 Touch Real-Time PCR Detection System

The CFX96 Touch System is a powerful, precise, and flexible system, consisting of amplification instrument with integrated LCD touch screen and CFX Maestro software. The instrument has advanced optical technology with precise temperature control to deliver sensitive, reliable detection for singleplex or multiplex reactions. The key features include setting up the system quickly, minimizing sample and reagent use, optimizing reactions in a single run, analyzing data faster, configuring the system to fit the needs, and so on.

6.1.4 Application of PCR for Microbiological Detection

In infectious diseases, PCR is widely used in analyzing the presence of pathogen in patients' specimens. PCR can detect pathogen's nucleic acid qualitatively or quantitatively, which can provide information for disease diagnosis, curative effect evaluation and prognosis.

In clinical microbiology, many bacteria are difficult to identify and cultivate, and it takes long time to complete detection. PCR is a very rapid and accurate method. Therefore, PCR technique has greater advantages in identifying some infectious agents than traditional microbiological methods. PCR can be applied to detect *Mycobacterium tuberculosis*, *Chlamydia trachomatis*, *Neisseria gonorrhoeae*, *Helicobacter pylori*, *Mycoplasma pneumoniae*, etc. In the diagnosis of viral infectious diseases, viruses can be identified by PCR, such as hepatitis A virus, hepatitis B virus, hepatitis C virus, human immunodeficiency virus-1, human papillomavirus, cytomegalovirus, severe acute respiratory syndrome coronavirus, EB virus, influenza virus, rubella virus, measles virus, Ebola virus, etc. Nucleic acid of Toxoplasma gondii detected using PCR plays a role of diagnosis of the diseases toxoplasmosis.

PCR amplification technique can also be used for the inspection and quarantine of animals and plants at China's import and export ports. With the rapid development of international trade and modern logistics, the risk of epidemic spread has increased significantly. China has strengthened the monitoring and detection of epidemic infectious diseases of animal and plant, such as canine parvovirus, classical swine fever virus, equine influenza virus and bean pod mottle virus. PCR is used to detect unknown pathogens or virulent subtypes of organisms.

In addition to microbiology, PCR is applied to analyze mutations occurring in many genetic diseases, such as sickle cell anemia, muscular dystrophy, etc. Many malignant tumors are also characterized by certain genetic mutation. The technology is especially useful in forensic science, only a few amounts of specimens obtained from subjects can meet the need for detection of DNA. PCR technique is applied to match transplanted tissues, explore relationships among species in the field of biological evolution, study cryopreserved fossil in archaeology, and other aspects of molecular biology and so on.

6.2   Matrix-Assisted Laser Desorption Ionization-Time of Flight Mass Spectrometer

The Nobel Prize in Chemistry 2002 was awarded "for the development of methods for identification and structure analyses of biological macromolecules" with one half jointly to John B. Fenn and Koichi Tanaka "for their development of soft desorption ionization methods for mass spectrometric analyses of biological macromolecules" and the other half to Kurt Wüthrich "for his development of nuclear magnetic resonance spectroscopy for determining the three-dimensional structure of biological macromolecules in solution" . Several decades ago, people began to use mass spectrometry to detect pathogenic microorganisms. Now the mass spectrometry technology is relatively mature. The Matrix-Assisted Laser Desorption Ionization-Time of Flight Mass Spectrometer (MALDI-TOF-MS) is a newly developed instrument that can be applied to the discovery of disease biomarkers. Currently, its employment in identifying pathogens is being advanced, exhibiting a promising prospect for clinical applications.

6.2.1   Principle and Components of MALDI-TOF-MS

The MALDI-TOF-MS is a combination of MALDI and time-of-flight (TOF) mass spectrometer. The principle of MALDI is to irradiate the eutectic film formed by the sample and the matrix with a laser. The matrix transfers the energy of the laser to the bio-molecules. In the process of ionization, the bio-molecule gains or loses a proton, and the bio-molecule is ionized. Therefore, the selection of matrix, solvent and sample preparation method is the key factor. The choice of matrix is of great importance. The matrix is an energy-absorbing compound that can convert laser energy into heat energy, facilitating the desorption/ionization process. The matrix usually has a conjugated pi system, such as α-cyano-4-hydroxycinnamic acid (CHCA), 5-dimethoxy-4-hydroxycinnamic acid (sinapinic acid, SA), 2,5-Dihydroxybenzoic acid (gentisic acid, DHB), nor-harmane. The conjugated pi system can absorb energy and blast the analyte molecules into gas phase. The bio-molecules are ionized by proton transfer with the nearby matrix. MALDI is a soft ionization technique by which molecular ions are mainly formed. The advantages of MALDI include no heated injection chamber, complete molecular ions remaining intact when ionized, sensitive molecules that decompose at high temperatures.

The time-of-flight mass spectrometer is a classical mass spectrometer with two flight modes, parallel flight mode and vertical flight mode. Most modern mass spectrometer products adopt vertical flight mode. Like most mass spectrometers, a time-of-flight mass spectrometer separates ions by mass-to-charge ratio. The mass analyzer of time-of-flight mass spectrometer is an ion drift tube. The ions leaving the source are accelerated to the same energy by a high-voltage electric field. Based on the formula, kinetic energy = $\frac{1}{2} mv^2$, the ions of different masses have different velocities, and therefore arrive at the detector at different times. According to this principle, ions of different masses can be separated according to the mass-to-charge ratio. Compared with other types of mass spectrometer, the time-of-flight mass spectrometer scans faster and the instrument structure is simpler. The resolution is the ability to generate separate signals from ions of similar mass, which is an important property of time-of-flight mass spectrometer. In general, the time-of-flight mass spectrometer is suitable for the detection of biological molecules, due to its satisfactory resolution and capability of detecting a wide range of molecular masses.

6.2.2　Application of MALDI–TOF–MS for Microbiological Detection

Due to the combination of MALDI and TOF mass spectrometer, MALDI-TOF-MS is easy to operate, and has short detection time as well. MALDI-TOF-MS can be used to detect peptides, lipids, nucleotides, saccharides, DNA, RNA, RNA-protein conjugates and other biomolecules. Microbial identification is the most mature and extensive application of this technology at present. The identification of microbial species level mainly consists of biological molecules with molecular weight ranging from 2 000 to 20 000 Da, such as ribosomal protein and a small amount of house-keeping protein.

Microbial ribosomes are composed of ribosomal ribonucleic acid (rRNA) and ribosomal proteins (RPs). RPs consist of small subunit and large subunit nuclear proteins. 52 different types of RPs exist in prokaryotes and 82 types in eukaryotes. Moreover, RPs are abundant in microorganisms. Therefore, the spectrum of these microbial RPs can be quickly collected by the MALDI-TOF-MS. This detection technique is revolutionary.

6.2.2.1　Microbial Mass Spectrometry

Microbial mass spectrometry is less affected by medium and metabolites, so it is not sensitive to the differential expression of microbial growth stage. But it is very stable in response to high abundance of protein expression. A stable peptide mass fingerprinting (PMF) specific at the species level can be formed at the later stage of logarithmic growth. According to certain statistical requirements and standards, multiple mass spectrograms of known genera and species should be collected to form standard mass spectrograms by statistical algorithm. Then, the mass spectrogram data-base can be constructed by several standard mass spectrograms. When identifying unknown strains, the obtained mass spectrogram can be compared with the spectrogram data-base to complete the identification. This method has good specificity and can be used to identify tens of thousands of species.

6.2.2.2　Procedures of MALDI-TOF-MS for Microbiological Detection

The microbial identification process of MALDI-TOF-MS is very simple and can be divided into four steps. The first step is to prepare the matrix solution. The selected matrix is dissolved in water or acetonitrile aqueous solution. Sometimes a smaller amount of trifluoroacetic acid is added. Commercial matching matrix solutions are now available for purchase. The second step is sample preparation. Samples with volume less than 1 cubic centimeter are directly selected from the colony and evenly coated on the target plate, or use the extraction method to extract the protein for spot target. Then sprinkle about 1 μL of matrix solution on it. The solvent evaporates from the sample solution leaving behind a solid sample spot on the target. The third step is the analyses by mass spectrometry. The last step is data analysis and report writing. Mass spectrometry and principal component analysis (PCA) are performed by software. Recently, many mature mass spectrometry data-bases can be used directly, and some companies have also developed several handy programs, such as VITEKMS, SARAMIS, Bruker IVD MALDI biotyper, Andromas, etc.

6.2.2.3 Advantages and Disadvantages of MALDI-TOF-MS

Compared with traditional microbial identification methods, MALDI-TOF-MS has many advantages. Although for some biochemical tests, it merely takes a few minutes to complete, it typically takes about 24-48 hours to get a complete identification report for vast majority of microbial specimens, and even much more time for some caustic bacteria or slow-growing bacteria. Different from traditional methods, MALDI-TOF-MS is easy to operate and has relatively short detection time. Generally, MALDI-TOF-MS is more suitable for routine clinical detection than molecular biological methods in detecting some microorganisms.

The MALDI-TOF-MS is widely used in clinical laboratory and has attracted more and more attention. At present, the accuracy of bacterial species identification using MALDI-TOF-MS is above 90%. The application of MALDI-TOF-MS in the identification and classification of bacteria with multiple serotypes has been preliminarily applied, and it shows good typing ability in salmonella typing. The MALDI-TOF-MS can also be used to detect different drug resistance strains, fungi and so on. Blood, urine, other sterile body fluids and stool samples can be tested by the MALDI-TOF-MS.

It is worth noting that some MALDI-TOF-MS of domestic brands have begun to be used with good performance, such as CMI-1600, Autof ms1000, microTyper MS, Ebio Reader TM 3700, etc. These enterprises have broken the monopoly of foreign enterprises on the market of MALDI-TOF-MS. In recent years, the research and development capabilities of Chinese enterprises have been increasing, and we hope that Made-in-China will flourish in the MALDI-TOF-MS field.

Glossary

amplification *n.* 扩增 using the base sequence of a gene as a template, many identical gene sequences are copied

template *n.* 模板 a model or standard for making comparisons

thermocycler *n.* 热循环器 a processor-controlled heat block

quantitative *adj.* 定量的 relating to the measurement of quantity

qualitative *adj.* 定性的 relating to or involving comparisons based on qualities

Electrophoresis *n.* 电泳 the motion of charged particles in a colloid under the influence of an electric field

gradient *n.* 梯度 a graded change in the magnitude of some physical quantity or dimension

in-situ *n.* 原位 being in the original position, not having been moved

ionization *n.* 电离 processes by which neutral atoms or molecules are converted to charged atoms or molecules

mass-to-charge ratio(m/Q) 质荷比 a physical quantity that is widely used in the electrodynamics of charged particles

spectrum *n*. 谱 an ordered array of the components of an emission or wave

spectrogram *n*. 光谱图 a photographic record of a spectrum

（李琴　安康）

新形态教材网·数字课程学习……

📺 教学 PPT　　　　📝 自测题　　　　💬 推荐阅读

Chapter 7
Disinfection and Sterilization

Learning objectives
- Know the utilization of disinfection and sterilization.
- Understand the definitions of disinfection and sterilization.
- Be familiar with the factors that will affect the disinfection and sterilization.
- Master different methods of disinfection and sterilization.

Microorganisms are ubiquitous in the environment. Air, soil, rivers, lakes, oceans, and other places are home to different numbers and species of microorganisms. A variety of microorganisms are also found on the surface of human, animal and plant bodies and in the cavities they communicate with the outside world. Pathogenic microorganisms can cause infectious and non-infectious diseases. In the process of human struggle with pathogenic microorganisms, disinfection and sterilization are the most direct methods in the process of killing and controlling harmful microorganisms in the external environment, and also effective to control nosocomial infection.

7.1 Terms for Disinfection and Sterilization

In health care, disinfection and sterilization, although both refer to the killing or removing of microorganisms from the transmission media, represent two different concepts.

Disinfection refers to the killing or removal of pathogenic microorganisms on the vector and making it harmless. The vector, also called intermedium, refers to solid, gaseous and liquid substances contaminated with pathogenic microorganisms in the living and working environment, including contaminated human body surface and superficial body cavity. The term "pathogenic microorganisms" here includes various pathogenic microorganisms other than bacterial buds, such as bacterial propagules, fungi, viruses, rickettsia, and chlamydia, etc. Disinfection is aimed at pathogenic microorganisms, not to kill or eliminate all microorganisms. Chemicals used for disinfection are called disinfectants. Which reduce the number of harmful microorganisms to a harmless degree. The disinfection process must reduce the survival probability of microorganisms to 10^{-3}.

Disinfection includes two categories according to the purpose of disinfection: preventive disinfection and disinfection of epidemic focus. Preventive disinfection refers to the disinfection of equipment/instruments, places, and human bodies without obvious sources of infection but may be contaminated by pathogenic microorganisms. For example, the disinfection of public places, tableware, materials, drinking water, and the disinfection of containers, isolation places especially for transportation, storage places of animals and related products, and so on, all belong to preventive disinfection. Disinfection of epidemic focus refers to the disinfection of places where there are or have had infectious sources (patients or carriers) and places that have been contaminated by pathogens. It aims to kill or eliminate pathogens expelled from infectious sources. Disinfection of epidemic focus includes the disinfection of patients' excreta, contaminated articles, and wards performed by infectious disease hospitals or infectious disease departments of general hospitals, as well as the disinfection of patients' homes performed by personnels of disease control.

Disinfection of epidemic focus includes concurrent disinfection and terminal disinfection. Concurrent disinfection refers to the disinfection of the environment and articles that may be polluted by pathogens when there are infectious sources, such as the disinfection of the patient's feces, pollutants, and secretions. Disinfection must be quick at any time, so it is characterized by repetition. Terminal disinfection refers to the last thorough disinfection of the epidemic focus after the infectious source has left (such as after the inpatient isolation, transfer, or death). In principle, terminal disinfection is only performed once, but the concentration and dose of disinfectants should be increased compared with concurrent disinfection to assure complete elimination of pathogens.

Sterilization is the treatment that kills or removes all microorganisms from the transmission media to make them sterile. All microorganisms mentioned here include all pathogenic and non-pathogenic microorganisms, such as bacterial propagules, bacterial spores, fungi and their spores, viruses, rickettsia, chlamydia, spirochetes, etc., and even protozoa and algae. The requirements of sterilization are strict, and the items must be completely sterile after inactivation. It will not be considered to meet the requirements of sterilization even if there is only one bacterial colony. The concept of sterilization is absolute, which means the complete elimination of microorganisms on the transmission media. However, it is difficult to achieve such a goal realistically. Accordingly, in massive industrial production activity, sterilization qualification standards should be stipulated. The probability of the presence of live microorganisms per unit of the product after sterilization is called the sterility assurance level (SAL), which is usually expressed as 10^{-n}. Generally, for medical sterilization, the SAL is set at 10^{-6}, i.e., if a million copies of an item are sterilized, only one copy at most is allowed to have live microorganisms.

Antisepsis is the destruction of undesirable microorganisms, such as those that cause disease or putrefaction.

Cleaning is the removal of visible foreign material on the surface of objects and is normally performed manually or mechanically.

Asepsis is the state of being free from disease-causing contaminants (such as bacteria, viruses, fungi, and parasites) or preventing contact with microorganisms. The term sepsis often refers to those practices used to promote or induce asepsis in surgery operations or in medical cases for disinfection.

The operation technique of preventing microorganisms from entering the body or objects is called aseptic operation.

7.2 Methods of Disinfection and Sterilization

There are many methods of disinfection and sterilization, which can be broadly summarized as physical, chemical and biological methods. An appropriate method should be selected according to the actual disinfection and sterilization work in order to achieve better results.

7.2.1 Physical Disinfection and Sterilization Methods

The methods of using physical factors to kill or eliminate pathogenic microorganisms and other harmful microorganisms on objects or places are called physical disinfection and sterilization methods. Those methods are easy to implement, reliable, and without toxic residues. Commonly, physical disinfection and sterilization methods are natural air purification, mechanical decontamination method, thermal disinfection and sterilization, ionizing radiation disinfection and sterilization, ultraviolet disinfection, microwave disinfection, infrared disinfection, and plasma sterilization, etc. The followings are brief descriptions of several common physical methods.

7.2.1.1 Thermal Disinfection and Sterilization

Thermal disinfection and sterilization are the earliest, most common and most reliable methods to inactivate all microorganisms, including bacterial propagules, fungi, viruses, and the most bacterial spores. Thermal disinfection and sterilization is divided into two categories: dry heat, and wet heat methods.

Dry heat disinfection and sterilization can cause oxidation, denaturation, charring of bacteriophage proteins and concentration of electrolytes, causing cellular toxicity, thus causing microbial death. But its inactivation ability of microorganisms is not as good as that of wet heat disinfection. Dry heat disinfection and sterilization methods include dry baking, incineration, cauterization, infrared and other methods. Wet heat disinfection can make the protein in bacterium coagulated and denatured, which leads to the death of the microbiome. Wet heat disinfection and sterilization methods include boiling, circulation steam, pasteurization disinfection, intermittent sterilization, pressure steam sterilization and so on. The penetrating power of dry heat is much less than that of wet heat; therefore, the time required for dry heat sterilization is longer, and the temperature is higher; generally at 160°C, for 2 hours, and mainly used for sterilization of

67

items that are not resistant to moisture. Compared with dry heat disinfection, wet heat disinfection has stronger penetration and provides higher efficiency in sterilization and disinfection. The commonly used wet heat disinfection methods include boiling disinfection, pressure steam sterilization, circulation steam disinfection, and pasteurization, etc..

The commonly used thermal methods: (1) Pasteurization disinfection: mainly used in dairy products and other food industries; (2) Boiling disinfection: mainly used for disinfection of tableware, milk bottles, and bottle stoppers; (3) Pressure steam sterilization: mainly used for sterilization of medical instruments (surgical instruments and medical instruments) and experimental articles (glassware and culture medium); (4) Dry heat sterilization: mainly used for sterilization of surgical instruments, glassware, powder and grease; (5) Incineration sterilization: mainly used for sterilization of clothes, paper, and bacterial inoculation rings contaminated from pathogens.

7.2.1.2　Ionizing Radiation Disinfection and Sterilization

The method that uses y-rays and high-energy electron beams generated by electron gas pedals to penetrate the items to kill the inside microorganisms is called ionizing radiation disinfection and sterilization, which is a normal temperature sterilization method applicable to heat-labile items, also called "cold" sterilization. Ionizing radiation can achieve the purpose of sterilization. Its advantages are: (1) intense penetration, so for controlling the irradiation dose it can be packaged first and then disinfected or sterilized; (2) it can be carried out at room temperature without raising the temperature of items; (3) it irradiated items do not produce radioactivity, so there is no harmful residue; (4) easy to operate; (5) save manpower, and material resources, so it is suitable for batch flow operation.

The common unit of ionizing radiation is Gray (Gy), which is equal to 1 Joule of energy absorbed per kg of material, i.e. 1 Gy = 1 J/kg. Disinfection and sterilization by ionizing radiation are influenced by fewer factors, so controlling the irradiation dose can ensure the sterilization effect. Most countries have a sterility assurance level (SAL) of 10^{-6} for irradiated items. The sterility assurance level is the possibility that an item is allowed to have live microorganisms after sterilization. Ionizing radiation can be damaging to humans, so it is important to take care of protective measures. Ionizing radiation can also cause some damage to irradiated items, mainly affecting their stability. Therefore, some large molecular solutions, polymers, etc. should not be disinfected and sterilized by ionizing radiation.

7.2.1.3　Ultraviolet Disinfection

Ultraviolet(UV) disinfection is mainly used for disinfection of object surfaces and air. UV is very effective in disinfecting air and inactivating airborne disease pathogens such as influenza virus, measles virus, rubella virus, and mumps virus, etc. When disinfecting the surface of an item, it is required that the surface of the item is smooth and clean. UV light is so weak that it cannot penetrate even a piece of paper. Therefore, when using UV disinfection, the parts that cannot be irradiated by UV light will not achieve the disinfection effect cannot be disinfected. At the same time, the disinfection effect of UV lamps is also affected by factors including the intensity of irradiation, irradiation time, surface condition of the object, air cleanliness, lamp usage time, temperature and humidity, irradiation distance, sensitivity of microorganisms, and the number of microorganisms. The higher irradiation intensity and/or the longer irradiation time, the better the effect of sterilization. Low irradiation intensity or UV lamps used for a long time should be replaced or used for a long time to improve the sterilization effect. Whatever the item being disinfected, 30W UV lamp irradiation intensity at a distance of 1m shall not be less than 70 W/cm^2; otherwise it should be replaced.

7.2.2   Chemical Disinfection and Sterilization Methods

The use of chemical drugs or preparations to kill pathogenic microorganisms or other harmful microorganisms is called chemical disinfection and sterilization. Its mechanism is to make the microorganism's body nucleic acid or protein coagulation denaturaed, or interfere with the metabolism of microorganisms, or inhibit the growth and reproduction of bacteria and lysis to make the microorganisms die and achieve the purpose of disinfection. The chemical disinfection method is easy to use, but the effect is less reliable than thermal disinfection. This method can be used when the conditions for thermal disinfection are not available or when the disinfected items are not tolerant of heat.

Disinfectants usually refer to the chemical substances used for disinfection, while the physical factors used for disinfection are called physical disinfection methods or disinfectors. Disinfectants are used to kill the microorganisms on the transmission media to meet the requirements of disinfection or sterilization of the system of the state. Disinfectants does not necessarily kill all microorganisms, especially resistant bacterial spores; it is less effective than sterilants, which can kill all types of life.

Sterilants are preparations that can kill all microorganisms (including bacterial propagules, bacterial buds, fungi, viruses, rickettsiae, chlamydiae, and spirochetes, etc.) and achieve sterilization requirements. At present, sterilants commonly used in medicine and industrial and agricultural production include aldehyde compounds, alkylated heterocyclic gases, etc. Some chlorine-containing compounds and iodine-containing compounds can also be used as sterilants under certain conditions, but they are still referred to as disinfectants in the international arena.

Disinfectants do not necessarily act as sterilants, but all sterilants are excellent disinfectants. Generally, the standard for sterilants is whether they can kill germ cells or not. A sterilant should have two requirements: kill and remove all microorganisms; meet the requirements of being feasible for use, without damaging to articles, and having no harmful effects on humans.

Common methods of chemical disinfectants include soaking, wiping, spraying or conducting aerosol sprays; fumigation with their gases or fumes: heterocyclic gas disinfectants, peroxyacetic acid, etc.; direct treating with pharmaceutical powders; mainly chlorine-containing disinfectants.

An ideal disinfectant should have the following qualities: wide sterilization spectrum; low effective concentration; fast action; stable nature; easily soluble in water; can be used at low temperature; not easily affected by organic matter, acid, alkali and other physical, and chemical factors; low corrosiveness to goods; colorless, tasteless, odorless, easy to remove residual drugs after disinfection; low toxicity, not easy to burn and explode; inexpensive, easy to transport, and can be supplied in large quantities.

At present, no disinfectant fully meets the above requirements, so the use of the appropriate disinfectant can be selected according to specific conditions.

7.2.3　Biological Disinfection

Biological disinfection is a method of using some organisms to kill or remove pathogenic microorganisms or other harmful microorganisms. In nature, some organisms are killed during growth and reproduction, often forming an environment unfavorable to the survival of other microorganisms. For example, in sewage purification, the growth of anaerobic microorganisms under anoxic conditions can be used to prevent the survival of aerobic microorganisms; the fermentation of manure and garbage (composting) can be used to kill pathogenic microorganisms with the heat generated when thermophilic bacteria reproduce.

In practice, synergistic disinfection (also known as enhanced disinfection) is often used, i.e., more than two disinfection methods or disinfectants are used to accelerate and improve the disinfection effect.

7.2.4　Evaluation of Disinfection Effect

To evaluate the effect of disinfection, sampling before disinfection, sampling after disinfection, and laboratory culture tests are generally adopted.

7.2.4.1　Effect Evaluation of Pressure Steam Sterilization

Indicator bacteria: *Bacillus stearothermophilus* (ATCC7953 or SSIK31), containing 5×10^5– 5×10^6 cfu/tablet, at 121 ℃, D_{10} value is 1.3–1.9 minutes, KT value is ≤19 minutes, ST value is ≥3.9 minutes.

Evaluation: In the same test, all the bromocresol violet peptone medium inoculated with each indicator piece does not change color, which is judged as qualified sterilization. If one piece of bromocresol violet peptone medium inoculated changes from purple to yellow, it is judged as unqualified sterilization.

7.2.4.2　Evaluation of Ultraviolet Disinfection Effect

Indicator bacteria: *Escherichia coli* (ATCC8099 or ATCC25922); *Bacillussubtilisblack variant* (ATCC9372)

Evaluation: ① Physical detection: ordinary 30W straight tube new UV lamp with the radiation intensity ≥10^7 μW/cm². High-intensity UV lamp with the radiation intensity ≥200 μW/cm². ② Biological detection: the killing rate of indicator bacteria is ≥99.90%, which can be judged as qualified disinfection.

7.2.4.3　Evaluation of Disinfection Effect of Liquid Disinfectant

Indicator microorganisms: ①Bacteria: *Staphylococcus aureus*(ATCC6538), *Escherichia coli* (ATCC8099), *Pseudomonas aeruginosa* (ATCC15442), *Staphylococcus albus* (ATCC8032), *Mycobacterium chelonae* (ATCC93326), Bacillus subtilis black variety (ATCC9372). ② Fungi: *Candida albicans* (ATCC10231), *Aspergillus Niger* (ATCC16404). ③ Virus: poliovirus type I vaccine strain.

Evaluation: The killing rate of bacteria and fungi is ≥99.90%, and the inactivation of poliovirus type I can be judged as qualified disinfection. The black variety buds of *Bacillus subtilis* are killed completely, which can be judged as qualified sterilization.

7.2.4.4   Evaluation of Radiation Sterilization Effect

Indicator bacteria: *Bacillus pumilus* (E601).

Indicating bacteria killing rate is≥99.90%, which can be judged as qualified disinfection. All the indicator bacteria are killed, which can be judged as qualified sterilization.

7.2.4.5   Evaluation of sterilization effect of ethylene oxide

Indicator bacteria: Bacillus subtilis black variety bud (ATCC9372).

Evaluation: the killing rate of indicator bacteria is≥99.90%, which can be judged as qualified disinfection. All the indicator bacteria are killed, which can be judged as qualified sterilization.

7.3   Commonly Used Disinfectants and Sterilants

Commonly used disinfectants and sterilants are classified into aldehyde sterilants, alkylated gas disinfectants, peroxide disinfectants, chlorinated disinfectants, phenolic disinfectants, alcohol-based disinfectants, and guanidine disinfectants, quaternary ammonium disinfectants, iodine-containing disinfectants, etc. according to their chemical composition.

Commonly used chemical disinfection and sterilization methods (Table 7-1) are briefly described as follows.

7.3.1   Aldehyde sterilants

Aldehyde sterilants are the earliest chemical sterilants in use. Formaldehyde is the representative of the first generation of chemical sterilants. Glutaraldehyde is known as the third generation of chemical sterilants after formaldehyde and ethylene oxide (second generation), and o-phthalaldehyde has been applied to disinfection in recent years. Aldehydes mainly kill bacteria by coagulating proteins, reducing amino acids, and alkylating protein molecules.

Formaldehyde gas and liquid are highly effective in killing various microorganisms, including bacterial propagules, bacilli, Mycobacterium tuberculosis, fungi, and viruses, but are irritating, especially to the ocular and nasal mucosa. Its disinfection is relatively slow and requires a longer disinfection time.

Table 7-1 Commonly used chemical disinfectants and application

Designation	Nature	Bactericidal action	Commonly used concentration (%)	Disinfecting time (minute)	Operation method	Disinfection object
Calcium hypochlorite	White powder, soluble in water, effective chlorine content 60%~65%, It is strong bleaching and corrosive	Wide spectrum disinfectant, for bacterial propagules,virus,fungi and spore all have the effect of killing	0.1~1.0	15~120	Soak, wipe, scrub, sprayer, stir evenly	Excretion, vomit, secretions, sewage, garbage, furniture, food utensils, walls, ground, etc
Clorox	Light yellow liquid, the solution is alkaline, effective chlorine content 8%~12%	Wide spectrum disinfectant, for bacterial propagules,virus,fungi and spore all have the effect of killing	2~10	15~120	Soak, wipe, scrub, sprayer, stir evenly	Excretion, vomit, secretions, sewage, garbage, furniture, food utensils, walls, ground, air, etc
Sodium dichloroisocyanurate	White powder, stable performance, soluble in water, the solution is acidic, effective chlorine content 55%~65%	Wide spectrum disinfectant, for bacterial propagules,virus,fungi and spore all have the effect of killing,The bactericidal effect is stronger than that in other chloramine disinfectants	0.2~2.0	15~120	Soak, wipe, scrub, sprayer	Furniture, food utensils, walls, ground, air, etc
Peracetic acid	Colorless transparent liquid,volatile,unstable, easy to decompose in case of heat or organic matter, heavy metal ions, etc. peracetic acid content of 15%~18%	A broad-spectrum disinfectant that can kill bacterial propagules, tuberculosis bacilli, spores, viruses and other microorganisms	0.2~1	10~60	Soak, spray, fumigate, wipe	Furniture, tableware, clothing, toys, glass, rubber, plastic products, walls, floors, air, etc
Hydrogen peroxide	Colorless,odorless,transparent liquid, unstable,highlyoxidizing,easily decomposed in case of organic matter or metal and alkali, hydrogen peroxide content of 25%~28%	Broad-spectrum disinfectant,can kill all kinds of microorganisms	3~6	10~30	Soak, wipe, spray	Furniture, tableware, clothing, toys, glass, rubber, plastic products, walls, floors, air, etc

(Continued)

Table 7-1 (*Continued*)

Designation	Nature	Bactericidal action	Commonly used concentration (%)	Disinfecting time (minute)	Operation method	Disinfection object
Formaldehyde	37%~40% of formaldehyde aqueous solution, colorless transparent liquid, in a cold place for a long time, can have partial polymerization, easy to turbidity, and water or ethanol in any proportion of miscible, the solution was acidic	Broad-spectrum disinfectant,can kill all kinds of microorganisms	8~25	30~360	Soak,fumigate	Furniture, clothing, glass, rubber, plastic products, walls, floors, etc
Ethylene oxide	10% ethylene oxide mixed with 90% carbon dioxide gas, flammable and explosive, pay attention to safety	Broad-spectrum disinfectant that kills a variety of microorganisms	50~100	24~72	Fumigate	Equipment, bedding, clothes, furniture, glass rubber, plastic products
Iodophor	The unstable combination of iodine and surfactant, non-irritating, non-corrosive, containing 0.5% of available iodine	Broad-spectrum disinfectant that kills a variety of microorganisms	0.01-0.2	1~5	Soak, wipe	Skin, mucous membranes
Potassium permanganate	Strong oxidant, dark purple crystal, stable, resistant to storage, soluble in water, but the aqueous solution is unstable under acid and alkali conditions	It can kill bacterial propagules, viruses and destroy botulinum toxin	0.1~1	10~60	Soak	Tableware, utensils, fruits, vegetables, etc
Glutaraldehyde	It is colorless oily liquid that contains weak formaldehyde odor and weak volatility. It can be mixed with water and alcohol in any proportion. The solution is weakly acidic. glutaraldehyde 25% to 50%.	Broad-spectrum disinfectant, it can kill bacterial propagules, spores, fungi, viruses, stronger than formaldehyde	2	20~40	Soak	Medical instruments

Glutaraldehyde is broad-spectrum, fast, less irritating and corrosive, less toxic, and more stable in aqueous solution. It is suitable for disinfection and sterilization of heat-resistant medical devices and precision instruments, especially for various endoscopes. For sterilization, 2% glutaraldehyde is commonly used for 10 hours, and for disinfection, 2% glutaraldehyde or 1% synergistic glutaraldehyde is commonly used to soak for 10–20 minutes. Neutral or acidic compound glutaraldehyde disinfectant products are also prepared with synergistic agents. The bactericidal effect of Glutaraldehyde is better in alkaline conditions (pH7.6-8.6), but the stability is poor. The continuous use period of its disinfectant solution should be determined with the use of the situation and generally should not exceed 14 days. Glutaraldehyde has strong irritation and toxicity; therefore, when preparing and using glutaraldehyde, protective measures should be taken to avoid direct contact.

Phthalaldehyde has good bactericidal efficiency, low corrosiveness, slight irritation, and good stability, etc. It has been reported more often in recent years and is a promising chemical disinfectant.

7.3.2 Alkylated Gas Disinfectants

Alkylated gas sterilization is a class of derivatives based on methane and ethylene oxide, which are mainly used for sterilization and disinfection, such as ethylene oxide, ethylene propylene lactone, and propylene oxide.

Ethylene oxide can be non-specific alkylation with microbial proteins, DNA, and RNA, so that the carboxyl, amino, sulfur amino, and hydroxyl groups are alkylated, preventing the normal chemical reaction and metabolism of bacterial proteins, thus causing the death of microorganisms. Ethylene oxide gas penetrates strongly, but the damage to the goods is slight, without residual toxicity, wide sterilization spectrum, and reliable disinfection effect. It is widely used in medical disinfection and industrial sterilization, and the goods that should not be sterilized by general methods can be disinfected and sterilized with ethylene oxide, such as electronic instruments, medical devices, precision instruments, biological products, etc. In medical disinfection, it can be used for the disinfection or sterilization of the following items, such as surgical equipment, endoscopes, thermometers, rubber gloves, anesthesia equipment, cameras, etc. Ethylene oxide is flammable and explosive and must be sterilized in a sealed ethylene oxide sterilizer. There are many factors affecting the sterilization of ethylene oxide, such as the dose and duration of action of ethylene oxide, the type of microorganism, the degree of contamination, the packaging of sterilized items, temperature, relative humidity, etc. The sterilization effect can be achieved only by strictly controlling the relevant factors. Ethylene oxide is toxic to humans, and the maximum allowed concentration in the air of the workplace is 0.002 mg/L. After sterilization, the residual ethylene oxide on the articles should be removed before use.

Ethylene propylene lactone has a stronger bactericidal effect than ethylene oxide, but because of its carcinogenic effect, it has not been promoted as a conventional disinfectant. In recent years, it has been used for the disinfection of serum and serum products. Propylene oxide has poor volatility, low penetration, and only half the biological activity of ethylene oxide, so it is mainly used for the disinfection of powdered food and food additives.

7.3.3 Peroxide Disinfectants

Peroxide disinfectants are a class of disinfectants with a strong oxidizing ability, which are used to kill microorganisms by destroying the molecular structure of proteins with their oxidizing ability. Peroxide disinfectants include peroxyacetic acid, hydrogen peroxide, ozone, oxygen dioxide, etc. Peroxide disinfectants have the advantages of having a wide sterilization spectrum, strong sterilization power, and short sterilization time, being easy to dissolve in water, and having non-toxic components after decomposition and no residual toxicity. However, it is unstable, easy to decompose, irritating or toxic before decomposition, and has bleaching and corrosive effects on articles.

With its powerful oxidation effect, peroxyacetic acid first destroys the permeability barrier of the budding cells, then destroys and dissolves the core of the budding cells, causing DNA, RNA, protein, and other substances are damaged and leaked out, resulting in the death of the budding cells. Peroxyacetic acid can be used to disinfect the surface of various articles, except for metal products without a protective layer that is prone to corrosion and textiles that fade easily, Peroxyacetic acid is easy to evaporate and decompose after atomization, so it should be freshly prepared when used. It is a strong irritant to skin and mucous membranes and can even cause burns.

Hydrogen peroxide is a strong oxidizing agent, which can directly oxidize the outer layer of cell structure, so that the permeability of the cell is destroyed; in addition, the free radicals generated by the decomposition of hydrogen peroxide can directly destroy the proteins and nucleic acids of microorganisms, leading to the death of microorganisms. Hydrogen peroxide disinfectant is mainly used for disinfection of the environment and objects' surface, equipment disinfection, skin mucous membrane antisepsis, air disinfection, etc. Hydrogen peroxide is corrosive to human skin and mucous membranes, and can cause poisoning if it is inhaled too much, and it has a corrosive effect on metals and fabrics when it is contacted for a long time, as well as bleaching and fading effects.

Ozone is a strong oxidizing agent that can kill all types of microorganisms and destroy botulinum toxins. Generally speaking, ozone has a strong killing effect on microorganisms in water and air, and a slow killing effect on microorganisms in the environment and on the surface of articles. It can be used for drinking water disinfection, sewage treatment, the surface of articles, and air disinfection. Ozone has a short duration of decomposition in water, cannot remove continuous pollution, has very poor stability, and can decompose into oxygen at room temperature, so it can only be used freshly. Similar to the general strong oxidant, it can damage a variety of items, especially rubber products, and has bleaching and fading effects.

7.3.4 Chlorinated Disinfectants

Chlorinated disinfectants are a class of chemical disinfectants that produce hypochlorous acid with bactericidal activity when dissolved in water and have a killing effect on germ cells. Its active ingredient for killing microorganisms is expressed as effective chlorine, a measure of the oxidizing capacity of chlorinated disinfectants. It is the ratio of chlorine contained in the chlorinated disinfectant to its oxidizing capacity and the total amount of disinfectant, not the amount of chlorine contained in the disinfectant, and is generally expressed as a percentage of mg/L. Commonly used chlorine-containing disinfectants and their applications are shown in Table 7-2.

Table 7–2　Commonly used chlorine–containing disinfectants and their applications (reagent: water)

Disinfection object	Chlorinated lime	Sodium dichloroisocyanurate	Method of application
Meal tea set	1 : 800	1 : 1 200	soak, scrub
Bathroom facilities, slippers	1 : 100~1 : 150	1 : 1 000	soak, scrub
Food processing appliances	1 : 1 500	1 : 5 000	soak, scrub
Fruit, vegetables	1 : 1 000	1 : 2 400	soak
The surface of the object	1 : 5 00	1 : 500	soak, scrub
Hepatitis B patient contaminated items	1 : 150	1 : 500	soak
Drinking water	Active chlorine 4 mg/L	Active chlorine 4 mg/L	Constant chlorine
Swimming pool water	Active chlorine 5~6 mg/L	Active chlorine 5~6 mg/L	Constant chlorine

Chlorine-containing disinfectants include inorganic chlorine disinfectants (such as sodium hypochlorite, calcium hypochlorite, and trisodium phosphate chloride), and organic chlorine disinfectants (such as sodium dichloroisocyanurate, trichloroisocyanuric acid, and ammonium chloride T). Chlorine-containing disinfectants have a wide bactericidal spectrum and can effectively kill bacteria, fungi, viruses, amoeba encapsulation, and algae with rapid action, simple synthesis process, and can be produced and supplied in large quantities. Besides, they are inexpensive and easy to be widely used in drinking water disinfection, preventive disinfection, disinfection of epidemic sites and hospital disinfection. However, they are susceptible to organic matter and acidity, have bleaching and corrosive effects on articles, and loss of their active ingredients due to light, heat and humidity.

Sodium hypochlorite is an inorganic chlorine disinfectant, commonly used in the disinfection of medical supplies, disinfection of tableware, relying on hypochlorite generators for water disinfection and aqueous solution spraying can be used for preventive disinfection of epidemic areas.

Bleaching powder is a compound, with the main component being calcium hypochlorite. Bleaching powder is a white granular powder containing 25% to 32% effective chlorine be dissolved in water, and other inorganic chlorine disinfectant characteristics and use the same method, poor stability, accelerated decomposition rate in the presence of light and heat, affected by acidity and alkalinity. Bleaching powder can be used for bleaching of cotton, flax, pulp, silk fiber fabrics, sterilization and disinfection of drinking water, swimming pool water, etc.

Chloramine T contains 24%~26% effective chlorine, which is more stable in nature. It is a broad-spectrum disinfectant and has the effect of killing bacteria, viruses, fungi, and budding cells. It causes little irritation to the skin and can be used for disinfection of drinking water, disinfection of eating utensils and various utensils, treatment of wounds, and rinsing and disinfection of nasal and oral mucous membranes.

Sodium dichloroisocyanurate has a strong oxidizing effect. The effective chlorine content is 55%~65%, and it is a broad-spectrum disinfectant and sterilizer. It has strong bactericidal efficiency, good stability, safety, and low toxicity, and does not produce pollution. It can rapidly kill viruses, bacteria, and their budding cells and is widely used for the disinfection of drinking water, medical supplies, surface disinfection of articles and environmental disinfection of various places.

7.3.5　Phenolic Disinfectants

There are more types of phenolic disinfectants, such as phenol (carbolic acid), coal phenol soap solution (Lysol water), and halogenated phenols etc. Phenolic disinfectants are stable, mildly corrosive, and basically harmless to humans when used in concentrations. However, it has a special odour, limited bactericidal power, and can only kill bacterial propagules and lipophilic viruses. In addition, it irritates to the skin and can stain textiles with long-term immersion and damage rubber items.

Phenol is corrosive and irritating to tissues, and its vapours are toxic to humans, so phenol is rarely used as a disinfectant.

Coal phenol soap solution, also known as lysol water, is a phenolic disinfectant commonly used in the past, mainly for disinfection of object surfaces, such as furniture, walls, floors, utensils, contaminated items in laboratories, and sanitation and epidemic prevention treatment. Phenols are gradually being replaced by other disinfectants because they can contaminate water sources and cause public hazards and have a certain irritating and corrosive effect on the skin.

Compared with phenolic disinfectants, halogenated phenolic disinfectants have a significantly stronger bactericidal effect but still have the special odor and toxic side effects of phenol. In recent years, several new disinfectants have emerged with better germicidal effects and fewer toxic side effects than halogenated phenolic disinfectants, so the use of halogenated phenolic disinfectants is gradually being restricted.

7.3.6　Alcohol–Based Disinfectants

Alcohol disinfectants have a long history and have an important place in hospital disinfection. They can kill bacterial propagules but not bacterial germ cells and are medium-acting disinfectants. They are mainly used for skin disinfection. Ethanol and isopropyl alcohol are commonly used, which are fast-acting, colorless, and inexpensive.

Ethanol is a widely used disinfectant for clinical and household use and has synergistic and synergistic effects on other disinfectants such as glutaraldehyde, iodine, and chlorhexidine. Ethanol can kill bacterial propagules, viruses and mycobacteria, but not bacterial budding cells. Therefore, it can only be used for disinfection but not for sterilization. Ethanol is less irritating to the skin and has no damage to other objects. It is commonly used for skin disinfection before injection, surgical hand washing, instrument soaking disinfection, and surface disinfection. 60% to 90% of ethanol has the most bactericidal effect. Isopropyl alcohol is a commonly used organic solvent with similar properties and effects as ethanol but with stronger toxicity and higher price than ethanol. Isopropyl alcohol will lose its antibacterial effect when its concentration falls below 35%.

7.3.7 Guanidine Disinfectants

Guanidine disinfectants are not able to kill bacterial buds but have a strong effect on bacterial propagules, and are generally used for disinfection of skin and mucous membranes and also for disinfection of environmental surfaces.

Chloroform is a cationic disinfectant with the characteristics of fast-acting, non-irritating to skin and mucous membranes, stable, resistant to storage, and influenced by organic matter. It is mainly used for surgical hand washing disinfection, skin and mucous membrane disinfection of surgical sites, etc. It is inefficient in terms of direct sterilization.

Polyhexamethylene is a new guanidine disinfectant with strong bactericidal power, fast action, good stability, and low toxicity. It is widely used in the disinfection and sterilization of medical boil health, disinfection of pipes and containers in beverage and food processing operations, disinfection of drinking water, and swimming applicable water, also can be used in the tide, water ponds, cooling towers, fountains to remove algae, etc.

7.3.8 Quaternary Ammonium Disinfectants

Quaternary ammonium disinfectants are a class of cationic surfactants, of which single-chain quaternary ammonium disinfectants are low-potency disinfectants, such as benzalkonium bromide (Bromo-Germaine), which are easily soluble in water and can produce a large amount of foam by shaking. They have stronger killing efficiency on Gram-positive bacteria than on Gram-negative bacteria. It is more sensitive to lipophilic viruses but has stronger resistance to hydrophilic viruses and acid-resistant bacilli. It is characterized by low toxicity without irritation to skin and mucous membrane and can be used for skin disinfection and mucous membrane rinsing. In addition , it has good stability without damage to disinfected articles, etc. It is very easy to be absorbed by many objects, so the concentration of the soaking solution decreases gradually with the number of disinfected articles and should be replaced in time. It should not be used in combination with soap or other anionic detergents and should not be used for disinfection of excreta such as faeces, urine, and sputum.

7.3.9 Iodine–Containing Disinfectants

Iodine-containing disinfectants include iodine and various preparations with iodine as the main bactericidal component, such as iodophor and tincture of iodine, which is medium-acting disinfectants.

Iodophor is an indefinite complex formed by iodine with surfactant and co-solvent. It has a good killing effect on bacterial propagules, Mycobacterium tuberculosis, phage, fungi, viruses, and protozoa, etc. It can kill bacterial budding cells, but it takes a longer time. It is mainly used for skin and mucous membrane disinfection and treatment of contaminated wounds. Other iodine disinfectants such as iodine solution, iodine tincture, and iodine glycerin are widely used clinically. The alcoholic solution of iodine has a better bactericidal effect than the aqueous solution, but the aqueous solution is less irritating. Generally, iodine tincture is available for skin disinfection, while iodine solution is appropriate for mucous membrane disinfection. Iodine glycerin is a compound preparation of iodine, potassium iodide, and glycerin, which has strong antibacterial, and anti-inflammatory, anti-swelling and anti-fungal effects. It is much less irritating and especially applicable for the disinfection of mucous membranes. Free iodine disinfectant can be used for the disinfection of surgical instruments.

7.4 Factors Affecting Disinfection and Sterilization Effect

Whether it is a physical method or a chemical method, their disinfection and sterilization effects are affected by many factors. Avoidance of misusing these factors can improve the disinfection effect; conversely, improper handling can lead to disinfection failure. The main factors affecting disinfection effectiveness are the following.

Dosage (including intensity and duration)

In thermal disinfection and sterilization, the dose refers to temperature and time. In ultraviolet disinfection, the dose refers to the irradiation intensity and time. In chemical disinfection or sterilization, the dose refers to the concentration and time.

Degree of Microbial Contamination

It is obvious that the greater the degree of microbial contamination, the more difficult disinfection and sterilization become, therefore the need to increase, the amount and duration of disinfectants and disinfectants.

Temperature

Generally speaking, in physical disinfection and sterilization, the higher the temperature, the better the effect. Within a certain range, the higher the temperature of chemical disinfection and sterilization is, the better the effect is. Therefore, there is an optimum range of temperature requirements for chemical disinfection. For example, when using ethylene oxide for disinfection, when the temperature is lower than $10.7\,℃$, the drug itself cannot volatilize into gas. At $4\,℃$, the output intensity of UV light is only 20% to 30% of that at $27\,℃$.

Humidity

Humidity has different effects on different disinfection and sterilization methods. The relative humidity of the air has a significant effect on fumigation disinfection. Direct spraying of dry powder for ground disinfection requires high relative humidity to make the drug damp to fully function. When irradiating with ultraviolet light, its penetrating power gradually decreases with the increase of relative humidity, which is not conducive to disinfection.

pH

The change in pH seriously affects the effect of disinfectants, and different disinfectants have different requirements for pH value. For example, quaternary ammonium salts have a greater effect in alkaline solutions, and the concentration required to kill microorganisms at pH 3 is about 10 times greater than that at pH 8. The bactericidal activity of glutaraldehyde solution increases gradually when the pH value increases from 3 to 8. When the pH of the hypochlorite solution increased from 3 to 8, the bactericidal activity decreased.

Chemical Antagonists

Under natural circumstances, microorganisms are often mixed with many other substances, especially organic substances, which often affect the disinfection and sterilization effects. For example, protein and oily organic matter, etc. surrounding the microorganisms will hinder the penetration of various disinfection factors, and will also consume a part of the disinfectant, especially for disinfectants with oxidative effect, and then affect the dose and concentration of the disinfectant on the microorganisms.

Penetration Power

Different disinfection and sterilization factors have obvious differences in penetration ability. For example, the penetration power of dry heat is worse than that of wet heat. The penetrating power of formaldehyde vapor is worse than that of ethylene oxide, and ionizing radiation can penetrate deep into various substances, while ultraviolet rays can only act on the surface of objects or microorganisms in shallow liquids.

Surface Tension

The small surface tension of the disinfectant is conducive to the contact of the drug with microorganisms and the killing effect. Therefore, on the one hand, a solvent with low surface tension is used to prepare a disinfectant to improve the disinfection effect. On the other hand, surfactants can be added to the disinfectant to reduce the surface tension of the solution.

Cleanliness

The cleanliness of the object to be disinfected has a certain influence on the disinfection effect. For example, when water is disinfected, the turbidity of the water has an impact on the disinfection effect because the suspended particles in the water can absorb the disinfectant and reduce the effective concentration of the disinfectant. During air disinfection, steam, smoke, suspended particles, and organic matter in the air can affect the disinfection effect of ultraviolet rays.

Surface Condition of the Object

When the surface of the object is disinfected, the smoothness degree has a certain influence on the disinfection effect, and the impact on ultraviolet disinfection is more obvious.

Glossary

disinfection *n.* 消毒 the thermal or chemical destruction of pathogenic and other types of microorganisms

sterilization *n.* 灭菌 destroys of all forms of microorganisms, usually with physical methods to achieve the purpose of sterilization

antisepsis *n.* 防腐 the destruction of undesirable microorganisms, such as those that cause disease or putrefaction

cleaning *n.* 清洁 the removal of visible foreign material on objects of surfaces, which is normally performed manually of mechanically

asepsis *n.* 无菌 the state of being free from disease-causing contaminants (such as bacteria, viruses, fungi, and parasites), or preventing contact with microorganisms

disinfection of epidemic focus 疫源地消毒 the disinfection of places where there are or have had infectious sources (patients or carriers) and places that have been contaminated by pathogens

preventive disinfection 预防性消毒 the disinfection of equipment/ instruments, places, and human bodies that have no obvious source of infection but may be contaminated by pathogenic microorganisms

physical disinfection 物理消毒 the method of using physical factors to kill or eliminate pathogenic microorganisms and other harmful microorganisms on objects or places is called

chemical disinfection 化学消毒 the method of killing pathogenic microorganisms or other harmful microorganisms with chemical drugs or preparations

（黄颖）

新形态教材网·数字课程学习……

💻 教学 PPT　　　📝 自测题　　　💬 推荐阅读

Chapter 8

Mycobacterium Tuberculosis and Examination

Learning objectives:

- Know pathogenicity and epidemiological characteristics of *Mycobacterium tuberculosis*.
- Be familiar with biological characteristics of *Mycobacterium tuberculosis*.
- Master laboratory examination of *Mycobacterium tuberculosis*.

8.1   Introduction to *Mycobacterium Tuberculosis*

Mycobacterium tuberculosis complex (MTC) is the pathogen of human tuberculosis. This organism belongs to the kingdom *Prokaryotes*, the phylum *Firmicutes*, the order *Actinomycetales*, the family *Actinomycetes*, the genus *Mycobacteriaceae*. The species that comprise MTC are *Mycobacterium tuberculosis* (*M. tuberculosis*), *M. bovis*, *Bacille Calmette-Cuerin* (BCG) vaccine strain, *M. africanum*, *M. caprae*, *M. microti*, *M. canetti*, *M. pinnipedii*, and recently identified *M. mungi* and *M. orygis*.

8.1.1   Epidemiology

According to WHO, one-third of the world's population is estimated to be infected with *M. tuberculosis* accounting for nearly 90% of tuberculosis. Recently, the overall incidence and prevalence of tuberculosis have been declining, with an 11% cumulative reduction in incidence rate between 2015 and 2020. In 2020, a total of 1.5 million people died of tuberculosis, and an estimated 10 million people suffered from tuberculosis worldwide. Eight countries account for two thirds of the total, which are India, China, Indonesia, the Philippines, Pakistan, Nigeria, Bangladesh and South Africa.

China is one of the 22 countries with high burden of tuberculosis worldwide, with the number of about 1.3 million prevalent tuberculosis cases annually, accounting for 14% of the global number of patients. Although our country has been making steady progress in tackling tuberculosis that the incidence and mortality of tuberculosis have been greatly reduced by 42% and 90% respectively over the past two decades, the serious problems of tuberculosis have become complex with the emergence of multidrug-resistant strains of *M. tuberculosis*, coinfection of HIV, cross infection among tuberculosis pathogens and so on. One of the health targets of the United Nations Sustainable Development Goals (SDGs) is ending the tuberculosis epidemic by 2030. In 2030, we will achieve the goal of sustainable development which is to establish a comprehensive tuberculosis prevention and treatment mode, strengthen the screening and monitoring of multidrug-resistant tuberculosis (MDR-TB), standardize the management of tuberculosis diagnosis and treatment, and continue to reduce the incidence of tuberculosis in China.

8.1.2　Pathogenicity

M. tuberculosis does not produce endotoxin, exotoxin, and invasive enzymes. The pathogenesis results from the infected host's responses to the organism, of which the most important is the immune response. After exposure, *M. tuberculosis* entering and penetrating the bodies are phagocytized by macrophages, and can evade the cells killing. However, the macrophages contacted with *M. tuberculosis* secrete the cytokines and induce inflammation.

Humans are the only natural reservoir and highly susceptible to *M. tuberculosis*. *M. tuberculosis* can enter patients through respiratory tract, gastrointestinal tract and skin injury. Tuberculosis bacteria spread from person to person through the air. A person inhales only a few aerosols carrying *M. tuberculosis* to become infected. The infections in patients are primarily restricted to the lungs, but disseminated extrapulmonary disease can appear following circulating spread. The microorganism can also invade bones, joints, central nervous system, kidney, etc.

Common symptoms and signs of active lung tuberculosis are bad cough lasting at least 3 weeks, coughing up blood or sputum, chest pains, weakness, weight loss, fever, and night sweats. Other parts of the body's symptoms depend on the area affected by *M. tuberculosis*. People with latent tuberculosis infection do not display any of the symptoms because of the bacteria being inactive. Tuberculosis is curable and preventable.

M. tuberculosis is an intracellular pathogen. Macrophages phagocytize the bacteria and secrete the cytokines IL-12 and TNF-α that in turn recruit T-cells and natural killer cells into the area of the infection and stimulate intracellular killing. The people carrying the pathogen can acquire immunity, known as immune carriers. A person infected with *M. tuberculosis* or its components existing in the body has immunity against the bacterium. Immunoprophylaxis with BCG vaccination is used in many countries, but the effect is limited.

8.1.3　Biological Characteristics

The main characteristic of *Mycobacterium* bacteria is that the cell wall contains a large amount of lipids, which accounts for 60% of the dry weight. Mycolic acid, consisting mainly of components, is closely related to its characteristics of staining, growth, pathogenesis, and resistance. The microorganism is not easy to color with Gram's stain. Ziehl-Neelsen technique is the commonly used acid-fast staining. Due to performing an acid-fast staining procedure they retain the primary dye carbol-fuchsin against decolorization with acid-alcohol, so it is also called acid-fast bacillus (AFB).

8.1.4 Morphology

M. tuberculosis is a rod-shaped bacillus with branching growth trend. The length of the microorganism usually ranges from 1 to 4 micrometers and the width is somewhere between 0.3 to 0.6 micrometers. *M. tuberculosis* is non-motile, non-spore-forming, acid-fast positive bacterium. In recent years, it has been found that there is a capsule outside its cell wall, which is usually destroyed during smear preparation and difficult to see. Dehydration and shrinkage of the capsule can be prevented, if smear was treated with glue before fixation for electron microscope detection.

8.1.5 Growth Characteristics

M. tuberculosis is a strictly aerobic microorganism, and the condition of 5% to 10% carbon dioxide is necessary for primary recovery from specimens. Its optimal growth temperature locates in the range of 32 to 37℃, and optimal pH is between 6.5 and 6.8. *M. tuberculosis*, a very fastidious organism, requires special nutritional and other growth factors for recovery. It can grow well only on special medium containing serum, egg yolk, potato, glycerol, and some inorganic salts. Lowenstein-Jensen (L-J) solid medium is commonly used, in which egg yolk can promote the growth of this bacterium and malachite green can inhibit the growth of miscellaneous bacteria. The organism is relatively slow-growing, typically requiring incubation for 2 to 6 weeks to form typical colonies. The colonies on L-J medium are rough, dry, granular and nonpigmented. In the liquid medium, the bacteria grow faster, generally cultivated 1 to 2 weeks. Interestingly, *M. tuberculosis* grows and precipitates at the bottom of the tube, and then rises to the medium surface to form a bacterial membrane.

8.1.6 Biochemical Characteristics

The biochemical reaction of *M. tuberculosis* is inactive. Sugars are not fermented. Most of strains are positive in catalase test, and the enzyme activity disappear after heating at 68℃, which can be distinguished from non-*tuberculous Mycobacterium*. Niacin test, nitrate reduction test and pyrazinamidase test of *M. tuberculosis* are positive, which is helpful to distinguish from *M. bovis*.

8.1.7 Resistance

Due to the rich lipid components in the cell wall, *M. tuberculosis* is more resistant to various physical and chemical factors than other bacteria. *M. tuberculosis* can remain infectious ability in the dust for 8 to 10 days and survive in dried sputum for 6 to 8 months. It can resist to be treated by 3% hydrochloric acid, 6% sulfuric acid or 4% sodium hydroxide for 30 minutes. Therefore, acids or alkalis can be employed to deal with viscous substances in samples polluted by undesired microbes and digest samples before isolation and culture. In addition, malachite green can be added to the culture medium to inhibit the growth of other bacteria since *M. tuberculosis* is resistant to 1 : 13 000 malachite green. *M. tuberculosis* is sensitive to damp and heat. It can be killed by heating in liquid at 62 to 63 ℃ for 15 minutes or boiling. Ultraviolet rays can well kill the mycobacteria, which is used to disinfect contaminated items of tuberculosis patients.

8.1.8　Variability

The variation of *M. tuberculosis* existes in colony, morphology, virulence, immunogenicity, drug resistance, and so on. BCG (Bacille Calmette-Guérin) is a live attenuated vaccine strain of *M. bovis* used to prevent tuberculosis. The vaccine is the most widely administered and recommended as a kind of the routine newborn immunization schedule in our country. BCG was developed by Calmette and Guérin by subculturing *M. bovis* in a medium containing glycerol, bile salt and potato for 230 times for 13 years that started from 1908. Finally, it was first administered to human in 1921. Virulence variation is often accompanied by variation of colony characteristics. The colony morphology of the attenuated strain can change from rough type (R type) to smooth type (S type).

M. tuberculosis easily incurs drug resistance due to genetic mutations. *M. tuberculosis*, which can grow in the solid medium containing the most effective first-line anti-tuberculosis drugs as isoniazid, streptomycin or rifampicin, is called drug-resistant bacterium. The strains of *M. tuberculosis* resistant to at least both rifampicin and isoniazid are called multidrug-resistant mycobacteria. Recently, multidrug-resistant strains have gradually increased all over the world, and even caused outbreaks. The serious public health problem is worsened by it. In 2006, the first reports of extensively drug-resistant tuberculosis (XDR-TB) began to appear, which is defined as resistance to both isoniazid and rifampicin, and to any fluoroquinolone, and to any of injectables (amikacin, capreomycin and kanamycin). In 2021, WHO's Global TB Programme revised the definitions. The new definition of pre-extensively drug resistant tuberculosis (pre-XDR-TB) is that *M. tuberculosis* stains are resistant to any fluoroquinolone, in addition to drugs by MDR-TB and rifampicin-resistant TB. The updated definition of XDR-TB is the strains that resist at least one additional drug of second-line medicines comprising levofloxacin, moxifloxacin, bedaquiline and linezolid on the base of MDR-TB. The new definitions will be expected to lead to better reporting, surveillance and monitoring of drug-resistant TB in countries.

8.2　Laboratory Examination

8.2.1　Laboratory Biosafety

Transmission of tuberculosis is a hazard to individuals exposed to infectious aerosols in the laboratory. *M. tuberculosis* has strong resistance to environment factors. The strains in specimens from clinical cases may survive and be aerosolized during the processing of identification. So, whatever *M. tuberculosis* may exist in specimens, they must be considered potentially infectious and paid appropriate attentions and tackled with protective measures. Standards recommended for all laboratories handling specimens are endorsed by WHO. These standards require administrative controls, controlled ventilation system, personal protective equipment, waste management procedures and laboratory safety procedures.

8.2.2   Specimen Collection

Different types of specimens are collected for microbiological examination. Proper specimen collection and handling is an important part of obtaining reliable and accurate laboratory test results.

Respiratory Specimen Collection

Collect 3 to 5 mL in volume sputum of expectoration in the morning, preferably an early morning specimen. If the patient is unable to excrete sputum, induced sputum can be obtained through atomization inhalation of hypertonic saline or oral ammonium chloride. Acceptable quality specimens are thick and contain mucoid or mucopurulent material. Other than sputum, respiratory specimens include bronchoalveolar lavage, bronchial wash/brush, endotracheal and transtracheal aspirate.

Non-respiratory Specimen Collection

Extrapulmonary specimens may be divided into those from non-sterile and normally sterile body sites, which include tissue, blood, stool, urine, gastric aspirate, cerebral spinal fluid, and other body fluids (pleural, peritoneal, pericardial, synovial fluid). Pleural and peritoneal fluids are collected aseptically for 10 to 15 mL optimally and transported to the laboratory for examination immediately. If delayed, sodium citrate can be added to the final concentration of 0.5% to prevent the specimen from solidification. Collect 10 to 15 mL of total urine volume or 24-hour urinary sediment in the morning for examination, and conduct sterile catheterization if necessary. All specimens should be collected in a sterile leak-proof container, and transported as soon as possible.

8.2.3   Specimen Processing

Respiratory specimens are processed with acids and alkalis to inhibit or even kill undesired microbes depending on the acid- and alkali-resistant characteristics of *Mycobacterium*. Mucolytic agent is also used to dissolve and liquefy sputum to release AFB. If necessary, specimens should be centrifuged for at least 15 minutes at $3000 \times g$, and then mycobacteria sediment is collected.

8.2.4   Staining Procedures

Staining followed by microscopic observation is applied to exam smear prepared from patient specimens or organisms growing in culture. This is a rapid procedure for detection of *M. tuberculosis* in clinical specimen, but sufficient microorganisms, such as 10^5 bacilli per mL of sputum can be detected.

8.2.4.1 Smear Preparation

Working in a biological safety cabinet, take a clean grease-free microscopic slide, pick out the specimen (or processed specimen) onto the slide directly using the sterile loop, and spread it over an area approximately 1 cm × 2 cm. Dry the smear in the air, and heat-fix smear on the burner flame.

8.2.4.2 Ziehl-Neelsen Acid-fast Staining

Ziehl-Neelsen Acid-fast Staining is an important differential staining method used to identify acid-fast organisms, mainly mycobacteria.

Primary Staining

Place slides on staining racks. Flood the smear with carbol-fuschin solution, and gently heat the slide until the stain begins to steam and stand for 3 to 5 minutes. Don't evaporate and boil the stain throughout the process, and add more stain if necessary. Then wash it off with water.

Decolorizing

Adding 3% acid alcohol (3% HCl+95% ethanol) to decolorize until the smear appears faintly pink (no more than 10 minutes). Wash off it with water.

Counterstaining

Flood smear with methylene blue dye and counterstain for 2 to 3 minutes. Rinse with water, drain, and air dry.

8.2.4.3 Auramine O Staining

The auramine O can bind to mycobacteria because of the affinity of mycolic acid in the cell walls for fluorochromes. Therefore, it can bind to mycobacteria. This method is recommended for specimen examination due to its high sensitivity and fast speed.

Flood the smear with auramine O solution and allow it to stain for 10 to 15 minutes. Then rinse the slide with water. Decolorize with 0.5% acid-alcohol for 1 to 2 minutes until no yellow comes out, and wash with water. Flood smear with 0.5% potassium permanganate and let it for 1 to 2 minutes, and rinse the slide with water. Air dry and examine the smear with a fluorescent microscope as soon as possible after staining.

8.2.4.4 Microscopic Examination

The staining microscopy is used to detect acid-fast bacilli in clinical sputa. The results of examination of stained smears are commonly reported according to the WHO and the International Union Against Tuberculosis and Lung Disease (IUATLD) system. The Ziehl-Neelsen stain smears are examined under the oil immersion lens of microscope. Acid-fast bacilli retain carbol-fuschin, and appear red or pink; non-acid fast organisms and the background debris take the color of methylene blue dye and appear blue. *M. tuberculosis* is acid-fast bacteria. All acid-fast bacteria stained by auramine O show bright yellow or orange yellow fluorescence against a dark background.

8.2.4.5 Reporting of Acid-fast Bacteria (AFB)

The Acid-fast stained smears should be observed at least for 300 High Power Fields (HPF). The Reporting is done according to the improved reports recommended by Center for Disease

Control and Prevention (CDC).

When no AFB is seen after examining 300 fields, the result is reported as "AFB not seen" . When any definite AFB is seen, the result is reported as "AFB positive" and given a grade as follows (Table 8-1).

Table 8-1   Reporting results of smear microscopic examination

Reporting	Ziehl-Neelsen acid-fast stain (1000 ×)	Auramine O stain (450 ×)
AFB not seen	0	0
Doubtful, repeat with another specimen	1–2 AFB per 300 fields	1–2 AFB per 70 fields
1+	1–9 AFB per 100 fields	2–18 AFB per 50 fields
2+	1–9 AFB per 10 fields	4–36 AFB per 10 fields
3+	1–9 AFB per field	4–36 AFB per field
4+	> 9 AFB per field	>36 AFB per field

8.2.5 Isolation and Culture

The isolation and culture of *M. tuberculosis* provides the gold standard for the diagnosis of tuberculosis. The specimens inoculated into both solid and liquid medium can be performed for the optimal recovery. Many formulations of media have been proposed for the cultivation of mycobacteria. The solid media more widely used are L-J medium, Ogawa medium, Middlebrook 7H10 and 7H11 medium. The broth media is Middlebrook 7H9 broth medium or Sauton's medium.

L-J medium in the past years was the most common egg-based medium. Due to limitation of the lower recovery rate, Middlebrook medium for mycobacteria is recommended now. Middle-brook 7H10 and 7H11 media contain agar, organic compounds, salts, glycerol, and albumin. In addition to these substances, 7H11 also contains 0.1% casein hydrolysate, which enhances the growth of mycobacteria. Middlebrook selective 7H11 medium is made with the 7H11 medium plus the addition of antibiotics and dyes, which include carbenicillin, polymyxin B, trimethoprim lactate, amphotericin B, and malachite green.

Various specimens are inoculated onto the surface of culture medium using a sterile transfer pipette, and the incubated plates should be placed at 37°C in adequate aeration and atmosphere of 5% to 10% carbon dioxide. *M. tuberculosis* grows slowly. The incubation for mature colonies should take more than 7 days. Young colonies can be observed at an early stage of growth with the aid of magnification instead of non-visible with the naked eyes. Generally, after 6 to 8 weeks, colonies of *M. tuberculosis* are typically rough, dry, granular, and nonpigmented. However, the colonies on 7H10 media are flat and rough. If the typical colonies are found and acid-fast staining is positive, most of them are *M. tuberculosis*. The inoculum shall be incubated at least for 12 weeks before they are discarded as negative. Amounts of growth from the solid culture are recorded as follows (Table 8-2):

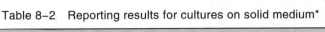

Table 8–2　Reporting results for cultures on solid medium*

Growth	Laboratory reporting
None	Not seen
1–9 colonies	Doubtful, repeat with another specimen
10–100 colonies	1+
>100–200 colonies	2+
>200 colonies (too numerous to count or confluent)	3+
Other mycobacterial growth	Positive for other mycobacteria
Contaminated	Contaminated
ZN^+ growth in presence of contamination	Positive for MTB and contaminated

*Reference from Mycobacteriology Laboratory Manual.

When colonies are observed, an acid-fast smear and subculture for identification should be done. The mycobacterial growth indicator tube (MGIT) system is one of conventional phenotypic methods, which consists of 7H9 medium, anti-tuberculosis drug, and fluorescent indicator. The principle of the system is that mycobacteria grow and consume oxygen, and the indicator compound excited emits fluorescent signals. The resulting fluorescence as a product of the reaction in each test can be examined. The automated system can continuously read and monitor the signals from tubes, in which bacteria to be detected are inoculated and grow. In addition to detecting whether mycobacterium grows, the system is used to perform the drug susceptibility testing. If the growth of specimen culture is equal to or greater than that of the control tube in the test, the strain is interpreted as "resistant" by the system.

8.2.6　Nucleic Acid Detection

In the past, the biological molecular methods for identification of mycobacteria were implemented for clinical and research uses. Generally, the number of bacteria in the specimen is required up to be 10^5 bacteria per mL for a smear examination, and 100 bacteria per mL for isolation and culture. The nucleic acid detection method taking advantage of less amount of specimen and less time compared with culture method can be carried out by rapidly detecting the organism.

8.2.6.1　Nucleic Acid Hybridization

cDNA probes, which are complementary to *Mycobacterium* specific rRNA, can hybridize with rRNA to form a stable DNA:RNA double stranded complex. The method has been employed in the rapid identification for *M. tuberculosis* in conjunction with culture methods.

8.2.6.2　PCR Technique

The target sequences for identification of mycobacteria are commonly used to determinate the sequences of 16S ribosomal DNA because of the molecule highly conserved, and the 16S-23S internal transcribed spacer (ITS) sequences supplied for identification of closely related species. PCR products are identified by reverse phase DNA hybridization or restriction-enzyme digestion analysis. Currently, the most reported methodology for mycobacterial identification is restriction-enzyme analysis, which discriminates between all mycobacterial species. The method with high sensitivity can detect 1 to 20 bacteria, and the results can be obtained in only 1 to 2 days.

Real-time PCR method for the detection of tuberculosis pathogenic organisms is recommended in our country (GB/T27639/2011). This standard method is TaqMan probe real-time fluorescence PCR technology. Specific amplification primers and probes for *M. tuberculosis* complex are designed with IS6110 and IS1081 inserted gene sequences as templates respectively.

8.2.7 Chromatographic Technique and MALDI–TOF Mass Spectrometry

Mycolic acids in the cell walls of different mycobacteria are different. These molecules or compounds can be identified in specimens through gas-liquid chromatography (GLC) and high-performance liquid chromatography (HPLC), as potential markers in diagnosis and surveillance of illnesses.

HPLC examines the mycolic acid profile of the bacteria and compares it with a database derived from standard mycobacteria. Matrix-assisted laser desorption ionization–time of flight (MALDI-TOF) mass spectrometry has changed the routine identification of microorganisms in the laboratory, and shown to be able to accurately identify *M. tuberculosis*. Recently, it has been widely employed in China. These technologies have limitations to require a pure culture. However, compared with conventional identification methods, they still have the advantages of fastness, traceability and high sensitivity.

8.2.8 Immunological Diagnosis

After entering the human body, *M. tuberculosis* can induce the body to produce specific cellular immunity and humoral immunity. However, it is generally believed that cellular immune and humoral immune responses can be separated in *M. tuberculosis* infection, that is, the cellular immune function is low and the antibody titer is increased in the active phase; the cellular immune function is enhanced and the antibody titer is reduced in the stable stage.

8.2.8.1 Detection of Antibodies for *M. tuberculosis*

The detection of anti-tuberculosis antibodies can be used as one of the rapid diagnostic methods of active tuberculosis. The positive rate of circulating antibodies existing in pulmonary tuberculosis patients is 80% to 90%. In the body fluid of pleural tuberculosis, abdominal tuberculosis and cerebrospinal fluid of tuberculous meningitis, the titer of anti-tuberculosis antibodies is significantly higher than that of blood samples. In recent years, immunochromatographic assay and protein chip have improved the sensitivity and specificity of detecting *M. tuberculosis* IgG antibodies.

8.2.8.2 Detection of *M. tuberculosis* Antigen

The exocrine specific antigen of *M. tuberculosis* in serum or body fluid samples can be detected using ELISA, which can be employed as markers to diagnose whether it is infected with *M. tuberculosis*, and the accuracy can reach more than 90%. For example, urinary antigen detection is based on the direct detection of lipoarabinomannan (LAM) in urine. This glycolipid is found in the urine of patients with active tuberculosis and can be detected using an ELISA.

8.2.8.3 Tuberculin Skin Test

When people have been exposed to *M. tuberculosis*, cell-mediated immunity usually occurs. The tuberculin skin test can evaluate the immune response mediated by T lymphocytes.

Tuberculin used in the test is the bacterial component of *M. tuberculosis*, including old tuberculin (OT) and purified protein derivative (PPD). At present, a standardized PPD is mostly used. In the routine test, PPD solution containing 5 units in 0.1 mL is injected into the inner skin of the forearm intradermally. Delayed-type hypersensitivity reaction to the administered tuberculin PPD protein is seen and measured. The reaction reaches a peak effect at 48 to 72 hours, after which erythema and induration are seen at the injection site and measured size and recorded in mm.

The result of the test is positive or negative according to the diameter of the induration. It is considered positive if the diameter is more than 5 mm, indicating that the subject is infected with *M. tuberculosis* or BCG vaccination. It is considered strongly positive if the diameter of induration is 15 mm and more, indicating that there may be active tuberculosis, which should be further examined. It is considered negative if induration is less than 5 mm, indicating that it has not been infected with *M. tuberculosis*, but false negative reaction should be considered. Inadequate response to PPD protein in the presence of *M. tuberculosis* infection may be seen in recent tuberculosis infection, the elderly, acquired immune deficiency, patients suffering from other infectious diseases.

The potential diagnosis of the positive PPD skin reaction may be made in active and latent tuberculosis infection, BCG vaccination in the past and infection with a variety of non-tuberculosis mycobacteria. Epidemiological investigation of *M. tuberculosis* infection in people without BCG vaccination and the cellular immune function of tumor patients are measured.

8.2.9 Interferon–γ Release Assay (IGRA)

When the individual is infected with *M. tuberculosis*, there are sensitized lymphocytes in the body. The lymphocytes may be rapidly induced to produce cytokines on encountering the same antigen that they recognize, such as IFN-γ. Therefore, IFN-γ can be employed as an index for the diagnosis of *M. tuberculosis* infection. At present, the specific antigens of *M. tuberculosis* mainly used are RD1 gene coding proteins such as early secreted antigenic targets (ESAT-6) and culture filtration protein (CFP-10). The determination methods include whole blood ELISA and enzyme-linked immunospot supplied with commercial kits.

8.2.10 Drug Susceptibility Testing

The drug susceptibility testing for *M. tuberculosis* isolated from patients is highly important for guiding clinical therapy and monitoring drug-resistance *M. tuberculosis*. Drug susceptibility testing methods for *M. tuberculosis in vitro* include absolute concentration method, proportional method, radiometric method and so on. The results of these conventional methods show that directly observation of the microorganism or the growth of the microorganism indirectly through color reactions. Subsequently, the resistance of the microorganism is identified through its growth in the presence of drugs. Proportional method is a standard drug susceptibility assay recommended by WHO and IUATLD. Absolute method is widely used in laboratories at all levels in our country. In addition to these conventional methods, determining by observation of the bacteria's growth and metabolic inhibition in media containing drugs, genetic mutations related to drug can be detected using molecular techniques.

8.2.10.1 Absolute Concentration Method

The method uses a concentration series of anti-tuberculosis drugs, mixed with culture medium. Then the isolates of *M. tuberculosis* from clinical samples are inoculated in them as 0.1 mL of bacteria to be tested at the concentration of 10^{-2} g/L and incubated at 37°C for 4 weeks. If colonies (the number is more than 20) grow on the culture medium, the result is marked as positive, then the minimum inhibitory concentration (MIC) of the drug against *M. tuberculosis* is determined according to the situation of growth. By comparing the ratio of MIC between the tested strain and the standard strain (H37Rv) under the same testing conditions, the strain is judged as susceptible or resistant. If the ratio is less than or equal to 2, it is judged as susceptible, and if the ratio is greater than or equal to 8, it is judged as resistant.

8.2.10.2 Proportional Method

The suspension of *M. tuberculosis* to be diluted into a gradient series of concentration are inoculated onto the culture medium containing anti-tuberculosis drugs, accompanied by non-drug medium as control, and incubated at 37°C for 4 weeks. The appropriate inoculation dilution is selected in which the colonies of inocula on the culture media appear and is countable, and in which, the colonies of the drug-containing medium and control medium inoculated with the bacteria are counted. The proportion of drug resistance mutations in the tested concentration is calculated according to the colonies counting results, which is expressed as the percentage of drug-resistance colonies to total number of control colonies. Less than or equal to 1% colonies existed are judged as susceptible, otherwise, it is drug resistance.

8.2.10.3 Molecular Method

Compared with phenotypic methods, the molecular methods for the identification of the susceptibility of *M. tuberculosis* to anti-tuberculosis drugs have the advantage of obtained results in a short time, without requiring the growth of the microorganism. The methods based on genetic determinants of drug-resistance include DNA sequencing, DNA microarray, line probes assay, single-strand conformation polymorphism, real-time PCR, fluorescence resonance energy transfer probes, amplification refractory mutation system, and so on.

Among the above methods, DNA sequencing is the "gold standard" method because it is the best and the most accurate one for the detection of gene mutations. In 2018, WHO released a series of documents to improve drug susceptibility testing for tuberculosis in laboratories worldwide. A technical guide on the use of next-generation sequencing technology is included in the documents, which is used to detect the mutations of genes associated with drug resistance in *M. tuberculosis*. Sequencing technology generates a huge amount of data to be analyzed and interpreted.

In addition to identifying *M. tuberculosis*, line Probe Assay is employed to determine resistance to anti-tuberculosis drugs. This test detects the frequent mutations in the genes resistant to drugs such as *rpoB*, *KatG*, *inhA*, *rpsL*, *gyrA* gene, etc. The detection of these genes is preformed through extracting DNA from specimens or strains isolated in culture, amplifying nucleic acid sequences using PCR, hybridizing amplified segment with immobilized specific oligonucleotide probes, and a color development system permitting to analyze the nucleic acid probe. The method can be developed from collecting specimens to obtaining results in 48 hours or less.

8.3 Prevention and Treatment

Identifying rapidly infectious source cases, interrupting person-to-person transmission, and protecting susceptible individuals are important measures for effective infection prevention and control. WHO recommends the guideline to achieve the global targets of ending the epidemics of tuberculosis. The guideline emphasizes the importance of building integrated, well-coordinated, and multisectoral action towards tuberculosis infections prevention and control across all levels of care. The recommendations include detecting more tuberculosis cases, detecting tuberculosis cases earlier, detecting and managing drug-resistant tuberculosis, and addressing TB/HIV coinfection.

The effective and successful control of tuberculosis depends on the early diagnosis, immediate treatment, and adequate and whole-course medication. To treat latent *M. tuberculosis* infection, the medications recommended include isoniazid (INH), rifapentine (RPT) and rifampin (RIF). WHO recommends that treatment regimens be short-course, rifamycin-based, 3- or 4-month therapy, that is, three months of once-weekly isoniazid plus rifapentine (3HP), four months of daily rifampin (4R), and three months of daily isoniazid plus rifampin (3HR). The patients with active tuberculosis disease are treated with a standard 6-month course of 4 antimicrobial drugs, the first-line anti-tuberculosis agents, including INH, RIF, ethambutol (EMB), pyrazinamide (PZA). If tuberculosis disease is caused by the strains of drug-resistant tuberculosis, MDR-TB, or XDR-TB, the treatment is very complicated and must be modified.

Glossary

tuberculosis *n.* 结核病 an infectious disease caused by *Mycobacterium tuberculosis*, mainly affects the lungs and other parts of the body

enzyme *n.* 酶 a substance that acts as a catalyst in living organisms, regulating the rate at which chemical reactions proceed without itself being altered in the process

exposure *n.* 暴露 the fact of being affected by something in a particular situation or place

inflammation *n.* 炎症 the immune system's natural response of the body to injury and illness

immunoprophylaxis *n.* 免疫预防 prevention of disease through vaccines or passive immunization through antisera

staining *n.* 染色 a method of imparting dyes to cells or microscopic components in order to visualize better under a microscope

microorganism *n.* 微生物 a living thing that is too small to be seen with the naked eye, such as bacteria, fungi, and protozoa

spore *n.* 芽孢，孢子 cells produced by some bacteria and fungi which can develop into new individuals

colony *n.* 菌落 a group of bacteria that is formed by growth and reproduction of single bacterium on solid media

culture *n./v.* 培养 growing a group of microorganisms

specimen *n.* 标本 a small quantity of blood, sputum, etc. from subjects to be tested

smear *n./v.* 涂片 spread a liquid or a thick substance over a surface of slide

sequence *n./v.* 序列 identify the primary structure of a target molecule, a set of genes or parts of molecules

susceptibility *n.* 敏感性 a term used when the isolated microbe can be killed or inhibited their growth in the antimicrobial drugs

（李琴）

Chapter 9

Respiratory Tract Infection Viruses and Their Detection

Learning objectives:
- Know the common types of respiratory viruses and their characteristics.
- Know nucleic acid detection methods, antigen detection methods, and antibody detection methods for respiratory viruses.
- Understand the similarities and differences in clinical symptoms caused by several respiratory viruses.
- Be familiar with treatment and preventive measures against respiratory viruses.

Respiratory tract infection is one of the most common clinical conditions and has a major impact on health. Viruses play an essential role in respiratory infections. Respiratory viruses are defined as viruses that invade the respiratory tract and proliferate in the mucosal epithelium of the respiratory tract, causing localised infections of the respiratory tract or lesions in tissues and organs outside the respiratory tract. Common respiratory viruses include influenza virus, respiratory syncytial virus, metapneumovirus, parainfluenza virus, coronavirus and rhinovirus. A single respiratory virus can often cause multiple respiratory diseases. Conversely, a single respiratory infectious disease can be caused by multiple pathogens. Respiratory viruses are extremely contagious, with fast transmission, short incubation periods and similar clinical symptoms; therefore, it is extremely critical to identify the pathogen of the infection. Rapid pathogenetic testing is not only the basis for confirming the etiology but also for selecting a rational treatment plan.

9.1 Influenza Virus

9.1.1 Introduction

Influenza viruses belonging to the *Orthomyxoviridae* family, are single-stranded, negative-stranded, segmented RNA viruses, which are classified into types A, B, C and D, also known as

Alpha-influenza virus, Beta-influenza virus, Gamma-influenza virus and Delta-influenza virus, depending on the antigenicity of the nucleoprotein and matrix protein. Influenza A virus is also divided into different subtypes based on antigenicity of haemagglutinin and neuraminidase. Among the four influenza virus categories, the influenza A virus induces the most fatal diseases. Moreover, influenza A virus mutates more rapidly and show a higher extent of variability in terms of antigenicity and virulence. Antigenic drift is the main reason that influenza emerges seasonally every year and antigenic shift has caused viral gene reassortment and the constant emergence of new influenza A viral strains. Influenza A and B viruses contribute to the annual influenza epidemic in humans. Influenza pandemics are attributed to influenza A virus, while influenza B virus is unlikely to cause a pandemic. The prevalence of influenza C virus is relatively low and influenza D virus is a novel discovered influenza virus.

9.1.2   Clinical Symptoms

Influenza is an acute viral infection and highly contagious, impacting 5%~15% of the population with up to 650,000 death annually. Fever and respiratory symptoms such as cough, rhinorrhea, sore throat and shortness of breath are the major symptoms of influenza. Influenza is more serious than common cold. The clinical manifestations of the common cold are usually runny and stuffy nose, and the symptoms are relatively mild which usually clear up within 1 week with rare complications. Although most people recover without medical attention within a week, influenza is organ-damaging and easily leads to serious complications or even death. Furthermore, the most commonly occurring complication of influenza is pneumonia. In general, secondary bacterial pneumonia is more frequently, with *Staphylococcus aureus*, *Haemophilus influenzae*, and *Streptococcus pneumoniae* being the most common.

9.1.3   Detection Methods

Cell Isolation Culture and Electron Microscopic Observation

Virus isolation is performed by inoculating infected samples with chicken embryos and sensitive cells. Influenza viruses can be propagated in 9-11 days old chicken embryos. Samples are inoculated into the amniotic and/or allantoic cavity of chicken embryos, incubated at a certain temperature and humidity and then amniotic fluid and allantoic fluid are obtained. Infection and typing of influenza viruses are determined by hemagglutination test and hemagglutination inhibition (HI) test. Influenza virus can also be propagated in sensitive cell lines such as the madin darby canine kidney (MDCK), A549, mink lung epithelial cell line (Mv1Lu) and rhesus monkey kidney (LLC-MK2). MDCK cell culture is more sensitive than chicken embryo culture for the isolation of influenza viruses, and therefore MDCK cells are the cell line of choice for culturing influenza viruses. Nevertheless, influenza virus isolation using chicken embryos or cells usually takes 3 to 5 days or more, making standard virus isolation methods hard to carry out in clinical applications.

Electron microscopy (EM) offers a long history of use in the identification and characterization of viruses. There is no need for organism-specific reagents to identify pathogens which is one of the major merits of employing EM for virus diagnosis. It is hard to obtain enough material to allow the production of commercial assay kits when virus grows poorly in vitro. EM enables rapid morphological identification and differential diagnosis of the viruses contained in the specimen. Some enveloped viruses such as orthomyxoviruses, paramyxoviruses and coronaviruses have surface protrusions that are long enough to be clearly identified. Other respiratory viruses such as adenovirus can also be visualized by EM in terms of their morphology.

Hemagglutination Assay and Hemagglutination Inhibition (HI) Test

The hemagglutination expressed in the envelope of the influenza virus binds to specific erythrocyte surface receptors and the virus is attached to the erythrocytes causing them to agglutinate, a phenomenon known as hemagglutination. The ability of the hemagglutination phenomenon to be inhibited by the corresponding antibody is known as the HI test (Figure 9-1). HI measures the presence of specific antibodies in the serum and is widely used to diagnose infections caused by influenza viruses. The test can be used to detect or quantify antibodies against influenza viruses. The HI test is a rapid and cheap approach for antibody quantification. It does not require expensive or unusual laboratory equipment, except for red blood cell sources, and results can be attained in a few hours.

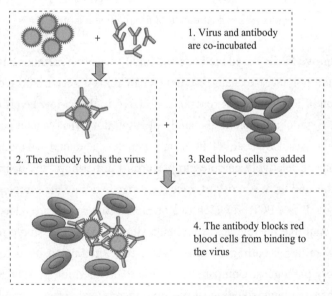

1. Virus and antibody are co-incubated

2. The antibody binds the virus

3. Red blood cells are added

4. The antibody blocks red blood cells from binding to the virus

Figure 9-1   Hemagglutination inhibition test

Nucleic Acid Test

Nucleic acid test is one of the main methods applied in the diagnosis of respiratory viral infections. The universal strengths of nucleic acid testing are the rapidity, specificity and convenience of the test. Polymerase chain reaction (PCR) is a technique used to "amplify" small segments of DNA. The implementation of DNA in vitro amplification is based on the principle of DNA semi-conserved replication and the principle of base complementary pairing. During replication, double-stranded DNA is unstranded, changing from double-stranded to single-stranded, usually at 95℃. After the temperature drops, the primers (they are short single-stranded DNA fragments, called oligonucleotides, which are complementary sequences to the target DNA region) bind to the DNA single strand. In the presence of DNA polymerase, the free dNTP (DNA bases, including A, C, G and T, are required for the construction of new DNA strands.) binds to the single strand in accordance with the principle of base complementary pairing, forming a new double-stranded DNA consisting of a hybridization of the old and new strands. This process can be summarized in three basic steps of "denaturing-annealing-extending" (Figure 9-2). As the PCR proceeds, the produced DNA itself is used as a template for replication, thus initiating the chain reaction.

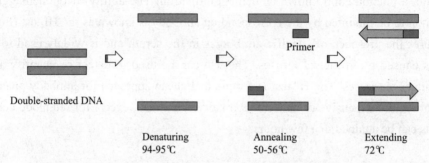

Double-stranded DNA

Primer

Denaturing 94-95℃　　　Annealing 50-56℃　　　Extending 72℃

Figure 9-2　Illustrations of the main steps of PCR

Numerous improved PCR-based methods and highly sensitive methods have been developed. Reverse transcription polymerase chain reaction (RT-PCR) is a very useful technique combining reverse transcription of RNA and PCR reactions of cDNA to detect low levels of respiratory viral genomes. RT-PCR is widely applied in the study of respiratory viruses as it can be performed on both live and dead viruses. However, RT-PCR-based nucleic acid analysis methods generally take at least 2 hours and are relatively complex to perform. Furthermore, the operator needs to have some analytical skills and there is a risk of infection when handling the samples.

Multiplex RT-PCR is a PCR in which two or more primer pairs are added to the same PCR system to amplify multiple nucleic acid fragments simultaneously. A single multiplex PCR can detect and identify multiple pathogens at the same time, making it ideal for the detection of groups of respiratory pathogens. Compared to single PCR, the multiplex PCR provides a faster and more comprehensive understanding of multiple respiratory viruses simultaneously. Despite a slight reduction in sensitivity, it has its unique advantages and high practical value in the differential diagnosis of clinical mixed infections.

Antigen and Antibody Test

Viral nucleic acid tests are highly sensitive, but they are difficult to carry out in a wide range of clinical settings because of the stringent requirements of the test, the complexity of the procedure and the fact that the specimen can easily be contaminated. Antigen test is a quick and easy test that can be performed as an early diagnosis of viral infections. Respiratory virus antigen test requires the collection of respiratory samples such as throat swabs and nasopharyngeal aspirates. A positive test result indicates active viral infection, while a negative result does not completely exclude viral infection. Antigen detection methods include immunofluorescence (IF), enzyme-linked immunosorbent assay (ELISA) and enzyme immunoassay (EIA).

The serum immunological antibody test is based on the principle of combining antigen and antibody to detect virus-specific antibodies in the patient's serum or plasma. On most occasions, blood samples should be taken at least twice in the course of the disease: during the acute phase and during the recovery phase. Antibody test is of little significance for the early diagnosis of cases but can be used as a complementary tool for retrospective confirmation of the diagnosis. Furthermore, the serological testing is considered a reference method in situations where many rapid antigen detection methods are inefficient. The methods used are IF, ELISA and gold immunochromatographic assay (GICA).

IF can be divided into direct immunofluorescence (DFA) and indirect immunofluorescence (IIF) methods (Figure 9-3). The DFA test, also known as the immunofluorescent antibody test (IFA), has been applied since the early 1960s and is commonly performed to diagnose influenza virus infections. DFA has a pair of antigen-antibody systems, a viral antigen with a corresponding fluorescein-labelled antibody. IIF has two pairs of antigen-antibody systems, the first pair being the viral antigen with the corresponding antibody and the second pair being the antibody and the corresponding fluorescein-labelled anti-human or animal antiglobulin antibody. DFA targeting the viral core antigen, is a simpler procedure than the IIF method and reduces the non-specific reaction of the secondary antibody in the latter method, thus greatly improving the specificity of the diagnosis. Besides, IIF is 5 to 10 times more sensitive than DFA, but is prone to non-specific fluorescence, and we should be very careful in handling and judging the results. IF has been widely utilized for many years to develop many rapid tests for the detection of respiratory viruses. However, this method is not applicable to viral respiratory infections caused by rhinovirus or coronavirus due to the lack of suitable reagents.

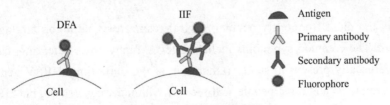

Figure 9-3   DFA and IIF

9.1.4 Prevention and Treatment

Despite the significant disease burden caused by respiratory viruses, only a few preventive and therapeutic interventions are currently available. Because the immunity gained from previous infections is not permanent, people would repeatedly infect influenza viruses each year. Numerous approaches are available to deal with seasonal influenza infections, including vaccines and antiviral treatments. Three types of vaccines are currently used worldwide, including inactivated influenza vaccine (IIV), recombinant HA vaccine and live attenuated influenza vaccine (LAIV). The dominant strain of influenza virus varies every year, so the composition of influenza vaccine changes annually and the development of a universal influenza vaccine is the ideal strategy to control influenza epidemics. Neuraminidase inhibitors (NAIs) are the primary anti-influenza drugs, but virus has developed resistance against old neuraminidase inhibitors, such as oseltamivir and zanamivir which would be slowly substituted by alternative small molecule inhibitors. New neuraminidase inhibitors will bring more options for anti-influenza virus treatment.

9.2 Human Respiratory Syncytial Virus

9.2.1 Introduction

Human respiratory syncytial virus (HRSV) is one of the most critical pathogens causing serious respiratory infections in infants and children, and human is the only host of HRSV. HRSV enters the host through the nasopharyngeal or conjunctival mucosa and can spread to the lower respiratory tract, which causes necrosis of the respiratory mucosa leading to airflow obstruction and develops an acute disease characterized by edema. HRSV belonging to the genus *Pneumovirus* of the family *Paramyxoviridae*, is a non-segmental, single-stranded, negative-stranded RNA virus. HRSV is originally divided into 2 subtypes, HRSV-A and HRSV-B, based on their antigenic differences. Both virus subtypes are highly contagious. Strains of these two subtypes often circulate together, but usually one subtype dominates. The viral particles are encapsulated by a lipid bilayer containing glycoproteins G, F and SH. G proteins on the surface of the HRSV envelope play a role in host cell attachment without coagulation activity and F proteins are responsible for fusion and cell entry, while SH proteins are not a necessary part of either process.

9.2.2 Clinical Symptoms

HRSV is the most frequently occurring viral respiratory pathogen among infants and young children. The common symptoms including fever, runny nose, wheezing, cough and loss of appetite are usually present in stages rather than at the same time. HRSV generally causes mild flu-like symptoms and most people will recover within a week or two, but HRSV can be a serious condition, especially in infants and the elderly. If HRSV involves the upper respiratory system, the symptoms are often relatively mild, similar to the common cold, while if HRSV involves the lower respiratory system, the symptoms are often more severe. Infants aged 2 to 6 months are particularly sensitive to the virus and face the risk of death if infection is severe. HRSV is the most commonly reported reason for bronchiolitis and pneumonia among children under 1 year old. Adults with underlying cardiopulmonary disease or immune deficiency are also susceptible to HRSV, presenting with severe or even life-threatening lower respiratory tract infections. Reinfection with HRSV is common and multiple HRSV infections may occur during an individual's lifetime. The illness caused by reinfection is usually mild with symptoms like the common cold, and it is mainly restricted to the upper respiratory tract. However, reinfection in the elderly can cause pneumonia.

9.2.3   Detection Methods

Cell Isolation Culture and Electron Microscopic Observation

Throat swabs, sputum and other respiratory specimens can be used for HRSV culture isolation. The cell lines commonly used are laryngeal carcinoma cells (Hep-2), human type II alveolar epithelial cells (A549) and human cervical cancer cell line (HeLa) cells. The culture conditions are 33-35℃, either static or rotating. When the virus is isolated in culture, the first generation of cytopathic lesions is often atypical, thus making it easy to misidentify false negatives. Typical lesions such as cell fusion can occur within 5 days of blind passages, but a positive cell isolation culture has a high degree of confidence. EM observation of HRSV can refer to the relevant section on influenza viruses.

Nucleic Acid Test

Nucleic acid detection method for HRSV is similar to that for influenza virus. Additionally, fluorescent quantitative real-time polymorphic chain reaction (FQ-PCR) is a nucleic acid quantification technique developed based on conventional PCR and is widely used in respiratory virus detection. FQ-PCR visualizes the entire PCR process in real time by adding a fluorescent group to the PCR reaction system and using the accumulation of fluorescent signals. FQ-PCR includes TaqMan chemistry (Figure 9-4) and SYBR Green I dye chemistry. The concepts of baseline and cycle threshold (CT) value are involved here. The baseline is the reference control

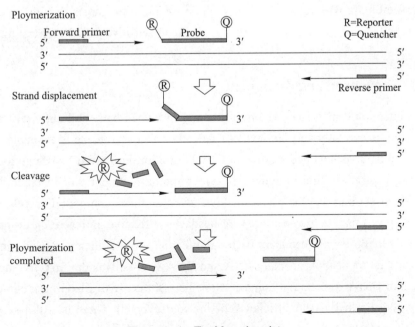

Figure 9-4   TaqMan chemistry

used to determine the fluorescence signal intensity of the background, which corresponds to the fluorescence intensity level before the PCR index amplification period. The CT value refers to the number of cycles that the fluorescence signal in each reaction tube undergoes when it reaches a set threshold. The technique has enabled the development of nucleic acid detection from qualitative to quantitative analysis. Compared to traditional PCR assays, it is not only sensitive and specific, but also effectively addresses the problem of cross-contamination.

Multiplex FQ-PCR has become a research hot topic for respiratory virus detection. This method combines the advantages of both FQ-PCR and multiplex PCR, allowing for both quantitative detection and high throughput detection in one reaction system. Influenza viruses can be successfully typed and subtyped using multiplex FQ-PCR. Furthermore, it is possible to simultaneously detect multiple respiratory viruses such as influenza, parainfluenza, respiratory syncytial virus and coronavirus.

With the rapid development of molecular biology techniques, in vitro nucleic acid amplification techniques are also advancing. Nucleic acid sequence-based amplification (NASBA) is a new technique developed on the basis of PCR, which can be implemented for the quantitative assay of RNA viruses and has many benefits such as great specificity and great sensitivity.

Antigen and Antibody Test

Antigen and antibody test for HRSV is also similar to that for influenza virus. Moreover, enzyme immunoassay (EIA) is a qualitative and quantitative analytical method that substitutes enzymes for radionuclides in radioactive skin-free assays, labelling antigens followed by immunoconjugation reactions to determine many biologically active substances. This technique has the benefits of reduced turnaround time for detection results and greatly simplifies the technical assembly, providing an effective method for rapid diagnosis of viral infections in a busy diagnostic laboratory, but is not nearly as specific or sensitive as DFA for testing respiratory viruses.

9.2.4 Prevention and Treatment

HRSV infection can't induce lasting immunity in human body and antiviral treatment for HRSV infection is currently very limited. No safe and effective vaccine is available. In addition to general treatment such as bed resting and drinking a lot during the febrile period, the main treatment for respiratory viral infections is symptomatic treatment. For instance, physical or pharmacological cooling may be given for high fever, and oral compound acetylsalicylic acid (compound aspirin) may be given for severe headache. Effective antibacterial drugs should be given promptly to those with secondary bacterial infections. Ribavirin, a nucleoside analogue that interferes with the replication of many RNA and DNA viruses, was the first drug approved for the treatment of HRSV infection in humans. Nonetheless, the use of ribavirin in clinical practice is currently very limited and its efficacy remains controversial. There is still a need for more effective antiviral drugs and a vaccine to protect the general population.

9.3   Coronaviruses

9.3.1   Introduction

Coronaviruses (CoVs), which belong to the *Coronaviridae* family, are enveloped, non-segmented, single-stranded positive-stranded RNA viruses. There are four genera classified based on serotype and genomic characteristics: α-CoV, β-CoV, γ-CoV and δ-CoV, of which α-CoV and β-CoV can infect humans. Coronavirus is one of the most prevalent pathogens of respiratory tract infection. Prior to the emergence of SARS, there are two prototype human coronaviruses, HCoV-OC43 and HCoV-229E, both of which are pathogens of the common cold. SARS has been shown to give rise to severe acute respiratory syndrome, which is the first instance of a critical human disease induced by a coronavirus. Since the identification of SARS, four novel human coronaviruses have been reported in succession in association with respiratory disease, which are named as HCoV-HKUI, HCoV-NL63, MERS and SARS-CoV-2. So, there are currently seven known coronaviruses that infect humans.

9.3.2   Clinical Symptoms

Individuals infected with SARS, MERS or SARS-CoV-2 present with severe lower respiratory tract infection accompanied by extrapulmonary involvement and a high mortality rate. However, the other four coronaviruses (HCoV-OC43, HCoV-229E, HCoV-HKU1 and HCoV-NL63) mainly cause mild, self-limiting upper respiratory tract infections such as the common cold. Symptoms mainly consist of runny nose, headache, cough, sore throat, fever and sometimes lower respiratory tract diseases such as pneumonia or bronchitis. Those infected with SARS-CoV-2 may develop symptoms within 2 to 14 days, including fever, dry cough, headache, fatigue, sneezing, sore throat and breathlessness. The patient's age as well as immune function are critical factors for the severity of the disease, which falls into three distinct categories: the most frequent symptoms (i.e. fever, fatigue and dry cough), the less frequent symptoms (i.e. pains, sore throat, conjunctivitis, headache, diarrhoea, loss of taste or smell, toes and skin rash) and the severe symptoms (i.e. chest pain or tightness, breathlessness or shortness of breath, and loss of words or movement). The risk of severe COVID-19 is higher in the elderly and some patients with underlying conditions (diabetes, cancer, heart diseases or lung diseases).

9.3.3   Detection Methods

Cell Isolation Culture and Electron Microscopic Observation

Vero cells, MDCK cells, Hela cells, Hep-2 cells and Huh7 cells can all be used to culture and isolate coronaviruses. Specimens of pharyngeal swabs or gargles treated with antibiotics are inoculated in cell culture plates for incubation. Cells are observed daily for 7 days and if no lesions are present, the cells are passaged blindly. If there are no lesions after 3 consecutive blind passages, the cells are discarded. EM observation of coronaviruses can refer to the relevant section on influenza viruses.

Nucleic Acid Test

Nucleic acid detection methods can refer to the relevant section on influenza virus and HRSV.

Antigen and Antibody Test

ELISA is a test that combines antigen and antibody immunoreactivity with efficient enzyme catalysis for the sensitive detection of minute amounts of viral antigens or antibodies (Figure 9-5). Specific viral antibodies (antigens) are adsorbed onto the surface of the solid phase carrier and then the corresponding antigens (antibodies) are added, followed by enzyme-labelled specific viral antibodies (antigens). Eventually, the amount of coloured product produced by the enzymatic reaction is directly correlated with the amount of antigen (antibody) present in the specimen, allowing qualitative or quantitative analysis of the presence and content of viral antigen (antibody) in the specimen. The high catalytic efficiency of the enzyme indirectly amplifies the results of the immuno-reaction resulting in a highly sensitive assay. ELISA can offer a simple, rapid and inexpensive approach for clinical or field use without the necessity of a highly contained laboratory. ELISA can be categorized into four various types, namely direct, indirect, competitive, and sandwich. Indirect, competitive and sandwich ELISA principles have been reported for serological assays used to detect coronaviruses.

Gold immunochromatographic assay (GICA) is a novel immunolabelling technique that uses colloidal gold as a tracer marker. Chloroauric acid (HAuCl4) can be polymerized into a certain

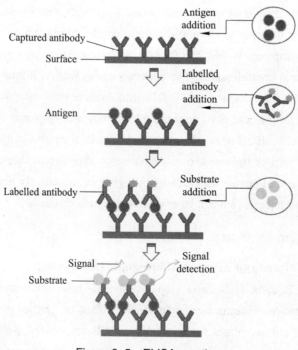

Figure 9-5 ELISA reaction

size of gold particles under the action of reducing agent, thus forming a negatively charged hydrophobic colloidal solution. The final formation of a stable colloidal state called colloidal gold. The specific antibody is fixed to the membrane in the form of a strip, and the colloidal gold labeling reagent is adsorbed on the gold pad. When the antigen to be tested is added to the sample pad, the sample moves forward by capillary action and reacts with each other after dissolving the colloidal gold labeling reagent on the gold pad. Afterwards, when the sample moves to the area of fixed antigen or antibody, the binding of the antigen to be detected and the gold labeling reagents are specifically bound to the sample and are retained, thus aggregating on the detection strip. The final color development result can be observed by the naked eye. The advantages of GICA consist of simple operation, inexpensive cost, wide range of applications and stable markers. The GICA method is less sensitive and the IFA method is more sensitive but less convenient than GICA. Therefore, neither the GICA method nor the IFA method is perfect alone as a test for respiratory pathogens, but their combined use is an important guide to clinical management and may be the preferred method for the early diagnosis of respiratory viral infections.

Virus neutralization test (VNT) is a method of incubating a mixture of virus and specific antibodies under appropriate conditions in vitro, allowing the virus to react with the antibodies, followed by inoculation of the mixture into a sensitive host, and then measuring the infectivity of the residual virus. VNT determines whether a person has neutralising antibodies in his sera, and thus whether he is immune to the virus. VNT is frequently used for serological testing of coronaviruses. VNT requires processing of live viruses in a dedicated biosafety level laboratory. In some cases, a pseudovirus can be used instead of a live virus.

9.3.4 Prevention and Treatment

The four common cold coronaviruses (HCoV-OC43, HCoV-229E, HCoV-HKU1 and HCoV-NL63) cannot yet be prevented by vaccines and there are no specific therapeutic drugs. The common cold is a self-limiting illness. Patients should drink plenty of fluids, rest in bed and take symptomatic treatment if fever develops. For SARS and MERS the emphasis is on local isolation and local treatment, thus preventing further transmission. Moreover, symptomatic supportive treatment and treatment for complications are mainly applied. At present there is still no effective treatment for COVID-19 and vaccination is considered an effective measure to prevent and control the outbreak, which plays a decisive role in the control of the global epidemic. Globally, multiple technical routes of COVID-19 vaccine development are advancing side by side. There are many types of SARS-CoV-2 vaccines currently in use, including inactivated vaccines, nucleic acid vaccines, adenovirus-based vector vaccines and recombinant subunit vaccines. The vaccine has been licensed and launched very successfully in numerous countries.

9.4 Human Metapneumovirus

9.4.1 Introduction

Human metapneumovirus (HMPV) is one of the major causes of acute respiratory infections and has become prevalent worldwide. In 2001, HMPV was first discovered in the Netherlands. Like HRSV, HMPV belongs to the genus *Pneumovirus* in the family *Paramyxoviridae* and the viral particles are encapsulated by a lipid bilayer containing glycoproteins G, F and SH. HMPV is an enveloped, single-stranded, negative-sense RNA virus. Two groups, A and B, are identified by phylogenetic analysis, and each group has two subgroups. In addition, these sublineages are often prevalent simultaneously. HMPV can be a cause of upper and lower respiratory illness in people of all ages, especially in young children, the elderly and those with immunodeficiency diseases.

9.4.2 Clinical Symptoms

Symptoms of HMPV are similar to those of HRSV or influenza, including cough, fever, nasal congestion and shortness of breath. Clinical signs of HMPV infection may progress to bronchitis or pneumonia, like other viruses that cause upper and lower respiratory tract infections. Many children are admitted to hospital with HMPV during the annual prevalence and lower respiratory tract infections are a common cause of hospitalization for them. The most frequent symptoms in children comprise cough, fever, runny nose and wheezing. Up to 50% of children with MPV-associated respiratory infections will develop a fever. Furthermore, acute otitis media is a common complication of MPV. Infected young people usually present with only flu-like symptoms, including cough, nasal congestion, hoarseness and breathlessness. However, in older or immunocompromised patients, the infection probably becomes more severe.

9.4.3 Detection Methods

Cell Isolation Culture and Electron Microscopic Observation

HMPV is characterized by slow growth replication and long culture times, making HMPV relatively difficult to culture. HMPV can be isolated from respiratory specimens in culture using either LLC-MK2 cells or Vero cells. LLC-MK2 cells are considered to be the best host for culture isolation of HMPV, followed by Vero cells. Culture isolation is performed by passaging LLC-MK2 cells or Vero cells into cell culture plates for culture. The cells are observed for cytopathic lesions every 3 days. Furthermore, the results are identified after 18 days of culture and if negative, the cells are passaged in blind for 2 generations. EM observation of HMPV can refer to the relevant section on influenza viruses.

Nucleic Acid Test

Nucleic acid detection methods can refer to the relevant section on influenza virus, HRSV and coronavirus.

Antigen and Antibody Test

Antigen and antibody test methods can refer to the relevant section on influenza virus, HRSV and coronavirus.

9.4.4 Prevention and Treatment

At present, there is neither specific antiviral therapy for HMPV nor any vaccine to prevent HMPV. Because HMPV usually clears on its own, treatment is mainly aimed at relieving symptoms. In general, this means using over-the-counter medication to control pain and fever (such as acetaminophen and ibuprofen) as well as decongestants. Patients with more severe wheezing and coughing may need a temporary inhaler, which may include inhaled corticosteroids. Individuals can assist in preventing the spread of HMPV and other respiratory viruses by washing their hands frequently with soap and water for at least 20 seconds; avoiding touching the eyes, nose or mouth of patients with unwashed hands; and avoiding close contact with patients. Up to now, as a last resort for the treatment of severe HMPV and HRSV infections, only immunoglobulin and ribavirin have been employed in humans.

9.5 Human Parainfluenza Virus

9.5.1 Introduction

Human parainfluenza virus (HPIV) is an enveloped, single- and negative-stranded RNA virus belonging to the genus *Paramyxovirus* of the family *Paramyxoviridae*. HPIV is classified into four types based on antigenicity, of which HPIV-4 can be subdivided into two subtypes, HPIV-4A and HPIV-4B. Many different animals can be infected naturally and under experimental conditions by HPIV. The incubation period for HPIV is usually around 3-5 days. The epidemiological characteristics of the different subtypes of HPIV vary somewhat. Among them, HPIV-1 and HPIV-2 are most likely to infect preschool children aged 3-5 years in autumn and winter. HPIV-3, which has the highest detection rate, is disseminated throughout the year, especially in summer, and the infection rate is the highest in young infants under one year of age. HPIV-4 is reported in only a few studies, and HPIV-4 infection is associated with milder symptoms.

9.5.2 Clinical Symptoms

Healthy adults generally have a well-established immune system making them less susceptible to the virus and even when infected the symptoms are mild. Patients usually recover on their own. HPIV usually causes upper and lower respiratory illness in infants, young children, the elderly and people who have weakened immune systems. Symptoms may include fever, runny nose and cough. The severity of respiratory infections caused by HPIV infection is related to the subtype of HPIV. Both HPIV-1 and HPIV-2 contribute to upper and lower respiratory tract illnesses, as well as flu-like symptoms. The most typical clinical feature is the croup (acute laryngotracheobronchitis). HPIV-3 is more commonly associated with bronchiolitis and pneumonia, mostly in children under the age of 12 months. HPIV-4 in adults and children usually gives rise to only mild symptoms of upper respiratory tract infections such as nasal congestion, runny nose and sneezing. However, it can also cause serious lower respiratory tract diseases such as capillary bronchitis and pneumonia in small infants and immunocompromised people.

9.5.3   Detection Methods

Cell Isolation Culture and Electron Microscopic Observation

HPIV can grow on diploid fibroblasts from a variety of primary animals and humans, commonly such as LLC-MK2 cells, Vero cells, and MDCK cells. Apart from HPIV-4, other subtypes of HPIV grow well in chicken embryos. In addition, HPIV is more easily isolated in epithelial cell lines than in fibroblast cell lines. EM observation of HPIV can refer to the relevant section on influenza viruses.

Nucleic Acid Test

Nucleic acid detection methods can refer to the relevant section on influenza virus, HRSV and coronavirus.

Antigen and Antibody Test

Antigen and antibody test methods can refer to the relevant section on influenza virus, HRSV and coronavirus.

9.5.4   Prevention and Treatment

Currently, there is no vaccine against HPIV. Nevertheless, researchers are making efforts to develop a vaccine. Minimizing visits to crowded public places, personal hygiene, good personal protection, frequent hand washing and better ventilation in the living room are the points of emphasis in the prevention of various respiratory infectious diseases. Close attention must be paid to various control measures to reduce the spread of the disease. No specific antiviral treatment is available for HPIV disease. Most people with HPIV disease will get well spontaneously, so symptomatic treatment is the mainstay of clinical practice.

9.6   Human Rhinovirus

9.6.1   Introduction

Human rhinovirus (HRV) belonging to the family of small RNA viruses, genus *Rhinovirus*, is the main cause of the common cold in humans. Humans are the main hosts of HRV present in nature. Until now, more than 120 serotypes have been isolated, making it the most serotyped virus among human infections. HRV contains specific surface antigens and there may be some cross-reactivity between serotypes, which makes it hard to find a validated serological test in the clinic.

HRVs are a large group of genetically diverse RNA viruses that are phylogenetically divided into three species (HRV-A, HRV-B and HRV-C). One hundred classical serotypes have been identified in HRV-A and HRV-B, and there are around 50 newly identified serotypes belonging to HRV-C. HRV is often co-infected with other respiratory viruses, such as respiratory syncytial virus, adenovirus, parainfluenza virus, coronavirus and enterovirus.

9.6.2　Clinical Symptoms

HRV infection often presents with flu symptoms. Clinical symptoms consist of runny nose, congestion, sneezing, headache, sore throat and cough, with no or a slight increase in body temperature. Symptoms occur mainly within 16h of HRV infection and will peak within 3-4 days, with a duration of illness lasting up to a week. Individuals usually recover in 3-7 days and HRV infection is a self-limiting disease. It is well known that HRV is a major trigger of asthma attacks or exacerbations in children and patients of all ages. It is also clear that the newly described HRV-C is a significant proportion of HRV-related diseases, including asthma and wheezing exacerbations. Research has found that, like HRV-A and HRV-B, the most common clinical manifestations in HRV-C patients are fever, headache, chills, pharyngeal congestion, cough, myalgia and sore throat. Similar to HRV-B, patients with HRV-C infection have a lower rate of upper respiratory symptoms (such as runny nose, sore throat and sneezing) than patients with HRV-A infection. Also, similar to HRV-A, patients infected with HRV-C strains have systemic symptoms (such as myalgia and chills) less frequently than those infected with HRV-B. Besides, co-infections with additional respiratory viruses are usually observed in patients with HRV.

9.6.3　Detection Methods

Cell Isolation Culture and Electron Microscopic Observation

HRV can be cultured with human diploid embryonic lung fibroblasts, common cells such as WI-38 cells and MRC-5 cells, or with Hela cells. Culture conditions are 33 ℃ or 34 ℃ and preferably under rolling drum conditions. Cytopathological effects can be observed readily after cultures are sustained for 10 to 14 days. EM observation of HRV can refer to the relevant section on influenza viruses.

Nucleic Acid Test

Nucleic acid detection method for HRSV is similar to that for influenza virus. Additionally, gene microarray technology refers to the orderly immobilization of a large number of oligonucleotide sequences on a modified vector, followed by hybridization with a labelled nucleic acid sample. The hybridization signal obtained is then used by a signal processing system such as a computer to obtain the results of the sample assay. Gene microarray technology has been applied by many scholars in China and abroad for the detection of various respiratory viruses because of its high throughput, parallelism and rapid detection. Establishing a genetic microarray assay for respiratory viruses allows for simultaneous parallel surveillance of multiple respiratory viruses. However, the shortcomings of gene microarrays are their high costs, long lead times, complex steps and poor reproducibility.

Antigen and Antibody Test

Antigen and antibody test methods can refer to the relevant section on influenza virus, HRSV and coronavirus.

9.6.4　Prevention and Treatment

HRV infections that are self-limiting usually resolve in about a week and do not require special treatment. Immunity can be acquired after infection, but it is short-lived. There is also little cross-protection between different types of HRV, which means that individuals can get colds several times. HRV can cause infection in both children and adults and is easily transmitted within families. Furthermore, symptoms may vary in severity from one individual to another. So far, symptomatic treatment has been dominant, as there is no vaccination or approved antiviral drugs available. The complex antigenicity of HRV, with over 120 serotypes, poses a major challenge in developing a vaccine. The development of antiviral drugs for the treatment of HRV infection is an essential and unmet medical need, which is particularly vital for high-risk patients, including infants.

Glossary

immunofluorescence *n.* 免疫荧光 the labelling of antibodies or disease-causing agents with a fluorescent dye in order to identify or locate them in a tissue sample

neuraminidase *n.* 神经氨酸酶 enzymes that cleave sialic acid (also called neuraminic acid) groups from glycoproteins

double-stranded *adj.* 双链的 double-stranded DNA consists of two polynucleotide chains whose nitrogenous bases are connected by hydrogen bonds

hemagglutination inhibition test 血凝抑制试验 the test to detect the ability of the hemagglutination phenomenon to be inhibited by the corresponding antibody

antigenic drift 抗原漂移 a small variation in antigen caused by the mutation of the genome

（张定梅）

新形态教材网·数字课程学习……

🖥 教学 PPT　　　📄 自测题　　　💬 推荐阅读

Chapter 10
HIV Infection and Laboratory Detection

Learning objectives:

- Know HIV prevention and treatment.
- Be familiar with the epidemiological characteristics and laboratory testing of HIV.
- Master clinical manifestations and specimen collection of HIV.

Human immunodeficiency virus (HIV) is the causative agent of acquired immune deficiency syndrome (AIDS). According to the latest report released by the United Nations AIDS programme in 2020, there were 1.5 million new AIDS virus infections worldwide, a decrease of 31% compared with 2010. In 2020, about 680,000 people died of AIDS related diseases in the world, a decrease of 48% compared with 2010. By the end of October 2021, there were 1.14 million cases of HIV infection reported in the Chinese Mainland (excluding Hong Kong, Macao and Taiwan). From January to October of 2021, 111 thousand cases of AIDS were reported nationwidely, 97% of which were sexually transmitted, and heterosexual transmission accounted for more than 70%.

HIV belongs to the lentivirus of the family Retrovirus, it was first identified From gay people in the United States in 1981. According to serological reaction and nucleic acid sequence determination of the virus, it can be divided into two types: HIV-1 and HIV-2. Only 45% of the sequences are homologous between HIV-1 and HIV-2 type. Within HIV-1 type, according to the homology of *env* gene encoding envelope protein and *gag* gene sequence encoding shell protein, it can be divided into three groups: group M, group O and group N.

HIV has weak survivability in the external environment and low resistance to physical and chemical factors. General disinfectants such as: iodine tincture, peroxyacetic acid, glutaraldehyde, sodium hypochlorite and other effective disinfectants for hepatitis B virus (HBV), also have a good inactivation effect on HIV. In addition, 70% alcohol can also inactivate HIV, but ultraviolet or gamma rays cannot. HIV is sensitive to heat and tolerates more low temperatures than high temperatures. Treatment at 56°C for 30 min could make HIV lose its infectivity to human T lymphocytes in vitro, but could not completely inactivate HIV in serum. Treatment at 100°C for

20 min can completely inactivate HIV.

10.1   The Morphology and Structure of HIV

Outside human cells, HIV virus exists in the form of spherical particles (also known as virus particles), which are 20 faceted, stereosymmetrical, spherical particles with glycoprotein spike structure on the surface, with a diameter of about 100~120 nm. Therefore, it is difficult to observe HIV virus particles with ordinary optical microscope, but it can be clearly observed with electron microscope. A typical HIV-1 particle consists of a core and an envelope. The viral envelope is a lipoprotein-like envelope that comes from the host cell and is embedded with the viral glycoproteins GP120 and GP41. GP120 is a viral surface antigen and is an envelope glycoprotein. GP41 is a transmembrane glycoprotein, and GP120 binds to GP41 through non-covalent interaction. The conical core of the virus is a semi-conical capsid formed by protein P24, which contains the viral RNA genome, core structural proteins and enzymes (reverse transcriptase, integrase, protease) necessary for viral replication.

10.2   HIV Genome and Function of Its Expressed Proteins

10.2.1   HIV Genome

The two positive strands of HIV genome formed a dimer at the 5' end through partial base complementation and pairing, with a genome length of 9.2 KB and high variation. There are 9 HIV genes in the middle of the proviral DNA, including 3 structural genes (*gag*, *env*, *pol*), 2 regulatory genes *tat* (trans-activator), *rev* (regulator of plasmid protein expression) and 4 auxiliary genes *Nef* (negative regulator), *VPR* (viral R protein), *VPU* (viral U protein) and *VIF* (viral infectious factor) encoding at least 9 proteins.

10.2.1.1   *gag* Gene and Core Protein of HIV

The viral core protein of HIV-1 is encoded by gag gene, including P17, P24 and P15, P17 and P24 constituting the inner shell of HIV particles and P17 constituting the inner membrane of HIV particles. P15 is further cleaved into nucleocapsid proteins P9 and P7 binding with viral RNA. The core protein of HIV-1 has good immunogenicity and is one of the most conserved proteins of HIV.

10.2.1.2   HIV *env* Gene and Membrane Protein

The *env* gene encodes an 88 kD viral envelope protein, which is glycosylated and its molecular weight is increased to 160 kD, which is the precursor of HIV envelope glycoprotein GP160. The precursor protein is cleaved by proteases into GP120 and GP41. GP120 is exposed outside the viral envelope and is called the outer membrane protein, which binds to the cell's CD4 receptor protein when it infects the cell. GP41 is a transmembrane protein, which is embedded in the lipid envelope of the virus. The outer membrane protein GP120 and transmembrane protein

GP41 of HIV bind by non covalent force. The envelope glycoprotein GP120 on the virus surface is a natural ligand of CD4 molecule. When HIV contacts target cells, GP120 binds with CD4 with high affinity, resulting in a conformational change of GP120 which can be recognized by CCR5. GP120 binds with CCR5, exposing the hydrophobic N terminal of GP41 and changing the conformation of GP41. Exposed GP41 can be inserted into the cell membrane and interact with the target cell membrane, which results in membrane fusion of HIV target cells and then the virus core can be introduced into the cell.

10.2.1.3   *pol* Gene and Main Enzyme Proteins of HIV

The gene *pol* encodes HIV replication enzymes, including reverse transcriptase, protease and integrase. Reverse transcriptase (RT), also known as RNA-dependent DNA polymerase, has the functions of polymerase and endonuclease (RNaseH). There are two forms: P51 and P66. They have the same amino terminal sequence but different hydroxyl terminal, and the termination region is different. It is speculated that the difference of hydroxyl terminal is also one of the reasons for the active mutation of HIV. Protease is an indispensable enzyme in the process of virus multiplication. It has the function of cutting off the precursor proteins of various structural proteins. Integrase (INT, P32) can integrate viruses with host cell chromosomes.

10.2.1.4   Non-structural Regulatory Genes and Coding Proteins of HIV

The non-structural genes of HIV-1 virus include two regulatory genes, *tat* and *rev* and the proteins encoded by them both have trans-activated effects on HIV replication. Tat protein with regulatory function is the first synthesized viral protein after the virus infected cells, earlier than gag protein after the virus infected cells. Tat protein is characterized by no immunogenicity, apoptosis induction and partial T cell activation. As a trans-activator, tat is a positive regulatory protein that can greatly improve the transcription and replication levels of HIV-1 genome. The rev protein encoded by *rev* gene is mainly located in the nucleus and nucleoli, which is an important trans-activator regulating HIV gene replication and has a negative regulation effect on HIV regulatory protein and a positive regulation effect on viral particle protein. Its main function is to promote the transformation of HIV gene expression from early (transcriptional regulatory protein mRNA) to late (transcriptional structural protein mRNA) and promote late transcription. Rev protein also interacts with its RNA sequence, rev protein response factor (RRE), to modulate the expression of HIV structural proteins at the post-transcriptional level.

10.2.1.5   Functional Cogenes and Their Coding Proteins of HIV

There are also amount of functional cogene-coding proteins of HIV that have received increasing attention for their roles in the virulence of HIV infection, including:

Vif protein: the *vif* gene encodes a 23 kD viral infectious particle (Vif protein). This protein suppresses the host's immune attack. Human lipoprotein BmRNA encoding enzyme APOBEC3G can inhibit retrovirus replication in cells. Vif can inhibit APOBEC3G ubiquitination, thereby inhibiting HIV-1 genome G-to-A mutation and thereby inhibiting viral variation and enhancing viral infectivity.

Vpr protein: the *vpr* gene encodes a protein with 96 amino acids and a molecular weight of approximately 14 kD. Vpr is highly conserved in HIV-1 and HIV-2. After HIV infects host cells, Vpr interacts with a variety of proteins in the cells and shows a series of biological functions on virus replication, host cell cycle and differentiation. Vpr protein plays an important role in HIV induced apoptosis, which can induce apoptosis of mitotic cells.

Nef protein: Nef protein is present in primate lentiviruses and is found in both HIV-1 and HIV-2. Nef protein is a 27 kD phosphorylated protein. It is produced in the early stage of viral infection and continues to be dispersed on the serous membrane and skeleton of infected cells in the late stage. It is an integrin of mature virus particles that binds to the membrane structure of cell. Nef protein is a negative regulator that inhibits the expression of HIV-1 proto-virus genes specifically transcribed by HIVLTR. Nef protein can also enhance viral infectivity.

Vpu protein: The *vpu* gene is unique to HIV-1, not HIV-2. HIV-2 has an unknown *vpx* gene. The gene encodes an 81-amino acid phosphorylated protein that maps to cell membranes. Vpu expression does not affect HIV replication, but reduces the release of virus particles from the cell membrane. The absence of Vpu can reduce the production of infectious virus particles by 5-10 times. Because HIV replication or protein translation is not inhibited, large aggregates of HIV particles can be found in cells. Vpu protein can disrupt the GP160-CD4 complex, thereby promoting more efficient degradation of GP160 into GP120 and GP41. It also induces the degradation of CD4, which is the main protein of HIV-1 down-regulating in host cells.

10.3   Mechanism of HIV Infection and Virus Replication

10.3.1   The Process of HIV Infection

HIV-1 infects specific CD4$^+$ cells in the human body. The specific susceptibility of the virus to CD4$^+$T cells is because that CD4 molecule is the HIV virus envelope glycoprotein GP120 receptor. GP120 binds to the receptor molecule on the surface of the target cell, making the virus attach to the target cell surface. The conformational changes of GP41 expose the fusion peptide at the N terminus of GP41 and insert it into the target cell membrane, damaging the membrane structure. The plasma membrane of the target cell and the viral membrane get close to each other, and then fuse. After fusion, the plasma membrane of the virus envelope and the target cell is cleaved, and the core protein and genetic material of the virus enter the host cell and release the viral nucleic acid. Viral RNA uses its own reverse transcriptase to reverse transcription and synthesize viral genome cDNA. The synthesized cDNA is in the form of DNA-RNA heterozygote, which is degraded by RNaseH activity of reverse transcriptase (RT) to synthesize a second strand of DNA. The double-stranded DNA is transported to the nucleus and, under the action of integrase, and the viral DNA genome is inserted into the host cell DNA. After the virus genes are integrated into the host genome, it is easy to lurk down and form persistent infection. HIV cannot replicate in stationary T cells.

10.3.2   HIV Replication and Release

Viral DNA integrated into the host cell is the template for viral RNA transcription. HIV RNA can be translated into regulatory proteins (tat, tev), functional auxiliary proteins (vif, vef, vpr, vpu or vpx), core proteins, enzymes and envelope glycoproteins of HIV. Under the action of viral protease, the capsid protein and enzyme of the virus are cleaved and processed. The viral RNA genome is packaged near the cell membrane and assembled into the virus core, which is assembled into virus particles. Then, by budding, the lipid capsule containing envelope glycoprotein is obtained from the host cell and secretes outside the cell to become mature virus particles.

10.4   Epidemiology of HIV

10.4.1   Sources of Infection

The source of HIV infection is AIDS patients and asymptomatic carrier. HIV exists in blood and various body fluids (such as semen, uterine and vaginal secretions, saliva, tears, milk and urine), which are infectious.

10.4.2   Transmission Route

Sexual Contact

This is the main route of transmission of the disease. HIV can be transmitted through unprotected sexual intercourse, including vaginal, anal and oral sex. The high-risk groups for HIV transmission through sexual contact include gay men, sex workers and the sexual partners of HIV-infected people. In Europe and the United States, homosexual and bisexuals transmissions account for 73%–80%, while heterosexual transmission only accounts for about 2%. Africa and the Caribbean are dominated by heterosexual transmission, accounting for 20%–70%. Among the reported infected persons in China in 2017, the proportion of heterosexual transmission was 69.6%, and that of male homosexual transmission was 25.5%. From January to October 2021, 97% of HIV was transmitted through sexual transmission, of which heterosexual transmission accounted for more than 70%.

Transmission Through Blood

High-risk groups susceptible to HIV infection through blood transmission include injecting drug users, informal paid blood donors and health care workers. People can contract HIV through transfusions of contaminated blood, contact with contaminated blood on broken skin, or sharing contaminated needles and other medical equipment.

Mother-to-child Transmission (MTCT)

HIV can be transmitted from HIV-infected mothers to newborns through the placenta, childbirth or breastfeeding. The 2017 report shows that the mother-to-child transmission rate of

AIDS in China decreased from 7.1% in 2012 to 4.9% in 2017.

Other Ways

When nursing people with AIDS, medical personnols were infected by syringes containing blood or contaminated damaged skin, but only 1% of them are infected. It can also be transmitted by organ transplantation or artificial insemination of virus carriers. Close living contact can also spread.

10.4.3 Susceptible population

Almost all population is susceptible. Homosexuals and promiscuous people, drug addicts, hemophiliacs and HIV-infected infants are at high risk. In addition, genetic factors may also be related to the disease, while HLADR5 is the most common type of AIDS.

10.5 Clinical Manifestations

HIV mainly invades the immune system of the human body, including $CD4^+T$ lymphocytes, macrophages and dendritic cells, etc. The main manifestation is a decrease in the number of $CD4^+T$ lymphocytes, which eventually leads to a defect in human cellular immune function and the occurrence of various opportunistic infections and tumors.

From the initial infection to the terminal stage of HIV, it is a long and complicated process. The clinical manifestations of HIV vary depending on the stage of the process. According to the clinical manifestations, symptoms and signs after infection, the whole process of HIV infection can be divided into acute stage, asymptomatic stage and AIDS stage. However, because the main factors affecting the clinical outcome of HIV infection are virus, host immunity and genetic background, it can be clinically manifested as three outcomes of typical progressors, rapid progressors and long-term slow progressors, and the clinical manifestations are also different.

The acute phase usually occurs 2 to 4 weeks after the first HIV infection. In medicine, it's called the "window period" for AIDS. Clinical manifestations of HIV viremia and acute impairment of the immune system occur in some infected individuals. The clinical symptoms of most patients are mild and be last for 1 to 3 weeks. Fever is the most common clinical manifestation, which can include a sore throat, night sweat, nausea, vomiting, diarrhea, rash, joint pain, lymph node enlargement, and nervous system symptoms. During this period, HIV RNA and P24 antigen can be detected in the blood, while HIV antibody appears about 2 weeks after infection. The number of $CD4^+T$ lymphocytes decreases transiently, and the ratio of $CD4^+/CD8^+T$ lymphocytes is also inverted. Mild leukopenia and thrombocytopenia, as well as abnormal liver function, may be present in some patients. People with rapid progression may develop severe infection during this period, developing from acute to asymptomatic. This period lasts between 6 and 8 years in most cases. The duration of infection is determined by the number and type of viruses, the path of infection, individual immune status differences, nutritional conditions, and living habits. In the asymptomatic period, due to the continuous replication of HIV in the body of infected person, the immune system is damaged, CD4$^+$T lymphocyte count gradually decreases, and symptoms or signs such as lymph node enlargement may occur. Persistent generalized lymphadenopathy may also occur, characterized by: (1) enlarged lymph nodes in two or more locations other than the groin, (2) lymph nodes $\geq$ 1 cm in diameter, without tenderness or adhesions, (3) lasting more than three months. AIDS stage is the terminal stage after HIV infection. The CD4$^+$T lymphocyte count is less than 200 μL, and the plasma viral load is significantly increased. During this period, the main clinical manifestations are HIV infection-related symptoms, signs and various opportunistic infections and tumors. Related symptoms and signs of HIV infection are fever, night sweat, and diarrhea lasting more than a month; weight loss of more than 10%. Some patients show neuropsychiatric symptoms, such as memory loss, apathy, personality changes, headache, epilepsy and dementia.

10.6   Collection and Preservation of HIV Samples

Determine the type of samples collected, the time limit, and method of processing, storage, and transportation, operate in accordance with the technical requirements of clinical blood collection, and comply with the relevant biosafety requirements, based on the specific requirements of the test items. Before sampling, check whether the required items are ready, whether they are within the validity period, whether they are damaged or they are sufficient. Check in particular, whether the examinee's information is consistent with the mark on the surface of the sample container, as well as the time of sample collection and the unique code.

10.6.1   Sample Classification and Collection

10.6.1.1   Collection of Blood Sample

Before blood collection, the test tube or filter paper shall be marked and coded after verification. It is recommended to use a preprinted, low temperature resistant label designed for refrigerated storage and to attach the label to the side of the test tube.

When drawing anticoagulated whole blood, disinfect the local skin, draw a proper amount of venous blood with a vacuum blood collection tube added with anticoagulant, or draw venous blood with a disposable syringe, transfer it to a test tube added with anticoagulant, gently reverse, and mix it for later use. Local skin should be disinfected when drawing peripheral whole blood. Prick the skin with a blood collection needle and wipe off the first drop of blood with sterile gauze. Collect the dripped blood for later use.

When drawing plasma, select a blood collection tube containing appropriate anticoagulant according to the test requirements, collect venous blood according to the instructions of the blood collection tube, and separate the plasma; or centrifuge the collected anticoagulant whole blood at 1500–3000 rpm for 15 minutes, and the upper layer is the plasma, which should be sucked out and placed in a suitable container for later use.

Collect venous blood according to the blood collection tube's instruction and separate the serum according to the test requirement; or use a vacuum blood collection tube without anticoagulant to draw a proper amount of venous blood, or use a disposable syringe to draw venous blood, transfer it to a test tube without anticoagulant or with coagulant, and place it for 1 to 2 hours. After blood coagulation and blood clot contraction, centrifuge it at 1500–3000 rpm for 15 minutes, suck out the serum, and place it in a suitable container for later use.

Centrifuge the collected anticoagulated whole blood at 1500–3000 rpm for 15 minutes when drawing the lymphocyte enrichment solution, draw the lymphocyte enrichment solution under the plasma layer, and place it in a suitable container for later use. Peripheral blood mononuclear cells (PBMC) are extracted by density gradient centrifugation with lymphocyte separation medium, and the PBMC layer is aspirated and placed in a suitable container for later use.

Appropriate anticoagulants shall be selected according to the test requirements, such as EDTA potassium or sodium salt, sodium citrate, heparin sodium (if the blood is not used for nucleic acid testing) or $CD4^+$ and $CD8^+$ T lymphocyte count determination, and EDTA potassium or sodium salt or sodium citrate for HIV-1 isolation and nucleic acid qualitative/quantitative testing. If dried blood spots are used for testing, the various blood samples collected can be prepared as dried blood spots if necessary. Dried blood plaques are most commonly prepared with anticoagulant whole blood, peripheral whole blood, and plasma. Siphon 100 μL of anticoagulant whole blood (or plasma) from the sample tube with a pipette, aiming at the center of the filter paper printing circle, drop the sample on the filter paper; or add the peripheral blood from the skin wound directly to the center of the filter paper printing circle. As needed, apply the sample to several rings at once. Dry naturally at room temperature for at least 4 hours (dry for at least 24 hours in humid climate), do not heat or stack blood spots, and do not contact with other interfaces. After the blood spots are fully dried, they are put into a sealed bag. Each dried blood spot is stored separately to avoid mutual contamination between blood spots. At the same time, a desiccant and a humidity indicator card are placed in the bag, sealed, packaged, and stored for later use.

10.6.1.2   Collection of Urine Samples

The results of the AIDS urine test are relatively accurate, so the results can be used as a basis for diagnosis. Collect the urine into a small cup and send the urine for examination. The window period of the method of urine test paper is three weeks to three months after high-risk contact. Patients can be tested at various times to improve the detection rate in accordance with their individual needs. It is generally recommended to test at the fourth week, the sixth week and the third month after high-level contact. HIV infection can be ruled out if the test results are negative. At the same time, if other types of test paper are used for detection at the same time, the accuracy can be improved. If there is a positive or suspected positive result on any occasion, it should be retested.

10.6.1.3   Collection of Oral Mucosal Exudate

Saliva contains a very small amount of HIV, and this test uses oral mucosal exudate to detect HIV antibodies. The sample used for the test is not actually saliva, but gingival crevicular fluid which is collected from the upper and lower gingiva. Scrape the upper and lower gums with a swab for 4 to 6 seconds, and then insert the sampling stick into the detection tube containing the diluent.

10.6.2   Preservation of Samples

Serum or plasma samples for antibody and antigen testing can be stored at 2–8°C for short-term testing, and stored below -20°C for more than one week. Plasma and blood cell samples used for nucleic acid detection can be stored at 2-8°C within 4 days; stored below -20°C within 3 months; stored below -70°C for more than 3 months. Oral mucosal exudate samples should be used immediately and stored in accordance with the product instructions. Urine rapid test samples must be stored in accordance with the product instructions. Urine samples can be stored at room temperature for 2 weeks with a special catheter; they should be stored at 2-8°C within three months; If the samples are to be stored for a long time (more than three months), preservatives must be added and the product instructions must be followed. Whole blood samples for CD4$^+$ T lymphocyte detection must be kept at room temperature for no more than 48 hours.

10.7   HIV Laboratory Testing

Laboratory testing is the primary basis for the diagnosis of HIV/AIDS infection. Depending on the level of detection, it can be divided into protein-level, gene-level, and cell-level detection. The main laboratory testing methods include HIV antibody detection, qualitative and quantitative detection of HIV nucleic acid. HIV-1/2 antibody detection is the gold standard for the diagnosis of HIV infection. HIV nucleic acid detection is also used for the diagnosis of HIV infection, and the quantification of HIV nucleic acid (viral load) is also the main index of disease progression, clinical drug use, efficacy, and prognosis.

10.7.1   HIV–1/2 Antibody Testing

As a protein level test, HIV-1/2 antibody detection is the mostly common used method in the diagnosis of HIV infection. Since HIV antibodies are contained in the urine, saliva, semen and tears of HIV infected individuals, the HIV antibody test can detect not only the blood samples, but also the above non-blood samples. HIV-1/2 antibody testing includes screening tests and supplementary tests.

10.7.1.1   Screening Tests

A negative response can issue a negative report of HIV-1/2 antibody, seen in people not infected by HIV, but the window period infection screening test can also show a negative response. If positive, original reagent double (quick test) / double well (chemiluminescence test or ELISA) or both reagents are needed to test; if negative, report HIV antibody negative; if one negative and the other one positive or two positive reaction, the supplementary test is required.

10.7.1.2   Enzyme-linked Immunosorbent Test (ELISA)

ELISA is the most commonly used HIV antibody screening experiment. The HIV antigen was coated in the Solid Matrix, the enzyme-labeled HIV antigen and the sample to be tested were added to make the substrate color. The amplification effect of enzyme catalyzed substrate reaction are used to enhance the sensitivity of antigen antibody reaction, and thus improve the HIV antibody detection rate. The ELISA test is not affected by hemolysis and lipid blood in the samples, and the stability is high. Data are obtained through the microplate reader to reduce the impact on the test results and ensure the accuracy of the test results. Moreover, it also has the advantages of high accuracy, low price, and is suitable for a large number of specimens. Through the continuous improvement and renewal of ELISA, its sensitivity and specificity are greatly improved, and the fourth-generation ELISA greatly shortens the window period and increases the detection of new isoforms, as shown in Table 10-1.

Table 10-1　The development of HIV antibody ELISA diagnostic reagents

ELISA reagent	Solid matrix	Lable	Test target	Window phase
First generation	Virus lysates	Antihuman-IgG	HIV-1 IgG antibody	6-8 weeks
Second generation	HIV-1/2 with recombinant antigens	Antihuman-IgG	HIV-1/2 IgG antibody	4-5 weeks
Third generation	HIV-1/2 with recombinant antigens	Antihuman-IgG	HIV-1/2/O IgM/ IgG antibody	About 3 weeks
Fourth generation	HIV-1/2 with recombinant antigens, p21 antibody	Antihuman-IgG	HIV-1/2/O IgM/IgG antibody,P24 antigen	About 2 weeks

10.7.1.3　Rapid Detection Test

At present, the universally used rapid detection methods mainly include spot ELISA and spot immunocolloidal gold or colloidal selenium, immunochromatography, particle coagulation test, percolation test, etc. Due to the need for specialized equipment and simplicity, rapid testing is suitable for emergency surgery, HIV screening in remote areas, and cases with high-risk behavior estimates and difficult to return. Rapid detection assays will couple different antigen combinations of HIV1-1/2 to different vectors to the corresponding antibodies in the sample, judge by visible changes, and generally color results within 30 min. Due to the subjective factors, different inspectors may draw different conclusions about the same result, especially the weak positive results, so the sensitivity and specificity of the rapid test need to be improved.

10.7.1.4　Authentication Experiment

The confirmatory test method includes Western blot and antigen detection.

Western Blot (WB)

Western blot is widely used in transmitted diseases, and it is also an HIV infection confirmation experiment. The principle is to use the HIV virus protein with sodium dodecyl sulfonate-polyacrylamide gel electrophoresis (SDS-PAGE) to separate the different molecular weight proteins, and then transfer the separated protein bands to the nitrocellulose membrane, react with the antibody in the sample, wash away the unbound serum protein, add the color development agent, and judge the results according to the band. The WB method is considered as the "gold standard" for screening to confirm HIV infection because of its good specificity.

Antigen Detection

Antigen detection plays an important role in the packaging and maturation process of the virus. The p24 antigen appears early in the serum, is generally detectable at 2-3 weeks after HIV infection, and peaks at 1-2 months. Later, as the body antibodies are gradually produced, the p24 antigen and the p24 antibody form an immune complex, and the antigen is no longer detectable. Later in the course of the disease, as the virus replication increases, the immune system is gradually destroyed, the p24 antibody titer decreases, and the p24 antigen can be re-detected. Therefore, p24 antigens exist in free form in early and late infection, while in most cases in the immune complex situation. Immune complex cleavage assay (immune complex dissociation, ICD) separates the antigen-antibody complex by acid or heat treatment, increasing the p24 antigen concentration, and thus improving the detection rate of the p24 antigen.

10.7.1.5   Nucleic Acid Test

With the continuous development of molecular biology techniques, the technology for detecting HIV from the gene level also continues to mature. Testing HIV nucleic acid by molecular biology techniques can not only qualitatively detect whether samples contain HIV, assisting in early diagnosis of HIV infection and shortening the window period; but also quantify the virus in the sample, namely, detecting viral load, for disease monitoring and predicting disease progression, etc. At present, the HIV nucleic acid detection technology commonly used in the laboratory is mainly: reverse transcription PCR (RT-PCR), branched DNA signal expansion system (bDNA), and nucleic acid sequence-dependent amplification system (NASBA). Comparisons of the three viral load methods are shown in Table 10-2. In addition, gene-level

Table 10–2   Comparison of different laboratory methods for the quantitation of HIV viral load

Technical principle	RT-PCR	bDNA	NASBA
Dynamic range	Standard: version 1.5 400-750 000 c/mL Supersensitivity :version 1.5 50-750 000 c/mL	The bDNA is version 3.0 50-500 000 c/mL	NucliSens HIV-1 Q T:176-3500 000 c/mL
Subtypes were amplified	Version 1.0:Only subtype B Version 1.5: B-G	A-H	A-G
Sample volume	Amplicor 0.2 mL Supersensitivity 0.5 mL	1 mL	10-2 000 μL
Anticoagulant agent	EDTA	EDTA	EDTA or heparin
Sample	Blood plasma	Plasma, peripheral blood mononuclear cells, semen, tissues, etc	Whole blood, plasma, peripheral blood mononuclear cells, semen, tissues, etc
Requirements	Plasma was isolated within 6 h and frozen at-20℃ or-70℃ prior to transport	Plasma was isolated within 4 h and frozen at –20℃ or –70℃ prior to transport	Plasma was isolated within 4 h and frozen at –20℃ or –70℃ prior to transport

testing can be used for viral epidemic characteristics and distribution, drug resistance testing, early diagnosis of infant HIV infection, etc. Based on traditional nucleic acid testing, emerging testing technologies such as nanotechnology, microfluidics, biosensors, and next-generation sequencing (NGS) can complement existing testing methods and improve the efficiency of HIV detection, diagnosis, and monitoring.

10.7.2 HIV Virus Isolation Experiment–PBMC Coculture Method

Peripheral blood mononuclear cells (PBMC) coculture method is a kind of HIV pathogen test, and the positive rate can reach 95%~99%, which can provide the early diagnosis and clinical AIDS stage of HIV infection, but due to its high operation technology and laboratory conditions, it is mainly used for scientific research. Two consecutive positive reactions of P24 antigen or reverse transcriptase in culture supernatant, increased p24 antigen content/reverse transcriptase activity, or accompanied by characteristic HIV cytopathic changes, are identified as HIV gene sequence and judged as HIV-1 isolation positive. The experiment must be operated in the biosafety cabinet of the biosafety tertiary laboratory, each batch of the normal donor PBMC alone to culture as a negative control, the culture process and detection method are completely consistent with the experimental samples. The negative control p24 antigen is tested negative, and the whole experimental data are valid.

10.7.3 HIV Laboratory Testing Strategy

The laboratory testing strategy for AIDS refers to the strategy used for epidemic monitoring, blood screening, and clinical diagnosis.

10.7.3.1 Detection Strategies Related to Epidemic Monitoring

Detection strategies related to epidemic monitoring include HIV anonymous unassociation testing and HIV real-name association testing. In the HIV anonymous unassociation test, all initially screened reactive samples are retested using different reagents with no reaction, and then "HIV antibody negative" result is reported; the results are reactive and "HIV antibody positive" result is reported. Real-name related epidemic monitoring requires clinical diagnosis-related testing procedures and results reports.

10.7.3.2 Detection Strategies Related to Clinical Diagnosis

In the clinical diagnosis for individuals, the HIV screening test is conducted first, and the reactive samples are then conducted with the HIV supplementary test, including the antibody confirmation test and the nucleic acid test. The results of supplementary test can make a diagnosis. HIV testing for high epidemic areas (more than 5%), high-risk groups (gay men, drug users, etc.) can use three enzyme-linked immune reagents or three rapid reagents or rapid reagents and enzyme-linked reagents for testing, and samples need to be further determined for supplementary tests.

10.7.3.3 Detection Strategies Related to Blood Screening

Detection strategies related to blood screening include HIV testing of blood donors and

HIV testing strategies for plasma donors and plasma products as well as testing related to early diagnosis of infant HIV-1 infection. Blood donor HIV blood screening should be tested at least once with nucleic acid and serological reagents, with blood screening markers including: serological markers HIV-1 antibodies and HIV-2 antibodies (anti-HIV-1 +2), or HIV-1 antibody, HIV-2 antibodies and HIV-1p24 antigen (HIV Ag/Ab1 +2); nucleic acid markers are mainly HIV-1 nucleic acid (HIV-1 RNA). Plasma donor and plasma product HIV serological tests are the same as donor HIV blood screening tests. For infants with AIDS infection, blood samples should be collected within 48 hours of birth, 6 weeks and 3 months after birth to conduct early diagnosis test for infant AIDS infection. Children with negative early diagnosis test results or no early diagnosis test should be screened for AIDS antibody at 12 months of age. The positive screening results should be followed up to 18 months. If the antibody test result is still positive at 18 months, supplementary tests should be conducted to clarify the infection status.

10.8   HIV Prevention and Treatment

10.8.1   Therapeutic Interventions

Modern antiretroviral regimens can effectively block HIV replication in people with HIV for decades, but these therapies are not curative and must be taken for life. HIV can be integrated into the host genome and persisted during the life cycle of the infected cells. Because they are largely transcriptionally silent, these latently infected cells are not identified as foreign cells, but contain replication-competent viruses that drive the recovery of the infection once the ART (antiretroviral therapy) is stopped.

Targeting the Provirus

Since the discovery that HIV can establish a latent infection with minimal HIV transcription, a range of approaches has emerged that specifically target latently infected cells. These include pharmacological modulation of epigenetic or signaling pathways involved in HIV transcription to reactivate latent HIV such that the cells can be targeted and eliminated ("shock and kill") or to permanently silence HIV transcription ("block and lock"). Recent reports have demonstrated that HIV latency is heterogeneous and that latency reactivation is stochastic, implying that a combination of agents targeting various pathways controlling HIV transcription may be necessary to achieve either robust silencing or latency reversal. A clear limitation of the "shock and kill" approach comes from the discovery that only a fraction of proviruses is intact and among these, only some are inducible by a potent stimulus such as T cell stimulation, let alone by far less potent latency-reversing agents (LRAs). Therefore, LRAs will likely need to be partnered with therapies that enhance the clearance of cells expressing viral proteins, such as immune-enhancing strategies or proapoptotic drugs, thus far, these approaches have yet to be successfully translated into human trials.

Targeting the Immune System

Significant progress has been made in the isolation and development of neutralizing antibodies for widespread clinical use, especially in the development of therapeutic vaccines, vaccine adjuvants and other immunotherapies. But when used alone, most of these methods have limited efficacy in humans. It is almost certain that AIDS treatment requires a combination of multiple therapies, see Figure 10-1. As HIV immunotherapy enters the clinic, careful attention must be paid to immune-related adverse events, including cytokine release syndrome and autoimmunity.

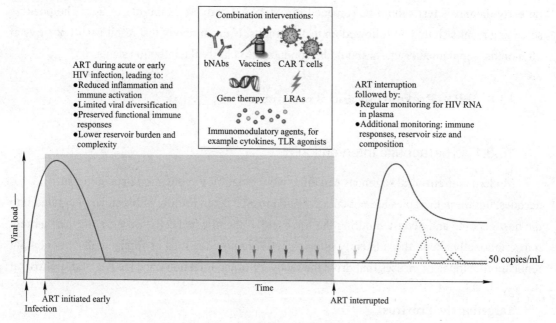

Figure 10–1   Strategies for immunotherapy

Strategies that will enhance immune-mediated clearance of latently infected cells include early initiation of ART and the administration of combined interventions at the time of suppressive ART (colored arrows) or during the treatment interruption phase, which will allow for increased antigen presentation. Given that there is no biomarker that can predict viral rebound, analytical treatment interruptions are used to determine whether the intervention has had a clinically meaningful impact. The overarching goal is to either delay viral rebound by at least months or years or reduce the set point of virus replication (that is, the stable level of viral load that the body settles at), preferably to a level of <200 copies/mL. The dashed colored lines represent different potential favorable outcomes from a cure intervention. [bNAbs, broadly neutralizing antibodies; LRA, latency reversing agent; TLR, Toll-like receptor]

Gene Therapy

Recently, gene therapy has shifted to creating effectors, such as the chimeric antigen receptor (CAR) T cells, which can recognize and eliminate HIV-infected cells (Figure 10-2). Other methods include gene delivery of new delivery systems to local tissues, leading to continuous production of antiviral drugs with systemic effects such as broad neutralizing antibodies and CD4 mimic. Continuous production of these antiviral drugs leads to continuous (and perhaps lifelong) control of the virus.

Examples of ex vivo (left) and in vivo (right) gene therapy approaches that have been tested in people with HIV on ART are shown in Figure 10-2. Ex vivo strategies include gene editing to either delete or inactivate CCR5 or HIV provirus in CD4-enriched T cells using gene-editing tools such as zinc finger nucleases (ZFN) or CRISPR–Cas9. Alternatively, autologous T cells can be modified to express a CAR that can recognize HIV envelope, and this can then be reinfused into the participant. In vivo strategies, on the other hand, do not require external manipulation of cells; nanoparticles or viral vectors [such as adeno-associated virus (AAV)], which encapsulate mRNA or DNA, respectively, for the relevant gene to be expressed are administered directly to the patient. These approaches have recently been successful using lipid nanoparticles that contain mRNA encoding CRISPR–Cas9135 or for expression of anti-HIV broadly neutralizing antibodies such as PG9 or VRC07. [PBMCs, peripheral blood mononuclear cells; PLWH, person living with HIV]

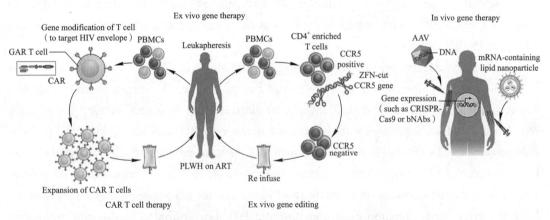

Figure 10-2   Strategies for gene therapy

10.8.2   Prevention of HIV

Due to the global genetic diversity of HIV, its diagnostic assays, viral load measurements, and response to antiretroviral treatment are all affected. HIV prevention is therefore of paramount importance.

Source of Infection

The source of infection of AIDS is mainly HIV/AIDS patients who have not been treated or failed to be treated, and they are divided into two categories: knowing their infection and not knowing their infection. Antiviral therapy (ART) can effectively reduce viral load and transmission in HIV/AIDS patients who are aware of their infection. For patients who do not know whether they are infected or not, infection risk assessment in the population and Pre-exposure prevention (PrEP) is necessary. Pre-exposure prevention (PrEP) is a prevention strategy that provides antiretroviral drugs to uninfected persons at risk of HIV, which reduces infection risk by more than 85% in some clinical trials.

Route of Transmission

AIDS is mainly transmitted through blood transmission, mother-to-child transmission and sexual contact. With the implementation of various HIV prevention and control strategies in China, mother-to-child transmission and drug use transmission have been effectively controlled, and sexual transmission has become the main route of HIV infection. Measures such as risk assessment and proper condom use can intervene to reduce the incidence of unsafe sex, thus effectively cutting off the sexual transmission of HIV. In addition, HIV infection can be avoided to some extent by raising awareness of the risks of infection, for example, in terms of choosing sexual partners, regular testing, informed dating or post-exposure prophylaxis.

Susceptible Population

The most vulnerable groups include high-risk sexual contacts, drug users, occupational AIDS exposure population, and infants born to HIV-positive mothers. Studies have shown that behavioral intervention through the Internet can reduce high-risk sexual behaviors and thus reduce sexual contact infections. In addition, the awareness rate of AIDS-related knowledge can also be improved through traditional media such as radio, newspapers, television and on-the-spot education in high-risk places.

In recent years, through the strict control of drug abuse in China, the possibility of HIV infection caused by drug abuse has been reduced at the source. Occupational AIDS exposure population refers to the medical staff engaged in diagnosis and treatment, nursing work by the blood, body fluids contaminated with the skin or mucosa, or by HIV containing blood, body fluids contaminated needle or other sharp device puncturing the skin, and may be infected by HIV. After the occurrence of HIV occupational exposure, the immediate and correct implementation of local treatment and timely prevention of medication is the key for the prevention of HIV infection. With the effective application of mother-to-child HIV prevention technology in pregnancy screening, the promotion of artificial feeding and the improvement of the application rate of antiviral drugs, the condition of infants being infected by HIV-positive mothers has also been improved.

Glossary

virus *n.* 病毒 an extremely small piece of organic material that causes disease in humans, animals, and plants

HIV 人类免疫缺陷病毒 abbreviation for human immunodeficiency virus: the virus that causes acquired immunodeficiency syndrome (AIDS, a serious disease that destroys the body's ability to fight infection)

infection *n.* 传染 a disease in a part of your body that is caused by bacteria or a virus

replication *n.* 复制 the process by which organisms and genetic or other structures make exact copies of themselves

gene therapy 基因治疗 exogenous normal genes are introduced into target cells to correct or compensate the diseases caused by defective and abnormal genes, so as to achieve the purpose of treatment

epidemiology *n.* 流行病学 study on the distribution and influencing factors of disease and health status in the population; and scientific research on strategies and measures to prevent and treat diseases and promote health

immunity *n.* 免疫 a physiological function that the body recognizes "self" and "non-self" antigens, forms natural immune tolerance to self antigens and repels non-self antigens

pre-exposure prevention (PrEP) 暴露前预防 a method of preventing HIV infection in persons who have not yet been infected with HIV by taking specific antiviral drugs before engaging in HIV-prone behavior

AIDS 获得性免疫缺陷综合征 abbreviation for acquired immunodeficiency syndrome: a chronic, potentially life-threatening condition caused by the human immunodeficiency virus (HIV)

（李祥　楼永良）

新形态教材网·数字课程学习……

教学 PPT　　　　自测题　　　　推荐阅读

Chapter 11
Food Microorganism

Learning objectives:
- Know the concepts related to food microbiology.
- Understand the types and sources of common food microorganisms, prevention strategies of microbial contamination in food.
- Be familiar with intrinsic and extrinsic factors that influence microbes in foods, food spoilage, foodborne disease.
- Master the detection of microbes in food.

Microorganisms are closely related to the food. For the most part, human are enjoying the benefits brought by microorganism, such as the delicious fermented foods which are inseparable from the role of microorganisms. However, some harmful microorganisms may cause food spoilage, and even food poisoning or other foodborne diseases. In order to better take advantage of the microorganisms, constantly develop new food microbial resources, and control harmful microorganisms, it is necessary to know the characteristics of microbes that grow in food and how food environment influences microbes.

11.1   Factors Influencing Microbes in Foods

Foods are ecosystems composed of the environment and organisms that live in them. The main microbial groups in foods are different due to the different habitat characteristics of various foods. The food environment is composed of intrinsic factors and extrinsic factors. Characteristics of the food itself are called intrinsic factors, which include nutrients, water activity (Aw), pH, osmotic pressure, oxidation-reduction potential, natural defense structures and antimicrobial substances. Extrinsic factors are external to the foods, such as temperature and gas composition. Both intrinsic and external factors to the food can be manipulated to preserve food.

Among the intrinsic factors, water is a major factor in controlling both microbial growth and chemical reactions in food. All kinds of foods contain a certain amount of water. Water exists in food as two forms of bound water and free water. Only free water, also called unbound or available water, can be used by microorganisms. The amount of available water determines whether microbes can grow. The measure of available water in foods is called water activity. Water activity is defined as the ratio of the vapor pressure of water in a food (P) to the vapor pressure of pure water (P_0) at the same temperature. Namely, $Aw=P/P_0$. Its value is between 0-1. Aw is mostly between 0.98-0.99 in daily food, which is suitable for the growth of most microorganisms. When Aw is lower than 0.90, bacteria can hardly grow. When Aw decreases to 0.88, the growth of yeast is seriously affected. The minimal Aw for most molds to grow is 0.80. It can be seen that the Aw required by mold is generally lower than that of bacteria and yeast. The Aw would be reduced in drying food to make it difficult for microorganisms to grow and reproduce, and thus the shelf life of the food could be prolonged.

Temperature is the main extrinsic factor influencing microbial growth and physiology. The temperature of food depends on its environment. Appropriate temperature can promote the growth and reproduction of microorganisms, while inappropriate temperature can weaken or inhibit the life activities of microorganisms. Temperature control is key for food safety since the influence of temperature on the growth rate of microorganisms is obvious. Food should be held below 4℃ or above 60℃, since 4-60℃ are the temperature ranges for microbial growth. There is an optimum temperature range for microbial growth. Above the optimal growth temperature, the growth rates decrease rapidly. Below the optimum temperature, growth rates also decrease, but more gradually. Microorganism can be classified as psychrophilic microorganism, mesophilic microorganism and thermophilic microorganism according to their adaptive temperatures for microbial growth. The three kinds of microorganisms can grow at 25-30℃, it is also the temperature at which food is easy to deteriorate. When food is stored at low temperature, the shelf life of food can be prolonged and the enzyme activity of fresh food can be reduced, and the freshness of food can be maintained. However, it should be noted that conventional refrigeration cannot avoid food spoilage because psychrophiles can still grow at the low temperature. The storage temperature must be below -20℃ if food would be preserved for a long time without spoilage.

11.2   Types and Sources of Common Food Microorganisms

The main microbial groups are different due to the diverse habitat characteristics in various foods. These food related microorganisms are called food microorganisms mainly including bacteria, actinomyces, yeasts, molds and viruses. Food microorganisms can be simply classified into "the good, the bad, and the ugly" . Bad microorganisms cause food spoilage. Food spoilage means the original nutritional value, texture, flavor of food are damaged, thus the food becomes harmful to people and unsuitable to eat. A product (i.e., meat, dairy and fruit) is considered spoiled if sensory changes make it unacceptable to the consumer. Sensory change is generally a result of food decomposition and the formation of metabolites resulting from microbial growth, and meanwhile enzyme activity within the food contributes to this change. While ugly microorganisms cause foodborne illness, which is closely related to food safety. Food safety is a scientific discipline describing handling, preparation, and storage of food in ways that prevent foodborne illness, which is related to the people's health.

There are two major pathways that food would be contaminated by microorganisms. One is called primary contamination, that is, foods are contaminated by the natural environment microorganisms (e.g. soil and plants) at raw materials phase, such as the pollution of grain, fruits and vegetables before harvest or the infection of livestock and poultry before slaughter. The other one is called secondary contamination, which means microorganisms are brought into food after the exposure to water, air, human, animals, production environment and food utensils during a series of processes including transportation, storage, processing, making finished products and sales.

11.3   Microorganisms Causing Food Spoilage in a Variety of Common Foods

The types of microorganisms involved in food spoilage and the characteristics of food changes are different in various foods. Food spoilage usually leads to color defects or changes in texture, the development of off flavors or odors, slime or other characteristics that make food undesirable for consumption.

11.3.1   Meat

The Aw of meat lean muscle tissue is 0.99, with a corresponding water content of 74% to 80%. Meat is rich in nutrients, containing high protein, fat and low carbohydrate. The composition of the meat affects the microbial growth. The pH of meat is from 6 to 7, it is suitable for the growth and reproduction of most microorganisms. The microbial contamination of fresh meat can be divided into pre-slaughter and post-slaughter stages. The muscle tissue of healthy livestock and poultry is sterile, and the structure of muscle tissues can prevent the invasion and diffusion of microorganisms. After slaughtering, meats generally go through four phases of stiffness, maturity, autolysis and corruption phase due to the action of tissue enzymes and external microorganisms. The meat of the first two phases is called fresh meat. At the maturity and autolysis phases, meat produce the decomposition products, which provide good nutrients for the growth and reproduction of spoilage microorganisms, and the large-scale growth and reproduction of microorganism result in the corruption and decomposition of meat.

The sensory characteristics of spoiled meat are mainly stickiness, discoloration and smelliness. Stickiness is an early phenomenon of meat deterioration because some microorganisms, such as *Pseudomonas*, *colorless bacilli*, *Flavobacterium*, *Proteus*, *Alkalogenes*, *Escherichia coli*, molds and yeasts, form mucus on the surface of meat. Discoloration means that the color of normal fresh meat changes after microbial contamination and growth. For example, the combination of myoglobin in the meat with hydrogen peroxide produced by microorganisms will make the color of meat turn green. *Flavobacterium* can produce yellow pigment to make the meat turn yellow. Odor change means that some microorganisms can produce ammonia, hydrogen sulfide, indole, mercaptan and stink when decomposing proteins to form a stink odor. Spoiled meat would become inedible and result in poisoning.

11.3.2   Milk

Milk is a good medium for many microorganisms because of its high water content, near-neutral pH, and variety of available nutrients. The major nutritional components of milk are lactose, fat, protein, minerals, and vitamins. Freshly collected milk contains various microbial growth inhibitors, such as lactoferrin, the lactoperoxidase system and lysozyme, which can maintain raw milk freshly within 36 h.

Microbial contamination pathway in fresh milk includes internal infection and external microbial contamination. The external environment pollution is an important source, mainly from animal skin, digestive tract, respiratory tract and excreta. In addition, the environmental hygiene condition of the milking place, the operation of food practitioners, even the milk storage apparatus are also microbial contamination origin.

Fluid milk is susceptible to spoilage by non-spore fermentative bacteria, mainly the lactic acid bacteria and coliform group. The genera of lactic acid bacteria involved in spoilage of milk include *Lactococcus*, *Lactobacillus*, *Leuconostoc*, *Enterococcus*, *Pediococcus*, and *Streptococcus*. Coliforms can spoil milk, but this is seldom a problem, since the lactic acid bacteria usually outgrow them.

The most common fermentative defect in fluid milk products is souring. This is mainly caused by the growth of lactic acid bacteria. Lactic acid itself has a clean, pleasant acid flavor and no odor. The unpleasant sour odor and the taste of spoiled milk result from small amounts of acetic and propionic acids. Other defects may occur in combination with acid production, e.g. protein in milk coagulates. Another defect associated with the growth of lactic acid bacteria in milk is ropy texture. Most dairy-associated species of lactic acid bacteria produce exocellular polymers that increase the viscosity of milk, causing the ropy defect. The polymer is a polysaccharide containing glucose and galactose with small amounts of mannose, rhamnose, and pentose.

The preservation of fluid milk relies on effective sanitation, pasteurization, timely marketing, and refrigeration. Raw milk is usually rapidly cooled immediately following collection and refrigerated until it is consumed. Obviously, there is often sufficient time for psychrotrophic bacteria to grow from milk collection to consumption, which could cause the flavor defects of milk. So it is important to prevent contamination of raw milk by the psychrotrophic bacteria. Psychrotrophic bacteria that spoil raw and pasteurized milk are primarily aerobic gram negative rod-shaped bacteria belonging to the family *Pseudomonadaceae,* mainly *Pseudomonas fragi*, *Pseudomonas putida*, and *Pseudomonas lundensis.*

11.4 Microorganisms for Food Poisoning

It may have the hazard for resulting in infectious diseases or food poisoning if pathogens or toxin producing molds exist in contaminated food. Food poisoning is the most common foodborne disease. It refers to non-infectious acute or subacute illness caused by the consumption of food or water contaminated with bacteria and/or their toxins, mycotoxins, virus or toxic chemicals. It does not include acute gastroenteritis caused by overeating, foodborne intestinal infectious, parasitic diseases, food allergy and gastrointestinal diseases of its own. Chronic toxic damage caused by toxic food also does not belong to food poisoning. According to the pathogenic factors, food poisoning can be classified into four categories including bacterial food poisoning, fungi and their toxins food poisoning, toxic animal and plant food poisoning, and chemical food poisoning. This section focuses on the first two categories.

11.4.1 Bacterial Food Poisoning and Its Common Bacteria

Bacterial food poisoning refers to the disease caused by eating food contaminated by pathogenic bacteria or their toxins with acute gastroenteritis as the main poisoning symptom. It is the most common type of food poisoning. Common bacteria causing bacterial food poisoning include *Salmonella*, *Vibrio parahaemolyticus*, *Staphylococcus*, *Escherichia coli*, *Clostridium botulinum*, *Bacillus cereus*, *Clostridium perfringens*, *Proteus*, etc.

Salmonella spp. are facultatively anaerobic gram-negative rod-shaped bacteria belonging to the family *Enterobacteriaceae*. They have more than 2,500 serotypes, but only a few are pathogenic to human beings, such as *Salmonella typhi* and *Salmonella paratyphi* causing human typhoid and paratyphoid. *Salmonella* are more pathogenic to animals, among them, some can also be transmitted to humans, causing enteritis, food poisoning and sepsis. *Salmonella spp.*, such as *S. typhimurium*, *S. enteritidis* and *S. choleraesuis*, are important pathogens as leading causes of foodborne bacterial illnesses in humans. A major outbreak of foodborne salmonellosis mainly involves contaminated meat, eggs and milk. Once a person eats food containing a large number of live bacteria, food poisoning can occur. *Salmonella* food poisoning can occur all year round, mostly in summer. Its incubation period is from several hours to 3 days, generally 12-24 h. The main symptoms are gastroenteritis symptoms such as nausea, vomiting, abdominal pain and diarrhea, accompanied by headache, fever and general weakness. Severe cases can cause spasm, dehydration and shock. The course of disease is 3-7 days, and the prognosis is generally good.

Vibrio parahaemolyticus is a gram negative bacterium, often presenting arc-shaped, rod-shaped, filiform and other shapes. It is a halophilic bacterium, so it widely exists in coastal seawater and seafood including marine fish, shellfish, shrimp and crab, also associated with a great variety of salted food such as salted bacon, eggs, pickles and cold dishes. A special consideration in the taxonomy of *V. parahaemolyticus* is the ability of certain strains to produce a hemolysin, called the TDH, or Kanagawa, which is linked to virulence in the species. A high percentage of seafood samples tested positive for species. Food poisoning can occur when someone eats these contaminated foods at a dose of 10^6-10^8 CFU/g. Gastroenteritis from *V. parahaemolyticus* is almost exclusively associated with seafood that is consumed raw, inadequately cooked, or cooked but recontaminated. *V. parahaemolyticus* infection occurs with seasonality, generally being greater during the warm-weather months between April and October. The most common symptoms of patients with *V. parahaemolyticus* infection are diarrhea, abdominal cramps, nausea and vomiting. The course of disease is generally 1-3 days. Mortality is extremely low.

Staphylococcus aureus belongs to gram positive cocci. It excretes a variety of virulence factors including the staphylococcal enterotoxins, which can cause staphylococcal food poisoning. This kind of food poisoning is common in China, second only to *Salmonella* and *Vibrio parahaemolyticus* food poisoning. One does not get staphylococcal food poisoning by eating live bacteria, one gets it by eating staphylococcal toxins that have already been made in the contaminated food. This form of food poisoning is known as an intoxication or poisoning because it does not require that the bacteria infect and grow in the patient. *Staphylococcal* toxin is unique because it is not destroyed by heating. Humans are the main reservoir of *S.aureus*. Animals are also *S.aureus* sources. In humans, the nose interior is the main colonization site. *S.aureus* also occurs on the skin. *S.aureus* spreads by direct contact, by skin fragments, or through respiratory droplets produced when people cough or sneeze. Most staphylococcal food poisoning is traced to food contaminated by humans during preparation. *S.aureus* is present in many foods. Staphylococcal food poisoning can occur all year round, mostly in summer. Incubation period is an average 2-4 hours, the shorter one will become ill within 30 minutes. The main symptom in patients is vomit, other common symptoms include nausea, cramps, diarrhea, headaches, and/or prostration. The lack of fever is consistent with the illness being caused by a toxin, not an infection. It is a self-limiting illness. Death due to staphylococcal food poisoning is rare.

11.4.2 Fungal Food Poisoning and Its Common Fungi

Fungi are widely distributed in soil, water, air, animals, plants and their debris. There are many kinds of fungi in nature. Among them, only a few (about 300 species) are harmful to people or animals. Food poisoning caused by consumption of food contaminated with fungi and fungal toxin (mycotoxin) is called fungi and their toxin food poisoning. Mycotoxin is the toxic metabolites produced by fungi, which can not only cause food poisoning, but also carcinogenicity. Therefore, it is of great significance in food hygiene. Fungi and their toxin food poisoning is mainly caused by moldy grain, oil or plants during storage, which are used as food without proper treatment, or the prepared food is moldy and deteriorated after being deposited for too long. Common foods are mainly peanuts, corn, rice, wheat, soybeans, millet, black spotted sweet potato, etc. However, only limited types of mold are able to produce mycotoxin.

11.4.2.1 Fungi

The most important group of toxicogenic molds is species of *Aspergillus*, *Penicillium*, and

Fusarium genus.

Aspergillus was an important genus in food firstly described nearly 300 years ago. The genus of *Aspergillus* is large, containing >100 recognized species. Although a few species have been used to make food (e.g., *Aspergillus oryzae* in soy sauce manufacture), most *Aspergillus* species occur in foods as spoilage or biodeterioration fungi. They are extremely common in stored commodities, such as grains, nuts, and spices, and occur more frequently in tropical and subtropical than in temperate climates. Almost 50 *Aspergillus* species can produce toxic metabolites, but the *Aspergillus* mycotoxins of greatest significance in foods and feeds are aflatoxins. *Aspergillus* species produce toxins that exhibit a wide range of toxicities and cause significant long-term effects. Aflatoxin B1 is perhaps the most potent liver carcinogen known for a wide range of animal species, including human.

At least 80 *Penicillium* species are reported to be toxin producers. Classification with the genus *Penicillium* species is based primarily on microscopic morphology. The range of mycotoxin classes produced by *Pencillium* species is broader than any other fungal genus. Toxicity of mycotoxin produced by *Pencillium* species is very diverse. However, most toxins can be classified into two groups, those that toxic to the liver and kidney and those that are neurotoxins. The most important toxin produced by a *Penicillium* species is Ochratoxin A.

Fusarium species are most often found as contaminants of plant-derived foods, especially cereal grains, seeds, milled cereal products, such as flour and corn meal, barley malt, animal feeds, and dead plant tissue. Many *Fusarium* species are plant pathogens, while others are saprophytic. Most can be found in the soil. In terms of human foods, they are most often encountered as contaminants of cereal grains, oil seeds, and beans. The most common characteristic of the genus is the production of large septate, crescent-shaped, fusiform, or sickle-shaped spores known as macroconidia, that generally range in color from white to pink, red, purple, or brown due to pigment production.

11.4.2.2   Mycotoxin

Mycotoxin is toxic metabolites produced by fungi. There are many fungi in nature, but not every fungus can produce toxins. Fungi that can produce mycotoxins are called toxin producing fungi. There is no strictly specific relationship between the type of toxin and the species of mold, that is, one mold species can produce several different toxins, and one toxin can also be produced by different molds. There are many kinds of mycotoxins, which are closely related to food contamination and important in food hygiene, such as aflatoxin (AF), ochratoxin (OT), trichothecenes, zearalenone (F-2 toxin), fumonisin and patulin etc.

Aflatoxin(AF) is both acutely and chronically toxic in animals and humans, producing acute liver damage, liver cirrhosis, and tumor induction. Acute aflatoxicosis in humans is rare. The greatest direct impact of aflatoxins on human health is their potential to induce liver cancer. Studies in several African countries and China have shown a correlation between aflatoxin intake and the occurrence of primary liver cancer. At present, more than 20 kinds of AF have been found, of which AF_{B1} is the most toxic and carcinogenic. Aflatoxins contamination mainly occurs in peanuts, corn, and other nuts and oilseeds, particularly in some tropical countries. Aflatoxins are among the few mycotoxins covered by legislation. Statutory limits are imposed by some countries on the amounts of aflatoxin that can be present in particular foods. Because of the strong toxicity and widespread contamination of AF_{B1}, AF_{B1} is mainly used as the contamination index in food hygiene supervision. The limit imposed by our country is 5 to 20 μg of AFB1/kg in several human foods, including peanuts and peanut products.

Ochratoxin (OT) is derived from isocoumarin linked to the amino acid phenylalanine including ochratoxin A, B, and C, mainly produced by *Aspergillus ochraceus* and *Penicillium verrucosums*. Among them, ochratoxin A(OTA) is the most important toxin for its toxicity is the strongest and the food pollution is the most serious. The target organ of toxicity in all mammalian species is the kidney. The lesions can be produced by both acute and chronic exposure. The major source of OTA in foods is corn, barley, wheat, oats, rice, and soybean, etc. Because OTA is fat soluble and not readily excreted, it also accumulates in the depot fat of animals that eat feeds containing the toxin, and from there it is ingested by humans eating, for example, pig meats.

11.5 Detection of Microbes in Food

Microorganisms inhabit our bodies and our environment. Therefore, it is not surprising to find many types of microorganism in food. Good microorganisms are those that are used in the production of food, bad microorganisms lead to food spoilage, and ugly microorganisms cause human illness. Determining the types and numbers of microorganisms in a food is an important guarantee for food safety. Food microbiological analysis refers to the National Food Safety Standard Food Microbiological Examination (GB4789) issued by the Food and Drug Administration.

11.5.1 Sample Collection and Processing

Sample collection is an important step in the process of food microbiological inspection. A sample will yield significant and meaningful information. So it is important that the collected sample can represent the mass of material being examined, the method of collection used protects against microbial contamination, and the sample is handled in a manner that prevents changes in microbial numbers between collection and analysis.

The number of samples collected must meet the needs of laboratory analysis and inspection, and repeated inspection if necessary. The specific sampling quantity shall be determined according to the type and quantity of food. The sample should be labeled timely and accurately with the sampler, sampling place, the name of the food, the date collected, source, batch number, quantity, preservation conditions and other information that may be useful in the analysis of results and tracking of the sample.

Once the sample is collected, it should be analyzed as quickly as possible to prevent a change in the microbial population. Samples shall be kept intact during transportation and stored at a temperature close to the original storage temperature.

Prior to analysis, some preparation of the sample is generally required. For meaningful results, the sample should be processed to produce a homogeneous suspension of bacteria so they can be pipetted. If the sample is solid, the food is generally mixed with a sterile dilution medium, such as phosphate buffer or 0.1% peptone water. To make a homogeneous suspension, the sample is added to a sterile plastic stomacher bag, diluent is added, and the sample is processed in a Stomacher (a device that has two paddles that move rapidly back and forth against the sample). A typical size food sample of 25 g is added to the sterile bag containing 225 mL of sterile diluent and mixed, and a 1 : 10 dilution of the food and associated bacteria is obtained. If the sample is liquid, a 1mL aliquot can be removed and added to 9 mL of buffer for direct preparation of serial 10-fold dilutions.

11.5.2 Microbiological Examination and Hygienic Standard of Food

Microorganisms might cause foodborne illness and spoiled food. To ensure a product has been produced under sanitary conditions and is microbiologically safe to consume, microbiological criteria need be established. Indicator organisms are usually used to assess either the microbiological quality or safety since pathogenic microorganisms are not easy to be detected directly. Examination of a product for indicator organisms can suggest the possibility of a microbial hazard about process failure, post-processing contamination, contamination from the environment, and general level of hygiene under which the food was processed and stored. Bacteriological examination items for food hygiene include standard plate-count bacteria, total coliforms, and specific pathogens. Mycological examination items include enumeration of yeasts and molds, fungi classification and identification, and mycotoxin detection. This section focuses on bacteriological examination.

11.5.2.1 Standard Plate-count Bacteria

Standard plate-count bacteria is commonly used as microbiological indicator for contaminant evaluation in food. It provides an estimation of the number of microorganisms in a food, which provide the evidence for hygiene evaluation of the test sample. Standard plate-count bacteria means the total number of forming colonies in 1 mL (g) treated food sample under certain condition (media, temperature, time, pH, and aerobic culture, etc.). The food sample is firstly homogenized 1 : 10 (weight: volume) in a buffer to give a 10-fold dilution. This is then diluted through a series of 10-fold dilutions to give 10-, 100-, 1 000-, 10 000-fold, etc. A measured aliquot (1mL) of the appropriate dilution is dispensed onto the surface of a sterile petri plate and sterile, melted, and tempered (46℃) agar is added to the plate. The agar medium and sample are mixed. Then after the agar solidifies, turn the plate over and incubate at 36℃ ± 1℃ for 48 h ± 2 h. Samples of aquatic products need incubate at 30℃ ± 1℃ for 72 h ± 3 h. Make 2 plates for each dilution. The isolated colonies known as colony forming units (CFU) are counted. In general, standard 90 mm-diameter plates should contain between 30 and 300 colonies. Fewer or more colonies per plate can affect accuracy. The average number of colonies per plate is determined and multiplied by the

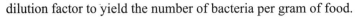

dilution factor to yield the number of bacteria per gram of food.

11.5.2.2　Total Coliforms

Total coliforms refer to the group of aerobic and facultative anaerobic gram-negative non-sporing bacillus that can ferment lactose, produce acid and gas under certain culture conditions. Coliforms mainly come from human and animal feces. So total coliforms are used as indicator of possible fecal contamination and therefore the potential presence of other enteric pathogens. Coliforms might be present in a food product at very low levels. Most probable number (MPN) method are used to estimate low numbers of organisms (<30 CFU/mL) in a sample and suitable for coliform determination.

11.5.2.3　Pathogens Detection

Contamination of food with pathogens has the risk of food-borne illness. Pathogens on the food would be warranted that has a low infectious dose. In China, pathogens in food hygiene inspection refer to enteric pathogens and pathogenic cocci, including *Salmonella*, *Shigella*, *pathogenic Escherichia coli*, *Vibrio parahaemolyticus*, *Yersinia enterocolitica*, *Campylobacter jejuni*, *Staphylococcus aureus*, *hemolytic streptococcus*, *Clostridium botulinum*, *Clostridium perfringens* and *Bacillus cereus*, etc. Pathogen detection should be carried out according to microbiological criteria including National Food Safety Standard Limit of Pathogenic Bacteria in Ready to Eat Food in Bulk (GB 31607—2021) and National Food Safety Standard Limit of Pathogenic Bacteria in Prepackaged Food (GB 29921—2021).

11.6　Prevention Strategies of Food Microbial Contamination

Food might be contaminated by microorganisms and their toxins in the process of food processing, transportation, storage and sales. Food microbial contamination could not only reduce the hygienic quality of food, but also cause various damages to consumers themselves. However, in nature, microbial contamination of food is inevitable. So it is necessary to strengthen food hygiene management to minimize the microbial contamination and the harm caused by it. The contamination prevention measures are proposed as follows according to the characteristics of various foods, microbial sources and pollution ways.

Prevent food microbial contamination. Many foods, such as fruits, vegetables, fish, meat, poultry and eggs, generally do not contain microorganisms inside, but their surfaces often contain various microorganisms in the process of cultivation, fishing, slaughtering and transportation. These microorganisms are easy to grow rapidly because they have adapted to the environmental conditions. As a preventive measure, the first is to clean the soil and dirt carried by some food raw materials to reduce or remove most of the microorganisms. Drying and cooling food to make the environment unsuitable for the growth and reproduction of microorganisms, which is also an effective measure. Aseptic sealed packaging is an effective method to prevent microbial contamination after food processing. Standardized operation and strict management in all links of food processing, transportation and storage are essential to avoid microbial contamination.

Reduce and eliminate existing microorganisms in food. Food and raw materials inevitably contain some microorganisms, including pathogenic organisms and spoilage microorganisms. Many methods such as washing, heating, sterilization, drying, adding preservatives, etc. can be used to reduce and remove microorganisms existing in food. It should be noted that the method selection should not damage the nutrition, flavor, apparent properties, internal texture and edible value of food.

Control the growth and reproduction of residual microorganisms in food. Some microorganisms may still remain in processed foods. The method such as low temperature, drying, anaerobic, anti-corrosion, etc. can be used to control the growth and reproduction of microorganisms in food in order to prolong the storage period of food and ensure the food safety.

Glossary

spoilage *n.* 腐败 something, usually food, decays or is harmed, so that it is no longer fit to be used

deterioration *n.* 退化，恶化 a symptom of reduced quality or strength, process of changing to an inferior state

actinomyces *n.* 放线菌 soil-inhabiting saprophytes and disease-producing plant and animal parasites

autolysis *n.* 自溶 lysis of plant or animal tissue by an internal process

pasteurized milk 巴氏杀菌奶，巴氏灭菌奶；巴氏消毒奶 milk that has been exposed briefly to high temperatures to destroy microorganisms and prevent fermentation

food poisoning 食物中毒 illness caused by poisonous or contaminated food

anaerobic *adj.* 厌氧的 living or active in the absence of free oxygen

enteritis *n.* 肠炎 inflammation of the intestine (especially the small intestine), usually characterized by diarrhea

mycotoxin *n.* 真菌毒素 a toxin produced by a fungus

homogeneous *adj.* 同质的 all of the same or similar kind or nature

（李迎丽）

新形态教材网·数字课程学习⋯⋯

🖥 教学 PPT　　　📝 自测题　　　💬 推荐阅读

Chapter 12
Microorganism of Public Places

Learning objectives:

- Understand the source, species and the hygienic standards of microorganisms in public places, and the prevention and control of microbial contamination in public places.
- Be familiar with the characteristics and significance of public places, and the health significance of the *Legionella pneumophila, Staphylococcus aureus* and the *Hemolytic streptococcus* of public places.
- Master the contents and techniques of microorganism detection for air, public articles and central air conditioning ventilation systems, and the detection principle and techniques of total bacterial count and total coliforms.

With the advancement of society and the improvement of living standards, public places, as an indispensable part of residents' life, are rapidly increasing both in types and numbers. While each public place has its unique characteristics that provides convenience for people, it also poses certain health risks due to differences in microbial species. Currently, there is a growing concern for health and safety in public spaces, leading to increased efforts by the government and regulatory agencies to improve health inspections. Therefore, it is crucial to continuously enhance public health inspections to prevent and control microbial contamination and infectious disease outbreaks in public areas.

12.1   Introduction of Public Places

Public places are artificial buildings where people gather together to meet various needs such as work, study, rest, recreation, sports, visit and tourism which include 28 public venues in seven categories according to *The Public Health Management Regulations*. Details are as follows:

Accommodation and social places: hotel, restaurant, car park, cafe bar, tea house, etc.

Bathing and beauty places: public bathroom, barber shop, beauty salon, etc.

Places of cultural entertainment: film and theater video hall (room), recreation hall (room), dance hall, music hall, etc.

Sports and recreation places: stadium (gymnasium), swimming pool (gymnasium), park, etc.

Cultural exchange places: exhibition hall, museum, art gallery and library, etc.

Shopping places: shopping malls (stores) , bookstores, etc.

Medical treatment and transportation places: waiting room, public transport, etc.

Public places today have shown a tendency to be multifunctional, and while it facilitates people's lives, it also has direct or indirect health implications due to the following reasons.

First, a public place is usually an environment crowded with people at short notice in a limited space. People who enter public places have different educational backgrounds, habits of life and different genders, ages and physical conditions, and they come into contact with each other frequently, which can easily lead to the spread of pathogenic microorganisms, and even cause the outbreak and epidemic of diseases through public articles and aerosols. In particular, in some hospital waiting rooms and branch clinics, healthy and unhealthy individuals coexist in the same place, which results in the occurrence of cross-infection once a carrier of the pathogen comes into temporal and spatial contact with a patient with compromised immunity. The COVID-19 pandemic in 2019-2022 is a typical case of transmission in public places. Of course, whether an infectious disease can be transmitted depends partly on population density or contact opportunities, and partly on the sanitary conditions of the environment.

Second, public utensils and articles used repeatedly by many people are often contaminated with pathogenic microorganisms, which can lead to the spread of disease if disinfection efforts are not thorough. Public goods such as communal cutlery, tea sets, towels, washbasins and bedding are vulnerable to contamination by enteric pathogens and contribute to the spread of enteric diseases. Also, certain contagious diseases are easily transmitted, such as conjunctivitis, which is easily transmitted by sharing pool water; tinea manus and pedis, which are often transmitted by sharing public bathing slippers and keyboards.

Last but not least, a large number of public spaces have been rapidly developed to meet the needs of residents' daily activities in recent years, many of them, however, have been rebuilt upon the foundations of the old town and sometimes, owing to their unreasonable choice of site and arrangement, as well as to their design, do not, as a rule, fully meet the hygienic requirements, which brings a greater tasks for sanitary supervision and management.

12.2 Sources and Types of Microorganisms in Public Places

Sources of microorganisms in public places are mainly from two aspects: nature and human activity. Natural environments are known to be rich in microorganisms, of which soil is the most abundant. Bacteria, actinomycetes, yeast, and fungi, which are primarily present in soil environments, can be sucked into the air along with dust, so the composition of microbes in outdoor air is essentially the same as in soil. The anthropogenic microorganisms are mainly derived from human activities, not only ground dust, but also human exhaled gases and metabolites, which may contain a variety of pathogenic microorganisms that can be discharged into the air. In addition, repeatedly used public goods contaminated with pathogenic microorganisms are also an important source, often leading to cross-infection between people. Meanwhile, central air conditioning and ventilation systems have been widely installed in public places to regulate the indoor air microclimate, so the air quality mostly depends on the hygienic status of the air conditioning system. All of these are mainly related to human health in public places.

12.2.1 Airborne Microorganisms

Airborne microorganisms include bacteria, fungi, actinomycetes, algae, etc. Of these, bacteria are the majority, and the rate of mold contamination shows an increasing trend. They are not only essential for ecological function, but also closely related to air pollution, environmental quality and human health. In fact, due to the relative dryness, UV exposure, lack of nutrients, and other disadvantages, the air is not an ideal place for microorganisms to live, so the microorganisms are mostly in the form of fungal and bacterial spores. Some respiratory infectious agents can be transmitted through droplets, droplet nuclei, and aerosols. Bacteria such as *Streptococcus aureus, Staphylococcus aureus, Tuberculosis Mycobacterium* and viruses such as influenza virus, rubella virus, measles virus, mumps virus and novel coronavirus have caused huge global public health problems in recent years.

12.2.2 Microorganisms of Central Air Conditioning Ventilation Systems

A central air conditioning and ventilation system is the sum of all the equipment pipes, fittings and instruments that centrally handle, transport and distribute air so that air temperature, humidity, cleanliness and airflow speed meet the set requirements of a room or confined space. It consists mainly of an air system and a water system. Microbial pollution factors in the air system are present in fresh air, supply air, return air pipes and fresh air units, while the parts of the contaminated water are cooling water and condensation water. Filters, ventilation ducts, cooling towers and inlet and outlet points will intercept certain indoor or outdoor air pollutants, including bacteria, fungi, viruses, particulate matter and organic matter. While microorganisms not only survive in central air-conditioning, they also multiply in these places. It is easy for them to become a medium for the spread and diffusion of pollutants, causing outbreaks of infectious diseases such as tuberculosis, *Legionella* pneumonia, influenza, COVID-19, rubella, mumps and so on. Since the *Legionella* pneumonia outbreak in the United States in 1976 and the first case reported in 1982 in China, the air pollution caused by centralized air conditioning and ventilation water systems aroused wide public concern, and the occurrence and prevalence of COVID-19 brought further attention to this health problem. Many countries have listed *Legionella* pneumonia as a national notifiable illness. The U.S. Centers for Disease Control and Prevention estimates there are between 8,000 and 18,000 cases of *Legionella* infection each year, with a 5%-10% fatality rate. Therefore, regular cleaning and inspection of central air conditioning systems is important to ensure the healthy quality of the indoor air environment.

12.2.3　Microorganisms on Public Article Surface

Public articles refer to a variety of articles, utensils, equipment and facilities, such as towels, bedding, cups, cutlery, etc., provided specifically for the guests repeated use or direct service by practitioners in public places. Once these items are not thoroughly disinfected, they can become vectors for certain infection diseases, with suspected microorganisms such as Intestinal pathogens, *Staphylococcus* (mainly *Staphylococcus aureus*), *Hemolytic streptococcus*, *Pseudomonas aeruginosa*, mold (penicillium and aspergillus), *Pseudomonas aeruginosa*, hepatitis B virus, parasite eggs, accompanied with the exceeding of total bacterial count, total coliforms, and fungal contamination, etc, with the consequence of health problems include intestinal infection, skin infection, and even hepatitis B virus infection and so on.

12.3　Sample Collection, Inspection Methods and Hygienic Standards for Microorganism of Public Places

Microbiological inspection in public places consists of two main aspects. One is microbial inspection and hygienic supervision of various habitats, such as air, water and public places, to make health assessments that can provide the basis for corresponding measures to prevent possible public health events. The other is to trace the source of infection and clarify the transmission routes and epidemic situation to control the epidemic and speed up the diagnosis and treatments. For these purposes, a series of management codes and sanitary standards have been formulated and promulgated to standardize the management and supervision of public places, such as *The Hygienic Management Specification for Public Places GB37487-2019*, *Hygienic Indicators and Limits for Public Places GB37488-2019*, *Examination Methods for Public Places,GB/T18204.4-2013*, *Standard Examination Methods for Drinking Water Microbiological Parameters GB/T5749-2022*, etc.

12.3.1　Microbial Detection on the Surface of Public Articles

12.3.1.1 Sampling Methods of Public Article Surface

According to the national standards of *The Examination Methods for Public Places-part 4:Microorganism on a Surface of Public Articles,* public articles include seven categories: cup utensils, cotton goods, sanitary ware, footwear, shopping carts, beauty and nail salon products and other items. Randomly sample the article surface where close contact with human body in the area of 5 cm × 5 cm (25 cm^2) as one sampling unit, at least gather two units at the same time. Soak the dry and sterilized cotton swab in 10mL sterile normal saline firstly, and then evenly smear back and forth on the sampling area, finally, put the cotton swab (with the touch part being cut off) into the remaining 9 mL saline (1 : 10 dilution). Then, samples are serially diluted and appropriate dilution will be applied for the following inspection items within four hours.

Examples for different articles sampling. For cup utensils: usually the sampling range is 1-5 cm in height around the inner and outer edges of the tea set in contact with the mouth, and the total sampling area is 50 cm². For towels: Fold the towel, pillow towel and bath towel in half, choose the central area of the front and back sides and evenly smear five times with the area of 25 cm² as one unit, and two units for each item. For foot wears: Evenly smear five times within 5 cm × 5 cm areas of each shoe on the foot contact surface, one pair of shoes is one unit, with a total sampling area of 50 cm². For sheets: Smear five times evenly on the upper and lower parts of the bed sheet with an area of 5 cm × 5 cm (25 cm²) as one unit and two units per item in total. For shopping carts (baskets): At the handle of the cart (basket), two 5 cm × 5 cm areas are selected and evenly smeared for 5 times of each, 50 cm² per item in total.

12.3.1.2　Microbial Detection of Articles in Public Places

According to the current national standard of *The Examination Methods for Public Places part four,* the microorganism detection items include total bacterial count, total coliforms, total fungi count, detection of *Staphylococcus aureus* and *Hemolytic streptococcus*, with methods of plate counting, multi-tube fermentation, plate counting, *Staphylococcus aureus* plate identification and *Hemolytic streptococcus* culture respectively.

Detection of total bacterial count

Total bacterial count is commonly used to determine the degree of microbial contamination or dynamic observation, and is also the hygienic limits of some samples.

Standard plate-counting method and spatula method are indirect counting methods to viable bacteria, while direct counting methods such as microscope direct counting and turbidimetric counting usually can not distinguish bacteria from living ones. Micro-colony rapid counting method, biochemical method, semi-quantitative method and other methods can also indirectly calculate the microbial biomass. Each method has its advantages and disadvantages, while the standard plate method and spatula method are most commonly used in national standards to evaluate the sanitary condition of inspection products.

The principle of the standard plate-counting method is aliquots of decimal diluted sample mixed with culture medium in Petri dishes. Colonies are counted after incubation at 36℃ ± 1℃ for 48 ± 2 hours and the number of microorganisms per gram or mL or cm² of the sample is calculated. Examine the plates carefully, if necessary with a lens, to avoid mistaking particle or precipitates for pinpoint colonies. Usually count all plates of the same dilution for colonies between 30 and 300, calculate the weighted mean and report the results after multiplying the dilution factors, with special treatment for other cases.

Detection of total fungi count

The method of sample treatment and inoculation procedure is the same as that of the total bacterial count, but the inoculation medium is Bengal red medium or Saber's medium, and the incubation temperature is 25-28℃. Start the observation after three days and keep observing for a week. Usually, colonies between 5-50 CFU on each plates are counted, and the total numbers of fungal count per mL original samples are calculated by averaging the colony numbers of the same diluted plates and multiplying the diluted factors. The counting and reporting methods are the same as that of the total bacterial count.

Detection of total coliforms (Multiple tube fermentation technique)

Coliforms are a large group of aerobic or facultative anaerobic gram-negative bacilli exist in the intestines of human and warm-blooded animals that can ferment lactose to produce acid and gas within 35-37℃ in 24 hours. The group includes four genera of *Escherichae, Klebsiella, Enterobacter* and *Citrobacter*. As the fecal pollution indicators, total coliforms are used to evaluate the hygienic quality of food, drinks, swimming pool water, public places and so on, indirectly indicating the possibility of intestinal pathogens contamination. The multiple tube fermentation method, also known as the most probable number (MPN) method, has been used for the detection of total coliforms more than 80 years. It can be described briefly as initial fermentation with lactose bile salt fermentation medium, EMB plate separation and refermentation confirmation test. The possible values of total coliforms count per 100 mL samples are reported by retrieving the MPN table. Another mostly used method is the filtration membrane method, which is very convenient to detect large volume of water samples with a higher sensitivity, reliability and quantification compared with the MPN method which can only be semi-quantified.

For public articles qualitative detection of total coliforms, the first step is lactose bile salt fermentation: pour 1mL sample into the double lactose bile salt fermentation medium, and culture it at 36℃ ± 1℃ for 24 ± 2 hours to observe the presence of acid and/or gas production. If these are both positive, take one inoculated loop culture medium to Eosin and Meilan agar plate, and culture it at 36℃ ± 1℃ for 18-24 hours, then observe the colony morphology and bacterial Gram staining. The last step is the confirmatory test: pick 1-2 suspected coliform colonies to inoculate at the same condition of the first step, and if acid and gas are both produced, total coliforms could be reported.

Detection of *Staphylococcus aureus*

Staphylococcus aureus, commonly existing in nature, is an important human pathogen that causes several diseases ranging from superficial skin infections to life-threatening diseases such as osteoarthritis and endocarditis. In addition, *S.aureus* is increasingly resistant to multiple antibiotics, thus becoming a growing threat to public health. *Staphylococcus aureus* is also an important food-borne pathogenic bacteria by its enterotoxin producing ability. According to the analysis of recent years, *Staphylococcus aureus* enterotoxin causes 33% of all bacterial food poisonings in the United States, while in Canada, it accounts for 45%. China also has a large number of such incidents every year. Therefore, it is of great significant to detect the *Staphylococcus aureus* on the surface of public places to reveal its ability of enterotoxin production and potential pathogenicity.

The detection methods of *Staphylococcus aureus* are as follows: add 1 mL sample into 9mL sodium chloride broth or tryptone soybean broth medium, and culture it at 36℃ ± 1℃ for 24 hours, then make one inoculating loop of enrichment bacteria solution inoculate it on

Baird-Parker plate or blood agar plate and have it incubated at $36°C \pm 1°C$ for 24 hours; The *Staphylococcus aureus* colonies are round, smooth, moist, convex, dark gray, with neat edges, cloudy surrounding, and a zone-pelluida outer layer on Baird-Parker plate medium, while on the blood plate, the colonies are rounded golden yellow bulge with a smooth surface and a clear hemolysis ring around it. Typical *Staphylococcus aureus* for microscopic examinations by smear staining is gram-positive and arranged in grape shape. The last step is the plasma coagulase test to indirectly reveal its ability of enterotoxin secretion. If there is typical suspicious colony growth on all the selected plates above, microscopic examination shows Gram-positive *Staphylococcus* and plasma coagulase test is positive, then confirmed the presence of *Staphylococcus aureus*.

Detection of *Hemolytic streptococcus*

Hemolytic streptococcus is widely distributed in nature, such as in water, air, dust, faeces, and in the mouth, nasal cavity, and throat of healthy people and animals. It can be transmitted through direct contact, airborne droplets or through infected skin and mucosal wounds, and cause suppurative inflammation of skin and subcutaneous tissue, respiratory tract infection, epidemic pharyngitis and neonatal septicemia, bacterial endocarditis, scarlet and rheumatic fever, glomerulonephritis and other allergic reactions. Contaminated foods such as milk, meat, eggs and their products can also cause food poisoning. Therefore, as an indicator bacterium, *Streptococcus haemolyticus* is used to assess the sanitary status of indoor air and environmental articles in public places.

Sampling procedure is the same as described above. When testing, add 1mL liquid sample into 9 mL glucose meat infusion broth; or directly streak inoculation on the blood agar plate. If the samples are contaminated seriously, 1mL liquid samples can be inoculated in Pick's broth at the same time, and culture it at $36°C \pm 1°C$ for 24 hours. Then the small round colonies with hemolysis are isolated and purified on the blood plate to confirm colony characteristics through hemolysis and bacterial Gram staining.

The bacterium has higher nutritional requirements, grows better in culture medium with blood and serum, poor in common culture medium. With flocculent or granular precipitation when growing in serum broth, small colonies with a diameter of 0.5-0.7 mm and a surface protrusion are formed on the blood agar plate. The colonies are transparent or translucent with smooth surface and opalescent light. Microscopic examination shows gram-positive non-spore coccus, round or oval, arranged in chain shape, and there are obvious colorless hemolysis rings with a clear limit of 2-4 mm around the colonies. The colony conforming to the above characteristics is *β-hemolytic streptococcus*. Streptokinase test and bacitracin sensitivity test are both positive for *Hemolytic streptococcus*.

12.3.2   Detection of Airborne Microorganism of Public Places

According to *The Examination Methods for Public Places: Airborne Microorganism* which came into effect on December 1, 2014, the total bacterial count and *Hemolytic Streptococcus* are usually used to indicate the cleanliness and the possible pathogenicity of the air.

12.3.2.1 Detection of Total Airborne Bacterial Count

The principle is sampling by impacting method or natural sedimentation method, counting and determining the total bacteria count of the air after culturing the sample in nutrient agar medium. The principle of Natural Sedimentation Method is to expose the nutrient agar plate to the air, and the microorganisms naturally settle on the plate according to its gravity. According to the room size, choose the representative position as sampling points. Usually three and five points are set with indoor area less than 50 m^2 and more than 50 m^2 respectively. The three points are set on the three equipartites of the indoor diagonal quarter, and five points are distributed to the five-point method of plum blossom. The points should be 1.2-1.5 m above the ground and at least 1 m distance to the wall with the doors and windows closed for 15-30 minutes, and the temperature, humidity, and weather conditions recorded when sampling. Expose the nutrient agar plates for 5 minutes at the sampling point, then turn the plates over and incubate them at 36℃ ± 1℃ for 48 hours. Count the total colony numbers on the plate and report the results.

The impact-based method is based on sampling by an impact-type air microorganism sampler that generates a high-speed flow through a slit or a small hole by pumping force, and then impinging on a nutrient agar plate with bacteria particles suspended in the air. After culturing them at 36℃ ± 1℃ for 48 hours, the number of bacterial colonies contained in each cubic meter is counted.

Sampling points are selected under the principle of uniform distribution: One, two, three or five sampling points are set for indoor areas of less than 50 m^2, 50-200 m^2, and more than 200 m^2, respectively. The room center, the indoor symmetrical point, the three equipartite points of a diagonal quarter and the plum blossom five points are sampled for one, two, three and five points, respectively, 1.2-1.5 m above the ground and at least 1 m from the wall, avoiding vents and air ducts when sampling.

Wipe and disinfect the entrance and edges of the six-stage sieve microbiological sampler, put the sterile petri dishes on the six-tier sieve rack in turn, open the flow device, and sample with a suitable flow rate (generally 28.3 L/min) for a certain time. Count the number of colonies after incubation at 36℃ ± 1℃ for 48 hours. According to the flow rate and sampling time, the number of colonies in the air is calculated and reported with the unit of CFU/m^3.

12.3.2.2 Detection of *Hemolytic Streptococcus*

The sampling methods is the same as that of the airborne bacteria detection but with the blood agar plate instead of the nutrient agar plate (Natural sedimentation method or six-stage sieve microbiological sampler), and detection process is the same as that of public place articles.

12.3.3 Microbial Detection in Central Air Conditioning Ventilation Systems

According to *The Requirements of Health Code for Centralized Air Conditioning and Ventilation System in Public Places* (WS394-2012), the total bacterial count, total fungal count, *Legionella* and *β-hemolytic streptococcus* are used to indicate the microbe pollution status of fresh air, cooling water and condensed water, and air supply system of the central air conditioning ventilation systems.

12.3.3.1   Sampling and Detection Methods for Microorganism in Air Supply

Sampling was performed using the impact method, where three to five air outlets were randomly selected for each air conditioning system, and one point was selected for each air outlet, which was generally located 15-20 cm below the air outlet and 50-100 cm out-of-plane. When sampling, a six-level sieve air impact sampler is used under aseptic operation with the air flow rate of 28.3 L/min for 5-15 minutes with the air conditioning ventilation system in normal running, and the doors and windows closed for more than one hour, and record the number of people indoor, temperature, humidity, and weather conditions at the same time. The sampled patri-dish should be cultured at 35-37℃ for 48 hours, and the total bacterial counts at each air supply port is recorded and converted to CFU/m^3 by dilution ratio and sampling volume, and the total bacterial counts in the air supply of central air-conditioning system is determined by the maximum value of all the air supply ports.

The sampled Salouraud culture medium should be cultured at 28℃ for five days, and observed everyday and the total fungi counts will be recorded on the fifth day. If there are too many colonies to count, then record it on the third day. The reporting rules are the same as that of the total bacterial count. The sampled blood agar plate should be cultured at 35-37℃ for 24-48 hours. The colonies conforming to the characteristics described at part of *Microbial Detection of Articles in Public Places-Detection of Hemolytic Streptococcus* are *β-hemolytic streptococcus*. The recording rules are the same as that of the total bacterial count. According to the *Health Code for Central Air Conditioning Ventilation System in Public Places* (WS394-2012), *Legionella pneumophila* is not a required item for licensing.

12.3.3.2   Sampling and Detection Methods for Microorganism on Air Duct Inner Surface

Sampling methods for the inner surface of air ducts include quantitative sampling robots and manual rubbing sampling methods. When robot sampling, three representative sampling sections should be selected for each air conditioning system (such as air supply pipe, return pipe and fresh air pipe), and one sampling point for each section. During manual test sampling, at least six sampling points should be selected for each air conditioning system and two representative sampling segments should be selected from the air ducts of each air conditioning system. One sampling point should be set on the upper and lower sides of the duct for each profile. If it is indeed impossible to sample in the duct, 3%-5% of all the air supply ports of the system, and not less than three, can be used as sampling points.

Depending on the amount of dust on the inner surface of the duct, sampling was performed using the scraping and wiping method. A quantized sampling robot or a 25 cm² sampling plate with 50 cm² or 100 cm² sampling area, respectively, should be used for specification. Collected samples should be added to a tween 80 sterile aqueous solution for a 10-fold gradient dilution, and 1 mL of the sample with appropriate dilutions is taken for the total bacterial and fungi count with standard plate count method, respectively, and the counting method is in accordance with that described above.

12.3.3.3 Sampling and Detection Methods for *Legionella Pneumophila* in Cooling Water and Condensed Water

Legionella pneumophila is commonly a contaminant of man-made water systems and water sources (natural water, artificial pipe water, cooling towers, water from hot and cold pipe systems, etc.), it is also often hidden in the cooling towers, and the water systems of large buildings, including hospitals, hotels, thermal baths, etc. These sites often become sources of infection and lead to constrained outbreaks. *Legionella pneumophila* is an obligate aerobic, spore-bearing, pod-free, gram-negative bacterium. *Legionella* requires cysteine and iron to grow, and stops growing with cysteine deficiency. Biochemical characteristics include absence of fermentation and oxidation of sugars, absence of nitrate reduction, negative or weakly positive oxidase tests, and negative urease. The optimum pH for growth is 6.9-7.0, and 2%-5% CO_2 may promote growth in some strains. *Legionella pneumophila* grows slowly and is easily covered by other colonies. The colony is neat, with a smooth surface, and displays fluorescence under UV light, often in a variety of colours, usually white, grey, blue, or purple, but also appearing dark brown, grey-green, and crimson. There are 41 species and 61 serotypes of *Legionella*, among which 15 serotypes are the main types of *Legionella pneumophila* (more than 80%). Legionellosis is an acute respiratory infectious disease. Clinical types currently include at least pneumonia and Pontiac fever. The disease is transmitted primarily by respiratory aerosols. Currently, there is no evidence that infected people or animals are the source of the disease.

When sampling, the cooling water sampling point is set 20 cm away from the tower wall and 10 cm below the liquid level, and the condensate sampling point is set at the drain pipe or condensate pan. The container can be a glass or polyethylene bottle with a screw or grated mouth and sterilized before use. Wide-mouth bottles are needed if sediment and ooze are collected, and about 200-500 mL of water sample (or sediment, sludge, etc.) should be collected from each sampling site under aseptic operation. If the sample was disinfected with chlorine or ozone, a solution of sodium thiosulfate was used to neutralize the oxides. All samples should be delivered to the laboratory within two days, not frozen, and protected from light and heat, and if stored at room temperature, no more than fifteen days.

The collected samples were deposited or centrifuged to remove impurities and then filtered through a 0.22-0.45 um aperture filter membrane to trap bacteria. The bacteria on the filter membrane were then sufficiently eluted in 15mL of sterilised water and followed by further heat and acid treatment. Finally, 0.1mL elution sample, heat treatment sample and acid treatment sample are inoculated on GVPC plate in 2.5% CO_2 incubator at 35-37℃. Typical *Legionella pneumophila* colonies grow slowly, and their characteristics are consistent with the description given above. To validate *Legionella pneumophila*, two suspected colonies were selected from each plate and inoculated with BCYE and L-hemionine deficient BCYE agar plates. After two days cultured at 35-37℃, those can grow on BCYE agar plates but not on L-hemionine deficient plates are *Legionella pneumophila* colonies. Colonies will be further identified by biochemical and serological experiments as described above.

To calculate the number of colony formation (CFU/mL) in the sample, the plate with the largest growth of *Legionella pneumophila* colonies will be selected from the three GVPC plate media, and the number of bacteria in the original sample is calculated according to the concentration ratio.

12.3.4 Hygienic Standards for Microorganisms in Public Places

The current series of public health standards specify the sanitary requirements for physical factors, indoor air quality, drinking water, swimming pool water, bathing water, central air conditioning ventilation system and articles in public places, in which microbiological parameters mainly include total bacterial count, total fungi count, total *Coliforms* count, *Staphylococcus aureus*, *Hemolytic streptococcus* and *Legionella pneumophila*. Detailed testing methods and quality requirements for different environment can be found in Table 12-1.

12.4 Prevention and Control of Microbial Contamination in Public Places

12.4.1 Government Supervision and Administration Departments Should Strengthen Supervision and Law Enforcement

In recent years, the demand for consumption of various services has led to a significant increase in the type and number of public places. However, there are potential dangers to public health due to the repeated use of public goods and the frequent turnover of people in these locations. Therefore, preventing the spread of disease and enhancing hygiene supervision in these places are the primary objectives of public health work. To further improve the level of health services, all commercial premises should carry out a comprehensive inspection of sanitary conditions before opening, such as disinfection facilities, health systems and knowledge training for all employees, and strictly implement all health management regulations and standards during working hours.

12.4.2 Enterprise Should Establish a Self–inspection System, to Ensure the Sanitation and Disinfection Effect of Public Places and Articles

The purpose of disinfection is to kill or remove pathogens in public places and on public articles. Disinfection should be listed as the first work for all the public places. Appropriate disinfection methods can be adopted according to the characteristics of the environment and public articles, and ensure the disinfection effect. For indoor air disinfection, natural ventilation and mechanical ventilation way can be adopted to let out foul air, and can also be physically sterilized by ultraviolet light. In the respiratory tract infectious disease epidemic periods or microbial pollution places, chemical disinfectant disinfection treatment, such as chlorine and peracetic acid spray disinfection, should be adopted.

Table 12-1 Health indicators and limit requirements for public places

Public places		Total bacterial count		Total coliforms count (MPN/100mL)	Total fungi count	Staphyloc-occus aureus	β-hemolytic streptococcus	Legionella pneumophila
		Impacting method (CFU/m³)	Sinking method (CFU/plate)					
Air	Sleeping/resting place	≤1500	≤20	/	/	/	/	/
	Underground air defense projects (hotels, dance halls, shopping malls, supermarkets, etc.)	≤4000	≤75	/	/	/	/	/
	Hotel, guest room, restaurant							
	3-5 star	≤1000	≤10	/	/	/	/	/
	1-2 star	≤1500	≤10	/	/	/	/	/
	General	≤2500	≤30	/	/	/	/	/
	Place of cultural and entertainment							
	Cinema, theatre, music hall, amusement hall, dance hall	≤4000	≤40	/	/	/	/	/
	Bar, tea house. coffee shop	≤2500	≤30	/	/	/	/	/
	Beauty salon	≤4000	≤40	/	/	/	/	/
	Gymnasium	≤4000	≤40	/	/	/	/	/
	Indoor swimming pool	≤4000	≤40	/	/	/	/	/
	Library	≤2500	≤30	/	/	/	/	/
	Exhibition hall	≤7000	≤75	/	/	/	/	/
	Shopping mall	≤7000	≤75	/	/	/	/	/
	Waiting room	≤4000	≤10	/	/	/	/	/

(Continued)

Table 12–1 (*Continued*)

Public places		Total bacterial count		Total coliforms count (MPN/100mL)	Total fungi count	Staphyloc-occus aureus	β-hemolytic streptococcus	Legionella pneumophila
		Impacting method (CFU/m³)	Sinking method (CFU/plate)					
Public transport waiting room	Waiting bus/train/ship room	≤7000	≤75	/	/	/	/	/
	Departure lounge	≤4000	≤40	/	/	/	/	/
Public transport means	Passenger train compartment	≤4000	≤40	/	/	/	/	/
	Ship cabin	≤4000	≤40	/	/	/	/	/
	Aircraft cabin	≤2500	≤30	/	/	/	/	/
Water	Domestic drinking water	≤100 CFU/mL		0*	/	/	/	/
	Artificial swimming pool water	≤200 CFU/mL		0	/	/	/	/
Public articles	Cups	≤5 CFU/ cm²		0	/	/	/	/
	Cotton fabrics	≤200 CFU/25 cm²		0	/	0	/	/
	Sanitary appliance	≤300 CFU/25 cm²		0	/	/	/	/
	Footwear	≤300 CFU/25 cm²		/	≤50 CFU/25 cm²	/	/	/
	Beauty / Hair tools	≤200 CFU/25 cm²		0	/	0	/	/
	Pedicure care	≤200 CFU/25 cm²		0	≤50 CFU/25 cm²	0	/	/
	Others	≤300 CFU/25 cm²		0	/	/	/	/

(*Continued*)

Table 12–1 （*Continued*）

Public places		Total bacterial count		Total coliforms count (MPN/100mL)	Total fungi count	Staphyloc-occus aureus	β-hemolytic streptococcus	Legionella pneumophila
		Impacting method (CFU/m³)	Sinking method (CFU/plate)					
Inner surface of air duct		≤100CFU/cm²			≤100 CFU/cm²			
Central air conditi-oning ventilat-ion systems	Cooling water\condensed water of central air conditioning		/	/	/	/	/	0#
	Air supply	≤500CFU/m³ (impacting method)		/	≤500 CFU/m³ (impacting method)	/	0 (impacting method)	0#(impacting method)

Note: *Refers to the total of coliforms count, thermotolerant coliform bacterial count and Escherichia coli count at the same time.

\# Not a required item for licensing.

All the data depend on the standard of *Hygienic Indicators and Limits for Public Places* (GB 37488-2019), *Health Code for Central Air Conditioning ventilation System in Public Places* (WS394-2012).

The disinfection methods of public appliances such as tea sets, hair dressing tools, towels (bath towels, face towels), slippers, bedding, toilets, etc. could be physical disinfection, such as high temperature, circulation steam, high efficiency ozone free ultraviolet disinfection box and other methods. In cases where these options are not available, chemical disinfectants can also be used for soaking and wiping disinfection. Common disinfectants, such as chlorine-containing disinfectant, iodoph, peracetic acid or glutaraldehyde, must be washed with clean water after disinfection.

12.4.3　Employees Should Undergo Regular Physical Examinations to Put an End to Bringing Illnesses to Work.

According to *the Regulations on the Administration of Health in Public Places*, those who serve customers must have a health certificate. Once they have contracted dysentery, typhoid fever, viral hepatitis, active tuberculosis, suppurative or exudative skin diseases, and other diseases endangering public health, they are not allowed to serve customers directly until they are cured.

12.4.4　The Whole Society Should Increase Investment to Improve the Sanitary Condition of Public Health Facilities and Equipment

Public health concerns the health and safety of everyone and also reflects the civilization of a country or region. Even public facilities in large and medium-sized places have improved in recent years, but some minor places such as inns, cultural and entertainment venues, public baths, beauty salons and other facilities remain poor. In these places, the sanitization of the environment is not strict, and the contamination of public goods is severe. Therefore, it is necessary to increase capital input to improve and create a proper environment for the recreation and fitness of the masses.

At the same time, health education should be vigorously carried out through various media to raise public awareness of disease prevention, help them build public health perceptions and ultimately shape their healthy lifestyles.

Glossary

aseptic technique 无菌操作 operation with medically clean or without contaminant

coliforms *n.* 大肠菌群 normal intestinal flora of human and animals,only a few of pathogen

staphylococcus *n.* 葡萄球菌 a species of Gram-positive bacteria that looks like bunches of grapes under microscope

strptococcus *n.* 链球菌 a species of bacterium, many types of which cause disease

legionella pneumophila 军团菌 aerobic Gram-negative bacillus, often exists in air conditioner coolers (towers), hot water pipes, shower heads and other places, and infects hosts in the form of aerosols, and *legionella pneumophila* is the most susceptible to disease.

enterotoxin *n.* 肠毒素 a kind of toxin produced by staphylococcus aureus

droplet nuclei 飞沫核 droplets lose water in the air and the remaining nuclei of proteins and pathogens

aerosol *n*. 气溶胶 a disperse system of solid or liquid particles suspended stably in a gaseous medium

habitat *n*. 生境 natural environment in which microorganism lives

inoculating loop 接种环 a kind of inoculation tool commonly used in bacterial culture

lactose fermentation test 乳糖发酵试验 a biochemical test used to examine the ability of bacteria to decompose lactose

lactose peptone broth 乳糖蛋白胨培养液 a kind of culture solution for determination of total coliforms

fermentation *n*. 发酵 the extraction of energy through anaerobic degradation of substrates into simpler

eosin methylene blue medium 伊红亚甲蓝琼脂培养基 a kind of culture medium for intestinal flora

central air-conditioning and ventilation system 集中空调通风系统 all equipment, pipes, accessories and instruments that centrally handle, transport and distribute air in order to meet the set requirements of temperature, humidity, cleanliness and airflow speed in a room or enclosed space

（杨红茹）

新形态教材网·数字课程学习……

教学 PPT　　　　自测题　　　　推荐阅读

PART IV
Physicochemical Analysis

Chapter 13

Instruments and Operation

Learning objectives:
- Know the basic classification of instruments of physicochemical analysis.
- Understand the basic concepts of instruments of physicochemical analysis.
- Master the basic principles and structures of pH meter, UV-vis, AAS, HPLC, GC, IC and MS.

13.1 Overview of Physicochemical Analysis and Related Instruments

Physicochemical analysis is a technical subject, using particular analytical methods, like physical or chemical techniques, or combined techniques, especially modern instrumental analysis, to detect the type and quantity of human health-related substance in the environment. To put it simply, it analyzes useful substances to find out whether they meet the appropriate legal standards, or harmful substances to identify whether they exceed certain limits. Physical and chemical analysis is of great importance in many respects. It can preliminarily illuminate the damage extent of physical and chemical hazards to human health, besides, it is an important means of providing scientific support for the formulation of standards and effective health measures. Physicochemical analysis covers a range of techniques and an even broader range of sample types and sources. Analysis may involve using a particular technique or a combination of methods and samples can be solids, liquids or gases. Physicochemical analysis is divided into different categories from different ways. According to the research field, it also can be divided into nutritional and food sanitation inspection, environmental sanitation inspection, and occupational health inspection. According to the object of detection, it can be divided into water quality inspection, food inspection, air inspection, cosmetic inspection, soil and substrate inspection, biological material inspection. According to the nature of detection, it can be divided into supervisory inspection, identification inspection, and entrusted inspection.

In the past, physicochemical analysis mainly relied on titration, weighing and other methods. These methods require a high degree of skill and long time to obtain accurate and precise results. Compared with traditional chemical analysis methods, instrumental analysis method has better accuracy, precision and lower limit of detection. The bias is the difference between the expectation of a test result or measurement result and a true value. The accuracy is closeness of agreement between the expectation of a test result or a measurement result and a true value. The precision is closeness of agreement between independent test/measurement results obtained under stipulated conditions. The limit of detection is output signal or value above which it can be affirmed with a stated level of confidence. For example, 95% indicates that a sample is different from a blank sample containing no determinand of interest. The limit of quantification is defined as multiple of the limit of detection. For example, when the concentration of determinand is twice or treble the limit of detection, it can reasonably be determined with an acceptable level of accuracy and precision. These are important indicators of evaluation methods. At present, physicochemical analysis increasingly relies on the use of precise instruments and equipment. These precise instruments have automated sample introduction, automated data processing, and even automated sample preparation controlled by computers.

According to the principle, these methods of physicochemical analysis can be divided into electrochemical analysis method, optical method, chromatography, mass spectroscopy, etc. Part of the instrument is relatively expensive. The structure is very precise and requires professional operation and maintenance. Mastering these techniques is fundamental to achieving top-quality physicochemical analysis.

13.2   Introduction to Electrochemical Analysis

Electrochemical analysis is an analytical method established according to the electrochemical properties and changes of the tested solution. Electrochemical analysis includes a variety of methods that are widely used in physicochemical analysis. According to different principles, electrochemical analysis is classified as shown in Figure 13-1.

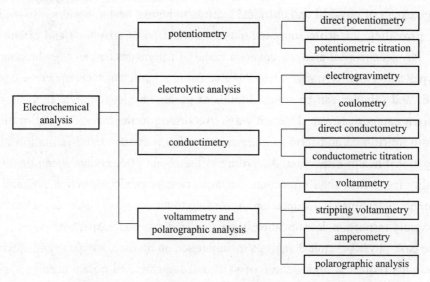

Figure 13–1   The classification of electrochemical analysis

13.2.1   Chemical Battery

Chemical battery is a device that converts chemical energy to electrical energy, including galvanic cell and electrolytic cell. In a galvanic cell, the electrode reaction occurs spontaneously and chemical energy is converted to electrical energy. The electrode reaction of the electrolytic cell cannot proceed spontaneously. An external voltage is needed to convert electrical energy into chemical energy so that electrode reaction can be carried out. The study of Daniell cell is very classical and is the basis of electrochemical analysis. The Daniell cell was invented in 1836 by John Frederic Daniell, a British chemist and meteorologist, and consists of a copper pot filled with copper sulfate solution, which is immersed in an unglazed earthenware container filled with sulfuric acid and a zinc electrode. He was searching for a way to eliminate the hydrogen bubble problem found in the voltaic pile, and his solution was to use a second electrolyte to consume the produced hydrogen.

A double electrode layer is formed at the interface between metal and electrolyte solution, and its value is called electrode potential, which can be calculated by Nernst equation. This alternating potential at the interface between metal and electrolyte solution is called the electrode potential. The electrode potential is relative. According to the International Union of Pure and Applied Chemistry (IUPAC), other electrodes are compared with hydrogen electrodes. Standard reduction potential is the voltage that would be measured when a hypothetical cell containing the desired half-reaction is connected to a standard hydrogen electrode anode.

A redox reaction involves transfer of electrons from one species to another. A species is said to be oxidized when it loses electrons. It is reduced when it gains electrons. An oxidizing agent, also called an oxidant, takes electrons from another substance and becomes reduced. A reducing agent, also called reductant, gives electrons to another substance and is oxidized in the process. The electrons involved in a redox reaction can be made to flow through an electric circuit. Electric charge is measured in coulombs (C). The magnitude of the charge of a single electron is 1.602×10^{-19} C, so 1 mole of electrons has a charge of 9.649×10^{4} C, which is called Faraday constant (F).

Various electrodes have been developed with electrical potential energy that responds very sensitively to changes in the concentration of a particular analyte in a solution or gas. These instruments range from straightforward galvanic cells to ion-selective electrodes, ion-sensing field effect transistor. Electrochemical analytical instruments are designed to be smaller and smaller.

13.2.2   Direct Potentiometric Method

The direct potentiometric method is a method to select the appropriate indicator electrode and reference electrode, immerse in the solution to be tested to form the galvanic cell, measure the electromotive force of the galvanic cell, and directly calculate the concentration of the component to be tested according to the Nernst equation. Reference electrode is one that maintains a constant potential against which the potential of another half-cell may be measured, such as saturated calomel electrode (SCE). The SCE is a reference electrode based on the reaction between elemental mercury and mercury chloride. The aqueous phase in contact with the mercury and the mercury chloride is a saturated solution of potassium chloride in water. Indicator electrode is one that develops a potential whole magnitude depends on the activity of one or more species in contact with the electrode. An ion-selective electrode (ISE), also known as a specific ion electrode (SIE), is a transducer (or sensor) that converts the activity of a specific ion dissolved in a solution into an electrical potential, which can be measured by a voltmeter or pH meter. The voltage is theoretically dependent on the logarithm of the ionic activity, according to the Nernst equation. Common ISE includes pH glass electrode, fluoride ion selective electrode, chloride ion selective electrode, etc. In use, the inert electrolyte is usually added as total ion strength adjustment buffer (TISAB), which can simultaneously control pH, eliminate cationic interference and control ion strength.

13.2.3　Voltammetry

Voltammetry is a category of electroanalytical methods used in analytical chemistry and various industrial processes. In voltammetry, information about an analyte is obtained by measuring the current as the potential is altered. The advantage of Voltammetry is that it can be applied in a wide variety of ways and can be measured simultaneously. The Voltammetry has a low limit of detection and a high sensitivity. Voltammetry is a very effective physicochemical analysis method for trace analysis and morphology analysis. The instrument of Voltammetry is simple in structure, cheap in price and low in operating cost. But Voltammetry requires a high level of skill and rigorous operations. Voltammetry requires external voltage control device, current measuring device and electrolytic cell. The cathode of the ordinary electrolysis process is replaced with a dropping mercury electrode (DME) with a smaller surface area and the anode with a SCE.

Square wave stripping voltammetry (SWASV) is a high sensitive electrochemical method to detect the trace metal ions. Stripping voltammetry is a method in which the material to be measured is enriched on the electrode surface by electrolysis and the enriched material is re-dissolved by applying a reverse voltage. Stripping voltammetry is analyzed according to the $I \sim \phi$ of the stripping process. Stripping voltammetry includes anodic stripping voltammetry (ASV) and cathodic stripping voltammetry (CSV). The enrichment process of anodic stripping voltammetry is electroreduction and its stripping process is electrooxidation. The enrichment process of cathodic stripping voltammetry is electrooxidation and its stripping process is electroreduction. The experimental device mainly consists of work electrode, reference electrode, auxiliary electrode, potentiometer, galvanometer, magnetic stirring apparatus and direct-current power supply.

13.3　Introduction to Spectrometer

The analytical methods based on light and other forms of electromagnetic radiation are widely used throughout physicochemical analysis. The interactions of radiation and matter are the subject of the science called spectroscopy. Spectroscopic analytical methods are based on measuring the amount of radiation produced or absorbed by molecular or atomic species of interest. Spectrometers have provided the most widely used tools for the elucidation of molecular structure as well as the quantitative and qualitative determination of both inorganic and organic compounds.

Spectroscopic analytical methods are classified according to the region of the electromagnetic spectrum involved in the measurement. The regions include ultraviolet (UV), visible, infrared (IR), microwave, γ-ray, X-ray, radio frequency (RF) and so on. According to the principle, spectroscopic analytical methods can be divided into absorption spectroscopy, emission spectroscopy, fluorescence spectroscopy. In absorption spectroscopy, the amount of light absorbed as a function of wavelength is measured, which can give qualitative and quantitative information about the target molecules. In emission spectroscopy and fluorescence spectroscopy, the intensity of emission and fluorescence is measured, which can give qualitative and quantitative information about the target molecules. According to the kind of examined species, spectroscopic analytical methods can be classified as atomic optical methods and molecular optical methods.

Beer-Lambert Law

The absorption law, also known as the Beer-Lambert law, indicates that the absorbance is proportional to the concentration of the target molecule, given the pathlength over which absorption occurs. The equation is as follows:

$$A = \lg^{(1/T)} = \varepsilon bc \qquad\qquad 13\text{-}1$$

Where A is the measured absorbance, T is transmittance, ε is the wavelength-dependent molar absorptivity coefficient with units of $M^{-1} \cdot cm^{-1}$, b is the path length, and c is the analyte concentration.

Therefore, the Beer-Lambert law is the theoretical basis for quantitative analysis of spectroscopic analytical methods. The Beer-Lambert law holds only in certain cases, mainly if the light is monochromatic and the sample solution is dilute. Some circumstances can lead to departures from the Beer-Lambert law, such as chemical deviations and instrumental deviations. Deviations from the Beer-Lambert law appear when the absorbing species undergoes association, dissociation, or reaction with the solvent to give products that absorb differently from the analyte. In practice, it is important to avoid chemical deviations. The need for monochromatic radiation and the absence of stray radiation are practical factors that limit the applicability of the Beer-Lambert law. To avoid deviation, it is advisable to select a wavelength band near the wavelength of maximum absorption of target molecules. Stray radiation, commonly called stray light, is defined as radiation from the instrument that is outside the nominal wavelength band chosen for the determination. Stray radiation will cause the detection results to deviate from the Beer-Lambert law. Therefore, it is very important to choose suitable light source and monochromator for spectrometer.

13.3.1   Spectrophotometry

Spectrophotometry is a widely used physicochemical analysis method for qualitative and quantitative analysis of target molecules. An absorption spectrum is a plot of absorbance versus wavelength. Most modern scanning spectrometers can produce such an absorption spectrum directly by computer. Different molecules have different absorption spectrums because of their outermost electron configuration. Therefore, Spectrophotometry can be used for qualitative analysis through the absorption spectrum, although the effect is not good. The components of a spectrometer include light source, sample cell, polychromator or monochromator, detector. The tungsten filament lamp provides a distribution of wavelengths from 320-2,500 nm. In the visible region, tungsten lamps or Tungsten/halogen lamps are used as light sources. The tungsten filament lamp provides a distribution of wavelengths from 350 to 400 nm. In the ultraviolet region, a deuterium lamp is usually used as a light source. The sample cell of spectrometer is cuvette, which has two transparent surfaces and two opaque surfaces. In the visible region, the cuvette is made of glass or quartz. In the ultraviolet region, the cuvette must be made of glass or quartz. The deviation is caused by mismatched cuvettes sometimes. If the cuvettes holding the analyte and blank solutions are not of equal pathlength and equivalent in optical characteristics, intercept will occur in the calibration curve. This error can be avoided either by using matched cuvettes or by using a linear regression procedure to calculate both the slope and intercept of the calibration curve. The monochromator is usually used as an optical grating or a dispersing prism. In general, the price and performance of optical grating are higher than dispersing prism's. Detectors include photocells, photomultiplier tubes, etc. Spectrophotometer with the traditional manual operation, also can be operated by computer control.

13.3.2   Fluorescence Spectroscopy

Fluorescence is a photoluminescence process in which molecules are excited by absorption of electromagnetic radiation. The intensity of the fluorescence produced by the molecule can be quantitatively analyzed, which is called molecular fluorescence spectrophotometry. Molecules are usually mainly in their lowest-energy state or ground state because it's more stable. The target molecules are stimulated by applying energy in the form of heat, electrical energy, light, particles, or a chemical reaction. The stimulus then causes the target molecules to undergo a transition to a higher-energy or excited state. The molecular fluorescence spectrometers obtain information about the target molecules by measuring the fluorescence emitted as it returns to the ground state as a result of excitation. The fluorescence spectrometer has the same structure as spectrophotometer. The components of a fluorescence spectrometer include light source, sample cell, monochromator and detector. In order to increase the energy of excitation light, the xenon lamp is usually chosen as the light source of fluorescence spectrometer. The xenon lamp provides a distribution of wavelengths from 250 to 600 nm. The sample cell of fluorescence spectrometer is different from the cuvette of spectrometer, which has four transparent surfaces. In most cases, cuvettes of fluorescence spectrometer are made of quartz. The monochromator of fluorescence spectrometer is the same as spectrophotometer's. But the monochromator of fluorescence spectrometer is not on the path of the excited light, it is perpendicular to the path of the excited light. This is the most obvious difference in the construction of fluorescence spectrometer and spectrophotometer. Due to the relatively low intensity of fluorescence, photomultiplier tubes are usually chosen as detector of fluorescence spectrometer.

13.3.3 Infrared Absorption Spectroscopy

Infrared absorption spectroscopy is also widely employed in physicochemical analysis for identification. The absorption of IR region radiation can give information about the identity of analyte, the functional groups, and the structure of molecules. Infrared absorption spectroscopy is one of the most powerful methods for determining the structure of both inorganic and organic compounds. In general, IR is not of sufficient energy to cause electronic transitions but can induce transitions in the vibrational and rotational states associated with the ground electronic state of the molecule. All molecules, organic and inorganic, absorb infrared radiation, without the homonuclear diatomic molecules. IR spectrum is the molecular energy selective absorption of certain wavelengths of infrared and causes the molecular vibrational energy level and rotational energy level transition. Material infrared absorption spectrum can be obtained by detection of infrared absorption, which is also known as molecular vibration spectrum or vibration spectrum. The vibration modes of a molecule are directly proportional to the number of bonds and atoms in it. The number of vibrations is large even for a simple molecule.

The IR spectrometer is made up of five components, a stable source of light, a wavelength selector, a sample container, a radiation detector which converts IR energy to a measurable electrical signal, a signal processing and readout unit. The stable sources for IR radiation are normally heated inert solids, such as a silicon carbide rod. Infrared radiation is emitted when the silicon carbide rod is heated to about 1,500 ℃ by the passage of electricity. The Nernst Glower and electrically heated spirals of nichrome wire also serve as IR sources. According to the different spectral devices, IR spectrometers are divided into dispersion and interference. Fourier transform infrared spectrometer uses Michelson interferometer to intervene with two complex infrared light beams whose optical path difference varies at a certain speed to form interference light, and then interacts with the sample. The detector sends the interference signal to the computer for mathematical processing of Fourier transform and restores the interferogram to IR spectrum. In recent years, Raman spectroscopy and magnetic resonance imaging (MRI) are increasingly used in physicochemical analysis.

13.3.4 Atomic Spectroscopy

Atomic spectroscopy is used for the qualitative and quantitative determination of more than 80 elements. Atomic absorption spectroscopy (AAS) currently is the most widely used of these techniques for detection of elements. Detection limit of AAS is usually in the range of

10^{-9} g/mL. In AAS, the analytes must be converted into an atomic vapor by a process known as atomization. In this process, the sample is volatilized and decomposed to produce atoms and perhaps some ions in the gas phase. Several methods are used to atomize samples. The two most important methods of these for AAS are flame atomization and furnace atomization. An atomizer is a part where the sample is atomized. The flame atomizer includes a nebulizer and a burner. The nebulizer atomizes the test liquid, and its performance has an impact on the precision, sensitivity and chemical interference. Therefore, it is necessary for the nebulizer to produce stable, evenly sized droplets with a high rate of atomisation efficiency. The nebulizer is one of the main factors affecting flame atomic absorption spectroscopy. The flame is produced by burning acetylene and air. By adjusting the ratio of acetylene to air, different properties of flame can be obtained. Flame atomization is easy to operate and reproducible. However, atomization efficiency is low, generally 10%-30%, and the residence time of the sample droplets in the flame is short, about 10^{-4} s. The atomic vapor is diluted in the flame by a large stream of air. All these factors limit the improvement of sensitivity.

Furnace performs better as an atomizer than flame. Furnace AAS is usually two orders of magnitude more sensitive than flame AAS. A multistep heating program is usually applied to remove the solvent of the sample, ash, or char the organic material present and then produce the atomic vapor. The purpose of ashing is to remove low boiling point inorganic and organic matter at higher temperature and reduce interference. Its temperature is generally 300-1,500°C, the time is about 0.5-10 s. The temperature range of atomization is 1,800-3,000°C, and the time is 5-10 s. Its disadvantage is poor precision, relative deviation of about 4%-12%. Hydride atomization is also a way of atomization. In addition, due to the characteristics of Hg, the Cold-Atom mercury testing system can be used to detect the content of Hg.

The AAS requires a line source of the element of interest, such as hollow cathode lamp. The hollow cathode lamp is a glass tube with a quartz window filled with a low-pressure inert gas discharge tube. Its anode is a tungsten rod with a titanium wire or tantalum piece welded to the end. Its cathode is a hollow cylindrical cathode made of the element to be tested. Generally, detecting an element requires a hollow cathode lamp made of that element.

Atomic fluorescence spectrometry is also widely used in the determination of mercury, arsenic, selenium and other elements. Its structure is similar to atomic absorption spectrometer. It usually uses hydride atomization. We are proud that the quality of China's atomic fluorescence spectrometer is very good and the market share of the atomic fluorescence spectrometer is very high.

Atomic emission spectroscopy (AES) was developed early on, but was eventually discontinued due to technical limitations. But with the emergence of inductively coupled plasma (ICP) technology, inductively coupled plasma-atomic emission spectrometry (ICP-AES), which can detect multiple elements at the same time, has been more and more widely used. The advantages of ICP-AES include good selectivity, low detection limit, high precision, fast analysis and simultaneous determination of multiple elements. The disadvantages of ICP-AES include

164

high requirements for standard materials, poor accuracy when the sample content is large, and can not guarantee the best sensitivity for most elements at the same time. Of course, the biggest disadvantage is the higher cost of ICP-AES and maintenance. As technology advances, newly developed spectroscopic methods will play a more important role in physicochemical analysis.

13.4 Introduction to Chromatography

Chromatography is a process used for separating mixtures by virtue of differences in absorbency. The word chromatography comes from the fusion of two words, *chroma* and *graphein*. The *chroma* is a Latin word meaning color, and the *graphein* is a latin word meaning graphing and writing. The original chromatography used calcium carbonate as a column to separate natural pigments, but now chromatography technology has developed very fast. Chromatography is a widely used method for the physicochemical analysis, because it has excellent performance in the field of material separation. The Nobel Prize in Chemistry 1952 was awarded jointly to Archer John Porter Martin and Richard Laurence Millington Synge "for their invention of partition chromatography" . There are many kinds of chromatography, but the common feature of all is to use of a stationary phase and a mobile phase. The stationary phase in chromatography is a phase that is fixed in place either in a column or on a planar surface. The mobile phase in chromatography is a phase that moves over or through the stationary phase, carrying with it the analyte mixture. The mobile phase may be a gas, a liquid, or a supercritical fluid. According to the different mobile phases, the chromatography is divided into liquid chromatography (LC), gas chromatography (GC) and supercritical fluid chromatography (SFC) and other types. By separation mechanism, the chromatography is divided into absorption chromatography, partition chromatography, exchange chromatography, etc. By stationary phase, the chromatography is divided into column chromatography, paper chromatography, thin layer chromatography, etc. In column chromatography, the stationary phase is held in a narrow tube, and the mobile phase is forced through the tube under pressure or by gravity. In planar chromatography, the stationary phase is supported on a flat plate or in the pores of a paper. Here the mobile phase moves through the stationary phase by capillary action or under the influence of gravity.

Components of a mixture are carried through the stationary phase by the flow of the mobile phase, and separations are based on differences in migration rates among the mobile phase components. Theories of chromatographic separation are numerous, such as the plate theory, Van Deemter rate theories, and others. The effectiveness of a chromatographic column in separating two solutes depends on the relative rates at which the two species are eluted. These rates are in turn determined by the rations of the solute concentrations in each of the two phases. In the selected chromatographic system, different components of the tested substance pass through the stationary phase at different times under the impetus of the mobile phase. The time elapsed from the beginning of sampling to the occurrence of the maximum concentration of the component after the column, that is, the time experienced from the beginning of sampling to the occurrence of the peak of the chromatographic peak of a component, is called the retention time of the component, expressed by RT, usually in minutes as a time unit. Retention time is the basis of chromatographic qualitative analysis. In chromatographic analysis, the retention time of the target molecule should be inconsistent with that of the interferent. This requires the selection of suitable mobile phase, stationary phase and other chromatographic conditions.

If a detector that responds to solute concentration is placed at the end of the chromatographic column and its signal is plotted as a function of time, a series of peaks is obtained. This plot, known as a chromatogram, is helpful for both qualitative and quantitative analysis. There are many peaks on the chromatogram, and different peaks represent different substances. The positions of the peaks on the time axis can be used to identify the components of the sample. In the chromatogram, the retention time is the time between injection of a sample and the appearance of a solute peak at the detector of a chromatographic column. Dead time is the time it takes for the sample to pass through the chromatographic system without being retained at all during the chromatographic process. The area of the chromatographic peak is positively correlated with the content of the component, so the area of the chromatographic peak can be used for quantitative analysis.

13.4.1　Gas Chromatography

Gas chromatography (GC) was a major scientific and technological achievement in the 1950s. This is a separation and analysis technology with good performance, which has been widely used in industry, agriculture, national defense, construction and scientific research. Gas chromatography can be divided into gas solid chromatography and gas liquid chromatography. In gas chromatography, the components of a vaporized sample are fractionated as a consequence of being partitioned between a mobile phase and a stationary phase held in a column. In performing a gas chromatographic separation, the sample is vaporized and injected onto the head of a chromatographic column. The mobile phase does not interact with the molecules of the sample and its sole function is to transport the sample species across the column. Due to the rapid transfer of the sample through the gas phase, the sample components can reach an instant equilibrium between the mobile phase and the stationary phase. Gas chromatography is a fast and efficient separation and analysis method. In recent years, the use of highly sensitive selective detector has enabled high sensitivity and wide applicability.

Gas chromatograph is composed of the following five systems: gas flow control system, sample injection system, chromatographic separation system, temperature control system, detection and recording system. The mobile phase in gas chromatography must be chemically inert, such as helium. Argon, nitrogen, and hydrogen are also used as mobile phases. These gases can be packed in pressurized tanks. Pressure regulators, gauges, and flow meters are needed to control the flow of gas. Column inlet pressures are usually range from 10-50 psi (lb/in^2) and flow rates are 25-50 mL/min. Sample injection system is very important for gas chromatography, and the injection speed will affect the detection result. Calibrated microsyringes are used to inject liquid samples through a rubber or silicone septum into a head sample port located at the head of the column. The sample port is ordinarily about 50°C above the boiling point of the least volatile component of the sample. Automated samplers, which are now widely used, greatly ease the work of inspectors. Whether the components can be separated depends on the column. Column size must be appropriate, too long waste of time, too short will lead to insufficient separation. The selection of chromatographic column type is also the key to complete separation. GC packed columns can be either packed or capillary columns. The GC packed column can accommodate larger samples and are generally more convenient to use than the former. Capillary columns have become of considerable importance because of their unparalleled resolution. In old days the vast majority of gas chromatography has been carried out on packed columns but capillary columns are becoming popular day by day. The function of column oven is to ensure the chromatographic process at an appropriate temperature, and the control of temperature has obvious effect on chromatographic separation.

At present, there are many kinds of detectors, which are commonly used: flame-ionization detector (FID), thermal conductivity detector (TCD), nitrogen phosphorus detector (NPD), flame photometric detector (FPD), electron capture detector (ECD) and other types. The FID is the most widely used and generally applicable of all detectors for gas chromatography. Most organic compounds, when they are pyrolyzed in a hot flame, produce ionic intermediates that conduct electricity through the flame. Detection involves monitoring the current produced by collecting electrons and ions produced by the combustion process at biased electrodes. The TCD, also known as a Katharometer, is a bulk property detector and a chemical specific detector. This device consists of an electrically heated source whose temperature at constant electric power depends on the thermal conductivity of the surrounding gas. The heated element may be a fine platinum, gold, or tungsten wire, or a small thermistor. The advantages of the TCD are its simplicity, its large linear dynamic range, its general response to both organic and inorganic species and its nondestructive character, which permits collection of solutes after detection. The ECD is a device for detecting atoms and molecules in a gas through the attachment of electrons via electron capture ionization. The ECD detectors are widely used because they selectively react to halogen-containing organic compounds.

GC is applicable to species that are appreciably volatile and thermally stable at temperatures up to a few hundred degrees Celsius. Many organic compounds meet this requirement, so gas chromatography is widely used in environmental monitoring, food testing, scientific research and other fields.

13.4.2   High–performance Liquid Chromatography

High-performance liquid chromatography (HPLC) is a powerful technique used to separate the components in a mixture, identify compounds in solution, and quantify each component. HPLC is considered an instrumental technique of physicochemical analysis. HPLC is particularly useful for analysis of large molecules and compounds that are either not very volatile or thermally unstable. The principles of HPLC are common to GC where separation is based upon chemical interactions with a mobile phrase and a stationary phase. In this case the mobile phase is a solvent and the stationary phase is made up of particles to which different chemical groups may be bound to allow selective separation of the required analyte. According to different stationary phases, the HPLC is divided into liquid-liquid chromatography, liquid-solid chromatography, ion-exchange chromatography, size-exclusion chromatography and affinity chromatography.

HPLC system is mainly composed of injection system, high pressure infusion system, separation system, detection system and data processing system. The product quality of pump is vital for the overall HPLC. The requirements for liquid-chromatographic pumps include the generation of pressures of up to 41.37 Mpa, pulse-free output, flow rate ranging from 0.1-10 mL/ min, flow reproducibility of 0.5% relative or better, and corrosion resistance to various solvents. At present, there are three types of pumps, including screw-driven syringe type, reciprocating pump, and pneumatic or constant-pressure pump. An elution with single solvent to constant composition is called isocratic elution. In gradient elution, two or more solvent systems that differ significantly in polarity are employed. The ratio of the two solvents is varied in a preprogrammed way, sometimes continuously and sometimes in a series of steps. Gradient elution frequently improves separation efficiency. Liquid-chromatographic columns are usually constructed from stainless steel tubing, 10-30 cm in length. It has inside diameters of 4-10 mm. Column packing typically has particle sizes of 5 μm or 10 μm. Most modern commercial instruments are now equipped with heaters to control column temperatures. HPLC has many kinds of detectors. The most widely used detectors for liquid chromatography are based on absorption of ultraviolet or visible radiation. Modern instruments use diode-array instruments that can display an entire spectrum as an analyte exiting the column. Of course, there are fluorescence detectors, evaporative light-scattering detector, differential refraction detector and so on. The detector used will depend on the nature of the sample. The combination of HPLC with a mass spectrometry detector is currently receiving a great deal of attention. Such HPLC/MS systems can identify the analytes exiting from the HPLC column.

13.4.3   Other Chromatography

Ion chromatography (IC), as a branch of HPLC, has also made great success in the physicochemical analysis. It is a process that allows the separation of ions and polar molecules based on their charge. It can be used for almost all kinds of charged molecule, including large proteins, small nucleotides and amino acids. According to the separation mechanism, ion chromatography can be divided into high performance ion exchange liquid chromatography, ion exclusion chromatography and ion pair chromatography. The composition of IC is the same as that of HPLC. The instrument consists of four parts, including the mobile phase transmission part, separation column, detector and data processing. In the case of background conductance suppression, MSM or similar suppressor is usually equipped. The mobile phase of IC is most commonly used in aqueous buffer, but sometimes organic solvents such as methanol and ethanol are mixed with aqueous buffer solution. Therefore, the pipes, valves, pumps, columns and joints through which the mobile phase passes should not be made of stainless steel, but the all-plastic IC system with polyether-ether-ketone material resistant to acid and alkali corrosion. The most important component of ion chromatography is the separation column. Tubular materials should be inert and are generally used at room temperature.

Supercritical-fluid chromatography (SFC), in which the mobile phase is a supercritical fluid, is a hybrid of gas and liquid chromatography that combines some of the best features of each. A supercritical fluid is formed whenever a substance is heated above its critical temperature. At the critical temperature, a substance can no longer be condensed into its liquid state through the application of pressure. The physical properties of a substance in the supercritical-fluid state can be remarkably different from the same properties in either the liquid or the gaseous state. For certain applications, it appears to be clearly superior to both gas-liquid and high-performance liquid chromatography. Instruments for supercritical-fluid chromatography are similar in design to high-performance liquid chromatography. At present, the most widely used mobile phase for supercritical-fluid chromatography is carbon dioxide.

13.5   Introduction to Mass Spectrometry

Mass spectrometry (MS) is an analytical technique that produces spectra (singular spectrum) of the masses of the molecules comprising a sample of material. The advantages of MS include the simultaneous quantitative and qualitative analysis, low limit of detection, high sensitivity and so on. Now, MS plays an increasingly important role in physicochemical analysis.

A MS can be obtained on samples as small as 10^{-12} g, which is smaller than any other spectroscopic method. The disadvantage is that the sample is destroyed. Molecular ion is when you have ionized your molecule in the simplest manner, you have removed an electron, while leaving the rest of your sample molecule intact. MS includes inlet, ion source, mass analyzer, detector, vacuum system.

13.5.1   Inlet and Ion Source

The system is under vacuum, and the inlet acts as a conduit between laboratory at atmospheric conditions to MS. An ion source is an electro-magnetic device that is used to create charged particles such as atomic and molecular ions. There are many types of ion sources, including electron bombardment ion source (EI), chemical ionization ion source (CI), Matrix-assisted laser desorption ionization (MALDI), electrospray ionization (ESI), and so on. EI ionizes the sample molecule through the direct action of electrons with certain energy. The high efficiency of EI contributes to the high sensitivity and resolution of mass spectrometers. The drawback of EI is that the molecular ion signal becomes weak or even undetectable. CI introduces a large amount of reagent gas, so that the sample molecules do not directly interact with ionized ions, and the active reaction ions are used to realize ionization. The thermal effect of CI may be low, so that the fragmentation of molecular ions is less than the electron bombardment ionization. Atmospheric pressure chemical ionization (APCI) is the chemical ionization reaction at atmospheric pressure with higher rate, higher efficiency, and can produce abundant ions. The ions produced under atmospheric pressure are transferred to a high vacuum by some means. In the early stage, it was a Ni63 radiation ionizing ion source, and another design was corona discharge ionization, allowing a flow rate of 9 L/S. ESI uses a strong electrostatic field with a voltage of 3-5 kV. The sample solution is made to form highly charged mist droplets. After repeated solvent volatilization and droplet splitting, a single multi-charged ion is generated. ESI is widely used in HPLC-MS.

13.5.2   Mass Analyzer

The function of mass analyzer is to separate mass by electric or magnetic field. The important component of the mass spectrometer, located between the ion source and the detector, is separated according to the mass-to-charge ratio (m/z) of the sample ions generated in the ion source in different ways. Under the action of magnetic field, the trajectory of the accelerated ion beam is bent to different degrees and separated. There are many types of mass analyzers, such as quadrupole, time of flight, ion trap, etc.

Magnetic analyzer includes magnetic field only (unit resolution) and double focusing (magnetic field and electric field). A quadrupole is a unit consisting of four precisely parallel rods with a direct current voltage (DC) and a superimposed radio-frequency voltage (RF). The opposite pair of electrodes is equipotential, and the potential between the two pairs is opposite. When a group of ions with different mass-to-charge ratio enter the electric field composed of DC and RF, only the ions meeting specific conditions oscillate stably through the quadrupole and reach the monitor to be detected. The TOF has an ion drift tube. All singly charged particles subjected to a voltage attain the same translational energy. The ions of different masses have different velocities, and therefore arrive at the detector at different times. Ions of different masses can be separated according to the mass-to-charge ratio. Ion trap consists of a pair of ring electrodes and two end cap electrodes. An RF voltage or dc voltage is applied to the circular electrode and the electrode is grounded at the end cap electrode. As the maximum RF voltage increases, the ions with the mass charge ratio from small to large are excluded and recorded to obtain the mass spectrum. Ion trap mass spectrometry (ITMS) can be used for multistage mass spectrometry analysis conveniently, which is very useful for the identification of material structures. In the use of MS, ion traps are considered to have a greater advantage in qualitative aspects, while quadrupoles have an advantage in quantitative aspects.

13.5.3   Detector

The function of detector is to measure ion currents and amplify signals. There are many kinds of MS detectors, the common ones are electron multiplier, ion detector, Faraday cup and so on.

13.5.4　Vacuum System

The operation of MS needs to maintain internal vacuum, so the role of vacuum system is very important. To prevent sample contamination, the system should be maintained at a low pressure of 10^{-9} torr. Simple vacuum pumps in lab only reach $10^{-2} - 10^{-3}$ torr. MS vacuum systems typically have Turbo Molecular pumps.

13.5.5　Mass Spectrum

A mass spectrum is a distribution of ions shown by a mass spectrograph or a mass spectrometer. The mass spectrum is a plot of ion abundance (y) vs m/z ratio (x). Mass spectrum can provide a lot of information about objects being measured, especially in qualitative analysis. The most abundant peak (and the tallest) is the base peak. The intensity of the base peak is set at 100%, and the intensity of the other streams is expressed as a percentage. Many ion peaks can be seen from the MS of organic compounds. The mass-to-charge ratio and relative strength of these peaks depend on the molecular structure and the type of instrument and experimental conditions. It is these ion peaks that provide abundant information for MS and provide the foundation for MS analysis.

13.5.6　Hyphenated Technique

With the development of technology, MS has been applied more and more in many detection fields. Modern chromatography and hyphenated techniques are important technique platforms in physicochemical analysis. Advances in interface technology have made it possible to combine chromatography with MS. Chromatography instruments provide a powerful ability to separate different substances, and MS provides precise qualitative and quantitative analysis. The hyphenated technique of chromatography and MS plays an important role in water quality monitoring, food safety, biomaterial analysis, omics research and other fields. ICP can be used as an ion source for inorganic mass spectrometry, usually linked to quadrupole mass spectrometry, to detect a wider range of elements at lower concentrations. In recent ten years, more and more national standards choose MS as the standard method of detection.

Glossary

physicochemical analysis 理化检验 a technical subject, using particular analytical methods, like physical or chemical techniques, or combined techniques, especially modern instrumental analysis, to detect the type and quantity of substance

bias *n.* 偏差 the difference between the expectation of a test result or measurement result and a true value

accuracy *n.* 准确度 the quality of being near to the true value

precision *n.* 精密度 the reproducibility of a measurement, the quality of being reproducible in amount or performance

electrochemical analysis 电化学分析 an analytical method established according to the electrochemical properties and changes of the tested solution

chromatography *n.* 色谱 a process used for separating mixtures by virtue of differences in absorbency, the solubility of a substance use, such as adsorption characteristics of physical and chemical separation methods

mass spectrometry 质谱 an analytical method that relies on the charge/mass ratio of molecules for separation and detection, an analytical technique that produces spectra (singular spectrum) of the masses of the molecules comprising a sample of material

direct potentiometry 直接电位法 a method of direct determination based on the relationship between potential and concentration

potentiometric titration 电位滴定法 a titration analysis method which determines the end point of titration according to the change of battery electromotive force during titration

voltammetry *n.* 伏安法 a category of electroanalytical methods used in analytical chemistry and various industrial processes

stripping voltammetry 伏安溶出法 an electrochemical analysis method combining electrolysis enrichment and dissolution determination

conductimetry *n.* 电导分析法 an analytical method for determining the concentration of the substance to be measured by measuring the conductivity of the solution, or directly expressing the measured result by the conductivity of the solution

coulometry *n.* 库仑分析法 an analytical method for determining the amount of matter transformed during an electrolysis reaction by measuring the amount of electricity (in coulombs) consumed or produced

amperometry *n.* 安培滴定法 a method of detection of ions in a solution based on electric current or changes in electric current

chemical battery 化学电池 a device that converts chemical energy and electric energy

redox reaction 氧化还原反应 a reversible chemical reaction in which one reaction is an oxidation and the reverse is a reduction

spectroscopy *n.* 光谱法 the use of spectroscopes to analyze spectra

quantitative *adj.* 定量的 expressible as a quantity or relating to or susceptible of measurement

qualitative *adj.* 定性的 relating to or involving comparisons based on qualities

ultraviolet *n.* 紫外线 radiation lying in the ultraviolet range, wave lengths shorter than light but longer than X rays

infrared *adj.* 红外线的 having or employing wavelengths longer than light but shorter than radio waves, lying outside the visible spectrum at its red end

absorption spectroscopy 吸收光谱法 a method for quantitative and qualitative analysis of substances according to their characteristic absorption of electromagnetic waves

fluorescence *n.* 荧光 light emitted during absorption of radiation of some other (invisible) wavelength

transmittance *n.* 透射比 the ratio of the luminous flux through a material or medium to the incident flux

functional group *n.* 官能团 an atom or group that determines the chemical properties of an organic compound

atomization *n.* 原子化 annihilation by reducing something to atoms

ashing *n.* 灰化 the process of converting to ash

plasma *n.* 等离子体 a fourth state of matter distinct from solid or liquid or gas and present in stars and fusion reactors; a gas becomes a plasma when it is heated until the atoms lose all their electrons, leaving a highly electrified collection of nuclei and free electrons

mobile phase 流动相 a phase that moves over or through the stationary phase, carrying with it the analyte mixture

chromatogram *n.* 色谱图 the recording (column or paper strip) on which the constituents of a mixture are adsorbed in chromatography

gas chromatography 气相色谱 a common type of chromatography used in analytical chemistry for separating and analyzing compounds that can be vaporized without decomposition

injection *n.* 进样 the act of adding a sample to an instrument

thermal conductivity 热导率 the property of a material to conduct heat

high-performance liquid chromatography 高效液相色谱 a branch of chromatography, the liquid as mobile phase, the use of high pressure infusion system, the mobile phase is pumped into the stationary phase of the column, in the column components are separated, into the detector for detection, so as to achieve the analysis of the sample

ion-exchange *n.* 离子交换 a process in which ions are exchanged between a solution and an insoluble (usually resinous) solid

pump *n.* 泵 a mechanical device that moves fluid or gas by pressure or suction

supercritical fluid 超临界流体 any substance at a temperature and pressure above its critical point, where distinct liquid and gas phases do not exist. It can effuse through solids like a gas, and dissolve materials like a liquid

ion source 离子源 an electro-magnetic device that is used to create charged particles such as atomic and molecular ions

mass analyzer 质量分析器 the important component of the mass spectrometer, located between the ion source and the detector, according to different ways to generate sample ions in the ion source according to the size of the charge-to-mass ratio m/z

ion abundance 离子丰度 the ion signal strength detected by detector in mass spectrometry analysis

（安康）

新形态教材网·数字课程学习……

💻教学 PPT   📝自测题   💬推荐阅读

Chapter 14
Nutrients and Harmful Substances Examination

Learning objectives:

- Understand the nutrients and common toxic substances in food.
- Be familiar with food sample collection methods.
- Master the principle of Kjeldahl method.
- Master the LC-MS/MS method for multiple pesticide residues.

14.1 Introduction to Food Nutrients and Harmful Substances

14.1.1 Food Nutrients

Nutrients are compounds in foods, providing us with energy and building blocks for repair and growth and substances necessary to regulate chemical processes. These nutrients are essential to life and health because the body cannot make them and must obtain them from food. There are six categories of essential nutrients: proteins, carbohydrates, lipids, vitamins, minerals, and water. Foods also contain other components such as fiber that are important for health.

14.1.2 Water

Water is essential. About 65% of the adult body is made up of water. Lack of water can cause death more quickly compared with the inadequacy of any other nutrients. All the chemical reactions that occur in the body take place in water. Water also reacts during the chemical processes, regulates body temperature, transports nutrients and wastes, and dissolves nutrients. An adult should drink six to eight glasses of water each day.

14.1.3 Protein

Proteins contain amino acid, sometimes referred to as the building blocks of protein. Dietary protein is supplied from plant and animal sources. We need proteins to build, repair body tissues and carry out the metabolic functions of our bodies.

The proteins are polymers of amino acids. The shape and thus the function of a protein are determined by the sequence of its amino acid. Proteins must be broken down (hydrolyzed) to amino acids before they can be used. Once absorbed, amino acids are utilized to make proteins, converted to energy, or stored as fat. About 20% of the human body is made of protein.

Functions of protein include: enzymes such as trypsin and pepsin; storage such as ovalbumin and ferritin; transport such as hemoglobin and lipoproteins; contractility such as actin and myosin; protection such as antibodies and thrombin; hormones such as insulin and growth hormone; structural such as keratin, collagen, and elastin; membranes.

14.1.4　Carbohydrates

The carbohydrates in our diet come from plant foods. Simple carbohydrates include the different forms of sugar (monosaccharides and disaccharides); complex carbohydrates (polysaccharides) include starches and dietary fiber.

Carbohydrates are called carbohydrates because they are essentially hydrates of carbon. Specifically they are composed of carbon and water and have a composition of $C_n(H_2O)_n$. The major nutritional role of carbohydrates is to provide energy; digestible carbohydrates provide 4 kilocalories per gram. No single carbohydrate is essential, but carbohydrates do participate in many required functions in the body.

Dietary carbohydrates include sugars and complex carbohydrates (starch and fiber). During digestion all carbohydrates except fiber are broken down into sugars. Sugars and starches occur naturally in many foods that also supply other nutrients. Examples of these foods include milk, fruits, some vegetables, breads, cereals, and grains.

Fiber is found only plant foods like whole-grain breads and cereals, beans and peas, and other vegetables and fruits. Individuals should choose a variety of foods daily because the types of fiber in food vary. Eating a variety of fiber-containing plant foods is important for proper bowel function. Fiber can also reduce symptoms of chronic constipation, diverticular disease, and hemorrhoids, and may lower the risk for heart disease and some cancers. Some of the health benefits associated with a high-fiber diet may come from other components present in these foods, not just from fiber itself. For this reason, fiber is best obtained from foods rather than supplements.

14.1.5　Lipids

Lipids include fats and oils from plants and animals. Cholesterol is a fat found only in animal products. Lipids are of special interest because they are linked to the development of heart disease, the leading cause of death among human.

Lipids are the substances in foods that are soluble in organic solvents. This category includes triglycerides, fatty acids, phospholipids, some pigments, some vitamins, and cholesterol.

In food, lipids (fats) provide a source of essential fatty acids, add caloric density (energy), act as carriers for flavors, and fat-soluble vitamins. Thanks to its contribution to texture and mouthfeel, it becomes precursors of flavor and provides heat transfer medium (in frying).

14.1.6   Vitamins

Vitamins are chemical compounds in our food needed in very small amounts (in milligrams or micrograms) to regulate the chemical reaction in our bodies. Based on the solubility, vitamins are divided into fat-soluble and water-soluble vitamins. Fat-soluble vitamins are stored in the fat cells and as the name suggests, these vitamins require fat in order to be absorbed. Vitamin A, D, E and K are fat-soluble vitamins. Water-soluble vitamins are not stored in our body as their excess gets excreted through the urine. Therefore, these vitamins need to be replenished constantly. Vitamin B and C are water-soluble vitamins. B vitamins include: thiamin, riboflavin, niacin, pantothenic acid, pyridoxine, biotin, folic acid and cobalamin.

Table 14-1 lists the fat- and water-soluble vitamins and their functions.

Table 14–1   Functions of some vitamins

Vitamins		Sources	Some functions
Fat-soluble vitamins	Vitamin A	Potato, carrots, pumpkins, spinach, beef and eggs	Needed for vision, healthy skin and mucous membranes, bone and tooth growth, immune system health
	Vitamin D	Fortified milk and other dairy products	Needed for proper absorption of calcium; stored in bones
	Vitamin E	Fortified cereals, leafy green vegetables, seeds, and nuts	Antioxidant; protects cell walls
	Vitamin K	Dark green leafy vegetables and in turnip or beet green	Aids in blood clotting
Water-soluble vitamins	Vitamin B_1 or Thiamin	Pork chops, ham, enriched grains and seeds	Coenzyme in energy metabolism; important to nerve function
	Vitamin B_2 or Riboflavin	Whole grains, enriched grains and dairy products	Coenzyme in energy metabolism; important for normal vision and skin health
	Vitamin B_3 or Niacin	Mushrooms, fish, poultry, and whole grains	Coenzyme in energy metabolism; important for nervous system, digestive system, and skin health
	Vitamin B_5 or Pantothenic Acid	Chicken, broccoli, legumes and whole grains	Coenzyme in energy metabolism
	Vitamin B_6 or Pyridoxine	Fortified cereals and soy products	Coenzyme in protein metabolism; helps make red blood cells
	Vitamin B_7 or Biotin	Fruits and meats	Coenzyme in energy metabolism
	Vitamin B_9 or Folic Acid	Leafy vegetables	Part of an enzyme needed for making DNA and new cells, especially red blood cells
	Vitamin B_{12} or Cobalamin	Fish, poultry, meat and dairy products	Part of an enzyme needed for making new cells; important to nerve function
	Vitamin C or Ascorbic acid	Citrus fruits and juices, such as oranges and grapefruits	Antioxidant; part of an enzyme needed for protein metabolism; important for immune system health; aids in iron absorption

14.1.7 Minerals

Minerals are elements or components which are present in food and are required by the body for developing and functioning properly. Some minerals assist in the body's chemical reactions and others help form body structures. Minerals are important for energy transfer and are the integral part of vitamins, hormones, and amino acids. Depending on the amount in the body, minerals in the diet are classified as macrominerals or microminerals (sometimes called trace minerals). The amount of the minerals that are needed for the body does not necessarily indicate its significance.

Microminerals are needed in small amounts. The list of the microminerals includes iron, iodine, copper, manganese, fluoride, zinc, cobalt, and selenium. If the microminerals are taken in excessive amounts, they can cause mineral toxicity and lead to numerous health issues like nausea, diarrhea, discoloration, etc.

The macrominerals are needed by the body in large quantities. Examples of macrominerals include calcium, chloride, sodium, potassium, magnesium, phosphorus, and sulfur. These minerals are essential for the metabolism and proper functioning of the human body. We don't produce these components and hence need to obtain them from different sources like food and supplements. The deficiency of macrominerals in the body has an adverse impact on human physiology.

Table 14-2 lists some of the macrominerals and microminerals and their functions.

Table 14–2 Functions of some minerals

Mineral	Sources	Some functions
Calcium	Almonds, carrots, milk, broccoli, canned fish, papaya, garlic, and cashew	Help blood clotting Help muscle contraction and nerve function Essential for building strong and healthy bones
Phosphorus	Mushrooms, meat, cashews, oats, fish, beans, squash, pecans, carrots, and almonds	Help the body to store and use energy Works with calcium in the formation of strong, healthy bones and teeth
Iron	Meat, eggs, beans, baked potato, dried fruits, green leafy vegetables, whole and enriched grains	Help in transporting oxygen to all parts of the body Produce and store the energy for further metabolisms
Copper	Crab, lobster, mussels, oysters, nuts, wholegrains and yeast extract	Formation of red blood cells Help with the functioning of the nervous system
Magnesium	Honey, almonds, seafood, tuna, chocolates, pineapple, pecans, artichokes, and green leafy vegetables	Provide structure for the healthy bones Produce energy from the food molecules Maintain proper functioning of muscle and nervous system
Sodium	Table salt, cheese, milk, soy sauce, and unprocessed meat	Maintain cellular osmotic pressure Help in maintaining blood volume and blood pressure and the fluid balance in the body

(*Continued*)

Table 14–2 (*Continued*)

Mineral	Sources	Some functions
Sulfur	Cheese, eggs, nuts, turnips, onions, fish, wheat germ, cucumbers, corn, cauliflower, and broccoli	Involved in protein synthesis Protect your cells from damage Help in promoting the loosening and shedding of Skin
Potassium	Spinach, apples, oranges, tomatoes, papaya, bananas, lemons, celery, mushrooms, pecans, raisins, pineapple, rice, cucumbers, strawberries, figs, brussels sprouts, and legumes	Control nerve impulses and muscle contractions Help in maintaining fluid balance in the body Maintain proper functioning of muscle and nervous system
Chloride	Table salt, soy sauce, liver unprocessed meat, milk and peanuts	Maintain proper blood volume, blood pressure, and pH of our body fluids
Zinc	Beef, pork, dark meat, chicken, cashews, almonds, peanuts, beans, split peas, and lentil	Aids in wound healing Support the immune system Help in the formation of strong bones Control the functioning of the sense organs in the nervous system Important and the essential process of cell division and reproduction
Iodine	Seafood, seaweed and iodised salt	Promote the normal functioning of the thyroid gland Help in the proper functioning of brain functions Promote normal growth and development of cells
Manganese	Cereals, nuts, oils, vegetables and wholegrains	Help maintain water balance Control nerve impulse transmissions

14.1.8 Harmful Substances in Food

Chemicals are used in every step of the process before food is being put on our table: production, harvesting, processing, packing, transport, marketing and consumption. Some of these chemicals remain in our food and many persist in the environment and our bodies for decades to come.

There are many harmful substances involved in food production. Herbicides, pesticides, chemical fertilizers are used on crops. Industrial level food processing uses a range of chemicals. Sterilising chemicals, preservatives are potentially harmful if their use is not regulated.

Pesticides are widely used in producing food to control pests such as insects, rodents, weeds, bacteria, mold and fungus. The toxicity of a pesticide depends on its function and other factors. For example, insecticides tend to be more toxic to humans than herbicides. Adverse effects from these pesticides occur only above a certain safe level of exposure. When people come into contact with large quantities of pesticide, this may cause acute poisoning or long-term health effects, including cancer and adverse effects on reproduction.

Preservatives are added to many processed foods including breads, cereals, and meat. Studies have found that additives are a source of headaches, nausea, weakness and difficulty breathing. New research has shown that they may damage human nerve cells. We do not fully understand all of the long-term effects that additives could have on our health because synthetic additives are a relatively new invention.

Certain fish contain toxic chemicals called Perchlorinated biphenyls (PCBs), which have been banned but still remain in our environment and end up in our food system. PCBs can damage the developing brain and have been linked to behavioral disorders.

Heavy metals are widely present in the environment and can get into our food. While environmental contamination (*e.g.* from soil and water) would be the main source, which can make heavy metals enter food through processing. Heavy metals are potent neurotoxicants that can impair children's normal brain development. While the levels in any one food may be low, the cumulative effect of dietary heavy metals can be significant. Below are key health concerns associated with exposure:

Mercury: impairing coordination of movements, vision, speech, and hearing, leading to muscle weakness, and lower IQs in children.

Lead: impairing brain development and leading to lower IQs in children, cardiovascular disease, and cancer.

Inorganic arsenic: impairing cognitive development in children, and leading to cardiovascular disease, diabetes, and cancer.

Cadmium: leading to kidney disease, cardiovascular disease, and cancer. It is neccesary to understand the neurological impacts of cadmium exposure.

Food packaged in plastic may contain phthalates or other harmful chemicals. As the chemicals can seep from the packaging into the food itself. Research has linked phthalates to behavioral disorders.

Table 14-3 lists some of the harmful substances and their adverse health effects.

Table 14–3   Adverse health effects of some harmful substances

Toxic chemical	Sources of exposure	Adverse health effects
Pesticides	Food residues; contaminated soil; agricultural settings; water contamination	Damage to the developing brain; loss of IQ; respiratory disease; non-Hodgkins lymphoma, childhood leukemia; early breast cancer; asthma; autoimmune disease; thyroid disease
Preservatives: propyl gallate, BHA (butylated hydroxyanisole) and BHT (butylated hydroxytoluene), sodium nitrite and sodium nitrate	Preservative-added food	Cancer
PCBs (banned substances)	Certain fish	Cancer, damage to the developing brain; loss of IQ; behavioral disorders
BPA (bisphenol A)	Canned food; many plastic containers	Damage to the developing brain; behavioral disorders

(*Continued*)

Table 14-3 (*Continued*)

Toxic chemical	Sources of exposure	Adverse health effects
Phthalates, adipates and organometals	Plastics; other forms of packaging	Behavioral disorders
Mercury	Fish; emissions from coal-powered electric plants	Damage to the developing brain; loss of IQ; behavioral disorders; lower overall function; visual and hearing impairment
Lead	Vegetables, meat, fruits, seafood, and wine (among many other foods contaminated with heavy metals)	Impaired brain development and lower IQs in children, cardiovascular disease, and cancer
Inorganic arsenic	Chicken, drinking water	Carcinogen; increased risk of cardiovascular disease and diabetes
Cadmium	Mushrooms, shellfish, freshwater fish, dried algae, and potable water, among others	Kidney disease, cardiovascular disease, and cancer. May impact nervous system

14.2   Food Sample Collection

A complete food sample analysis consists of the following steps: planning (identifying the most appropriate analytical procedure), sample selection, sample preparation, performance of analytical procedure, statistical analysis of measurements, and data reporting. Sample collection is very important to ensure that analytical data is reliable and to draw a representative sample.

14.2.1   Sample Plans

The criteria should be considered in formulating a sampling plan: type of food product, the size of food articles to be sampled, the degree of hazard to human health, the potential for fraud, acceptance and rejection criteria: adulteration, tolerance limits, compositional standards, net contents.

14.2.2   Sample Selection

The primary objective of sample selection is to ensure that the properties of the laboratory sample are representative of the properties of the population. Selection of a limited number of samples for analysis is of great benefit because it allows a reduction in time, expense and personnel required to carry out the analytical procedure, while it can still provide useful information about the properties of the population.

Populations, Samples and Laboratory Samples   It is convenient to define some terms used to describe the characteristics of a material whose properties are going to be analyzed.

Population   The whole of the material whose properties we are trying to obtain an estimate of is referred to as the population.

Sample   Only a fraction of the population is usually selected for analysis, which is referred to as the sample. The sample may be comprised of one or more sub-samples selected from different regions within the population.

Laboratory Sample   The sample may be too large to conveniently analyze using a laboratory procedure and so only a fraction of it is actually used in the final laboratory analysis. This fraction is usually referred to as the laboratory sample.

14.2.3   Sampling Method

In statistics, there are different sampling techniques available to get relevant results from the population. The two different types of sampling methods are: Probability sampling, non-probability sampling.

The probability sampling method utilizes some form of random selection. In this method, all the eligible individuals have a chance of selecting the sample from the whole sample space. This method is more time consuming and expensive than the non-probability sampling method. The benefit of using probability sampling is that it can collect the typical samples of the population.

Probability sampling methods are further classified into different types, such as simple random sampling, systematic sampling, stratified sampling, and clustered sampling.

The non-probability sampling method is a technique by which the researcher selects the sample based on subjective judgment rather than the random selection. In this method, not all the members of the population have a chance to participate in the study.

Non-probability sampling methods are further classified into different types, such as convenience sampling, consecutive sampling, quota sampling, judgmental sampling, and snowball sampling.

14.2.4   Sample Storage

Samples must be stored:

- In a suitable container, which may be security tagged/sealed, which is essential for legal samples.

- At a suitable temperature *e.g.* samples taken for testing of volatile chemicals, or unsaturated fatty acids, which may benefit from frozen storage. But conversely freezing may affect the outcome of microbial testing.

- Under conditions that prevent degradation of the sample, or the analyte to be tested. For example, many vitamins are light sensitive, so samples sent for analysis should be protected from light using dark packaging, or by wrapping the sample packaging in aluminium foil.

- In containers that prevent cross-contamination, *e.g.* if testing for: 1) metal elements, it would not be sensible to wrap samples in aluminium foil; 2) plasticisers, samples should not be placed in plastic bottles; 3) glass contamination, the sample must not be placed inside a glass container.

- For a suitable length of time. Samples kept for a long time before testing, may not be representative of the original product that was sampled.

Sample shipping and storage requirements should also be discussed and agreed with the receiving laboratory.

14.3   Determination of Nitrogen (Total) in Milk by Kjeldahl Method

14.3.1   Principle

Milk is digested in H_2SO_4, using $CuSO_4 \cdot 5H_2O$ as catalyst with K_2SO_4 as boiling point elevator, to release nitrogen from protein and retain nitrogen as ammonium salt. Concentrated NaOH is added to release NH_3, which is distilled, collected in H_3BO_3 solution, and titrated.

14.3.2   Determination

Digestion Burner Setting   Conduct digestion over heating device can be adjusted to bring 250 mL H_2O at 25℃ to rolling boil in circa 5-6 min. To determine maximum heater setting to be used during digestion, we would preheat 10 min (gas) or 30 min (electric) at burner setting to be evaluated. Add 3 or 4 boiling chips to 250 mL H_2O at 25℃ and place flask on preheated burner. We should determine heater setting that brings water from 25℃ to rolling boil in 5–6 min on each burner. This is the maximum burner setting to be used during digestion.

Digestion   Place flask in inclined position with fume ejection system on. We should start on setting low enough so that test portion does not foam up neck of Kjeldahl flask, and digest at least 20 min or until white fumes appear in flask. Next, we need to increase burner setting half way to the maximum burner setting and heat for 15 min before increasing heat to the maximum. When digest clears (clear with light blue green color), we would continue to boil 1-1.5 h at the maximum setting (total time circa 1.8-2.25 h).

To determine specific boil time needed for analysis conditions in laboratory, we should select a high protein, high fat milk test sample and determine protein content using different boil times (1-1.5 h) after clearing. Mean protein test increases with increasing (0-1.5 h) boil time, becomes constant, and then decreases when boil time is too long. And we should also select boil time that yields maximum protein test.

At the end of digestion, acid digest should be clear and free of undigested material and cool it to room temperature (circa 25 min). Cooled digest should be liquid or liquid with few small crystals. (Large amount of crystallization before addition of water indicates too little residual H_2SO_4 at the end of digestion and can result in low test values.) After digest is cooled to room temperature, add 300 mL H_2O to flask and swirl to mix (for 800 mL flasks add 400 mL H_2O). When room temperature water is added, some crystals may form and then go into solution, which is normal reaction. Let mixture cools to room temperature before distillation. Flasks can be stoppered for distillation at later time.

Distillation　Turn on condenser water, add 50 mL H_3BO_3 solution with indicator to graduated 500 mL Erlenmeyer titration flask and place flask under condenser tip so that tip is well below H_3BO_3 solution surface. For room temperature diluted digest, we should carefully add 75 mL 50% NaOH down sidewall of Kjeldahl flask with no agitation. NaOH forms clear layer under the diluted digest. Then we should immediately connect flask to distillation bulb on condenser, vigorously swirl flask to mix contents thoroughly and heat until all NH_3 has been distilled ($\geqslant 150$ mL distillate; $\geqslant 200$ mL total volume). Do not leave distillation unattended because flasks (500 mL) may bump at this point. We should lower receiving flask, let liquid drain from condenser tip and turn off distillation heater. After that, it's vital to titrate H_3BO_3 receiving solution with standard 0.1000 mol/L HCl solution to first trace of pink. And lighted stir plate may aid visualization of end point. Record mL HCl to at least nearest 0.05 mL.

14.3.3　Calculations

Calculate results as the following equation

$$Nitrogen\ (\%) = \frac{1.4007 \times (V_s - V_b) \times M}{W} \qquad (14\text{-}1)$$

where V_s and V_b is mL HCl titrant used for test portion and blank, respectively; M is molarity of HCl solution; and W is test portion weight, g.

Multiply percent nitrogen by factor 6.38, to calculate percent "protein". This is "protein" on a total nitrogen basis.

14.4　LC-MS/MS Method for Multiple Pesticide Residues in Foods of Plant Origin

The use of pesticides in agriculture has become unavoidable as technology becomes increasingly specialized, as they can increase productivity. However, the increasing use of pesticides threatens the environment and human and animal health through direct exposure. Pesticides enter the body through various channels, such as oral intake through food and water, as well as absorption through the skin. The degree of the adverse impact of exposure to pesticides depends on the exposure duration and quantity. Long-term exposure to pesticides has been associated with diseases, such as multiple sclerosis and cancer, as well as various chronic conditions. In addition, when the pesticide involved is highly complex, the associated toxicity may be much worse owing to interactions between substances. Hence, methods for analyzing pesticides should be continuously researched and developed to ensure the safety of agricultural products.

Various methods can be used to analyze pesticide residues, such as thin-layer chromatography (TLC) and mass spectrometry; however, simultaneous multi residue analysis is chiefly conducted using LC and GC coupled with mass spectrometry. GC-MS/MS is mainly used for such analysis because it advantageously minimizes signal interference from a complex sample matrix and can separate highly lipophilic substances, such as chlorothalonil and endosulfan. Some recently introduced pesticides have polar components. In addition, they are thermolabile and difficult to volatilize. Consequently, LC-MS/MS is used for such pesticides because it is difficult to accurately analyze them by high-temperature GC.

QuEChERS (quick, easy, cheap, effective, rugged, safe) is one such pretreatment method; it is a simple and rapid pretreatment method that uses a highly sensitive mass spectrometer and is mainly used for multiclass and multi residue analyses. Contrary to the existing pesticide residue analysis methods, the QuEChERS method can easily be developed and used to analyze pesticide metabolites. Many global studies are directed toward the development of further methods for the analysis of pesticide multi residues by the simultaneous application of GC-MS/MS and LC-MS/MS.

14.4.1   Principle

Pesticide residues in plant food samples are extracted and purified by QuEChERS, then the extract is concentrated, fixed volume and filtered, determined and confirmed by LC-MS/MS, and quantified by external standard method.

14.4.2   Sample Preparation

The sample is first homogenized using a grinder, and the resulting sample is used as the blank sample. After weighing 10 g of the pulverized sample, we would add 10 mL of acetonitrile to each weighed sample and shake for 1 min. Thereafter, 4g of anhydrous magnesium sulfate, 1g of sodium chloride, 1 g of sodium citrate, and 0.5 g of disodium citrate sesquihydrate are added to the sample solution, followed by vigorous shaking for 1 min using a rotary mixer. Subsequently, centrifugation is performed for 5 min at 3,700 r/min. For LC-MS/MS analysis, the centrifuged supernatant is filtered through a 0.2 μm syringe filter and used as the test solution.

14.4.3   Standard Solution Preparation

Individual standard solutions of pesticide residues are prepared in acetonitrile (CAN) at a concentration of 1,000-10,000 μg/L. Working solutions (10-100 μg/L) are prepared by diluting the stock solution with a blank sample. The matrix matching calibration standard solution is prepared by mixing the matrix matching working standard solution with an additional blank sample extract to reach a multi compound concentration of 0.005-1 mg/L. All standard solutions are stored in glass bottles at −20°C.

The method used to prepare calibration curves for standard substances match with metrics. Concentrations of 1-20 μg/L are used, and each calibration curve is prepared using five points. The interference effect is reduced by diluting the concentration by a factor of 10 for sample analysis.

14.4.4　Instrument Analysis Conditions

The analysis conditions for the LC-MS/MS instruments are shown in Table 14-4.

Table 14–4　Analytical conditions of LC–MS/MS

Instrument	AB Sciex Triple Quad 4500 LC/MS with Agilent 1290 series HPLC			
Column	Capcell core C18, 2.1 mm × 150 mm, 2.7 μm			
Mobile phase A	5 mmol/L ammonium formate & 0.1% formic acid in water			
Mobile phase B	5 mmol/L ammonium formate & 0.1% formic acid in methanol			
Gradient program	Time (min)	A (%)	B (%)	Flow (mL/min)
	Initial	85	15	0.3
	1	85	15	0.3
	1.5	40	60	0.3
	10	10	90	0.3
	12	10	90	0.3
	12.1	2	98	0.3
	16	2	98	0.3
	16.1	85	15	0.3
	20	85	15	0.3
Injection volume	10 μL			
Column temperature	40°C			
Sample tray temp	10°C			
Ionization mode	ESI positive			
Scan type	MRM mode			

14.4.5　Simultaneous Multi Component Analysis in Sweet Peppers

The sweet pepper samples are pretreated using the QuEChERS method. The pesticide residues are analyzed by LC-MS/MS. The results reveal that the simultaneous analysis method can effectively detect pesticide residues. The LOD values for LC-MS/MS are found to be 0.03-0.5 μg/kg, while the LOQ values are determined to be 0.6–1.5 μg/kg.

Glossary

amino acid 氨基酸 any of the substances that combine to form the basic structure of proteins

protein *n.* 蛋白质 a natural substance found in meat, eggs, fish, some vegetables, etc. There are many different proteins and they are an essential part of what humans and animals eat to help them grow and stay healthy

lipid *n.* 脂质，油脂 any of a group of natural substances which do not dissolve in water, including plant oils and steroids

carbohydrate *n.* 碳水化合物，糖类 a substance such as sugar or starch that consists of carbon, hydrogen and oxygen

vitamin *n.* 维生素，维他命 a natural substance found in food that is an essential part of what humans and animals eat to help them grow and stay healthy. There are many different vitamins

dietary fiber 膳食纤维 the part of food that helps to keep a person healthy by keeping the bowels working and moving other food quickly through the body

starch *n.* 淀粉；含淀粉的食物 a white carbohydrate food substance found in potatoes, flour, rice, etc.; food containing this

monosaccharide *n.* 单糖，单糖类（最简单的糖类）any of the class of sugars (e.g. glucose) that cannot be hydrolysed to give a simpler sugar

disaccharide *n.* 二糖，双糖 any of a class of sugars whose molecules contain two monosaccharide residues

polysaccharide *n.* 多糖；多聚糖 a carbohydrate (e.g. starch, cellulose, or glycogen) whose molecules consist of a number of sugar molecules bonded together

metabolism *n.* 新陈代谢 the chemical processes in living things that change food into energy and materials for growth

metabolite *n.* 代谢物，代谢产物 a substance formed in or necessary for metabolism

polymer *n.* （高分子）聚合物，多聚体 a natural or artificial substance consisting of large molecules (= groups of atoms) that are made from combinations of small simple molecules

hydrolyze *v.* 水解，使水解 to subject to or undergo hydrolysis

cholesterol *n.* 胆固醇 a substance found in blood, fat and most tissues of the body. Too much cholesterol can cause heart disease

pigment *n.* 色素，颜料 a substance that exists naturally in people, animals and plants and gives their skin, leaves, etc; a particular colour

phospholipid *n.* 磷脂 any of a group of compounds composed of fatty acids, phosphoric acid, and a nitrogenous base: important constituents of all membranes

precursor *n.* （尤指经新陈代谢形成另一种物质的）前体 a substance, cell, or cellular component from which another substance, cell, or cellular component is formed

coenzyme *n.* 辅酶 a nonprotein organic molecule that forms a complex with certain enzymes and is essential for their activity

preservative *n.* 防腐剂，保护剂 a substance used to prevent food or wood from decaying

additive *n.* （尤指食品的）添加剂，添加物 a substance that is added in small amounts to sth, especially food, in order to improve it, give it colour and make it last longer

residue *n.* 残留 a small amount of remains at the end of a process

pesticide *n.* 杀虫剂，农药 a chemical used for killing pests, especially insects

fungicide *n.* 杀真菌剂，杀菌剂 a substance that kills fungus

sampling *n.* 取样；抽样 the process of taking a sample

nitrogen *n.* 氮；氮气 a chemical element; a gas that is found in large quantities in the earth's atmosphere

catalyst *n.* 催化剂 a substance that makes a chemical reaction happen faster without being changed itself

ammonium *n.* 铵，铵盐，氨气 a salt made from ammonia containing nitrogen and hydrogen together with another element

titrate *v.* 滴定测量（液体中的物质）to find out how much of a particular substance is in a liquid by measuring how much of another substance is needed to react with it

distillation *n.* 精馏，蒸馏，净化；蒸馏法；精华，蒸馏物 the process of purifying a liquid by successive evaporation and condensation

flask *n.* 烧瓶 a bottle with a narrow top used in scientific work for mixing or storing chemicals

multiple *n.* 多个的，多种的 many in number; involving many different people or things

concentration *n.* 含量，浓度 the amount of a substance in a liquid or in another substance

chromatography *n.* 色谱法，色层分析法，层析法（利用混合物各部分在介质中的通透距离差异而将其分离的方法）the separation of a mixture by passing it through a material through which some parts of the mixture travel further than others

（吴淑春）

新形态教材网·数字课程学习……

💻 教学 PPT　　📝 自测题　　💬 推荐阅读

Chapter 15
Air Physicochemical Analysis

Learning objectives:

- Know the environmental and health impacts of air pollution .
- Understand the air composition and natural properties.
- Be familiar with the main air pollutants and steps in air sampling .
- Master the principle of gas chromatography/ mass spectroscopy and other methods for analyzing air pollutants.

15.1　Introduction

Air is a mixture, not a compound. It is essentially composed of nitrogen, oxygen and argon with small amounts of water vapor, carbon dioxide, and dust. Air can be liquefied and separated into its constituents by allowing the more volatile nitrogen to boil off first.

Nitrogen is an inert substance. It is a colorless, odorless, tasteless gas; does not burn and support combustion or respiration; is not poisonous. At high temperatures it combines with a few metals, such as magnesium, and also with oxygen and hydrogen. Argon comprises one-percent of the air by volume.

Carbon dioxide is introduced into air by combustion and respiration. It is removed by green plants, which get all their carbon from the carbon dioxide in the air and produce oxygen. The balance of plant and animal life keeps the amounts of oxygen and carbon dioxide in the air constant. The composition of a sample of dry air is as follows: nitrogen (78 vol%), oxygen (21 vol%), carbon dioxide (0.04 vol%), argon (0.94 vol%) and small amounts of other rare gases.

The chief factors in the air which affect human comforts are moisture, temperature, dust and small amounts of impurities given off by the human body. The human body is normally at a constant temperature 37 ℃, and this temperature is regulated by the evaporation of water from the surface of the body. The temperature and moisture of the surrounding atmosphere affect this process of evaporation. If the air is very hot and moist, the process of evaporation is very slow, and we feel uncomfortable. If the air is too dry, the evaporation from the body is too rapid, and we also feel uncomfortable. Thus it is very important to have a proper regulation of temperature and moisture. The presence of dust in the air causes a great deal of discomfort to the human body. Air in the countryside is far much clearer than that in the cities.

15.2　Air Pollution

Not so many years ago it was assumed that once a particular pollutant was admitted into the atmosphere its chemical composition did not change, and that an analysis of that pollutant would give an indication of the degree of contamination. However, it is now recognized that many chemicals undergo photochemical decomposition and reaction in the atmosphere, forming different pollutants that may be even more toxic than their precursors. The familiar smog, for example, is generally considered to be related to the interaction of nitrogen oxide, hydrocarbons, and sunlight.

15.2.1　Air Pollutants

Pollutants can be classified as either primary or secondary pollutants.

Primary pollutants are substances directly produced by a process, such as ash from a volcanic eruption or the carbon monoxide gas from a motor vehicle exhaust.

Secondary pollutants are pollutants produced through reactions between primary pollutants and normal atmospheric compounds. For example, ozone forms over urban areas through reactions of primary pollutants, sunlight, and natural atmospheric gases.

Air pollutants include toxic particles and gases emitted in large quantities from many different combustible materials. They also include particulate matter (PM) and ozone, and biological contaminants. The following are major air pollutants:

- Carbon oxides: carbon monoxide (CO), carbon dioxide (CO_2).
- Sulfur oxides: sulfur dioxide (SO_2), sulfur trioxide (SO_3).
- Nitrogen oxides: nitrous oxide (N_2O), nitric oxide (NO), nitrogen dioxide (NO_2).
- Hydrocarbons (organic compounds containing carbon and hydrogen); methane (CH_4), butane(C_4H_{10}),benzene (C_6H_6).
- Photochemical oxidants: ozone (O_3), PAN (a group of peroxyacylnitrates), various aldehydes.
- Particulates (solid particles or liquid droplets suspended in air): smoke, dust, soot, asbestos, metallic particles (such as lead, beryllium, cadmium), oil, salt spray, sulfate salts.
- Other inorganic compounds: hydrogen fluoride (HF), hydrogen sulfide (H_2S), ammonia (NH_3), sulfuric acid (H_2SO_4), nitric acid (HNO_3).
- Other organic (carbon-containing) compounds: pesticides, herbicides, various alcohols, acids, and other chemicals.
- Radioactive substances: tritium, radon, emissions from fossil fuel and nuclear power plants.

15.2.2   Global Air Pollution Problems

In both developed and rapidly industrializing countries, the major historic air pollution problem has typically been high levels of smoke and sulphur dioxide arising from the combustion of sulphur containing fossil fuels such as coal for domestic and industrial purpose. The major threat to clean air is now posed by traffic emissions. Petrol and diesel engine motor vehicles emit a wide variety of pollutants, principally carbon monoxide (CO), oxides of nitrogen (NO_x), volatile organic compounds (VOCs) and particulates (PM10), which have an increasing impact on urban air quality. In addition, photochemical reactions resulting from the action of sunlight on nitrogen dioxide (NO_2) and VOCs from vehicles lead to the formation of ozone, a secondary long-range pollutant. Acid rain is another form of long-range pollution influenced by vehicle emissions.

15.2.3   Indoor Air Pollution

In 1983, the World Health Organization (WHO) applied the term "Sick Building Syndrome" (SBS) to the clinical features observed in building occupants as a result of the indoor air pollution. Indoor pollution sources that release gases or particles into the air are the primary cause of indoor air quality problems. Inadequate ventilation can increase indoor pollutant levels by not bringing in enough outdoor air to dilute emissions from indoor sources and by not carrying indoor air pollutants out of the area. Human exposure to indoor air pollutants may occasionally be more than 100 times higher than outdoor pollutant levels, because a home's interior accumulates and concentrates pollutants given off by finishes, furnishings and the daily activities of the occupants. Actually, indoor air pollutants have been ranked among the top five environmental risks to public health. Thus, indoor air quality (IAQ) is recognized as an important concern to be addressed for the occupants' health and comfort. There are many sources of indoor air pollution. These can include:

- Fuel-burning combustion appliances.
- Tobacco products.
- Building materials and furnishings as diverse as:
  Deteriorated asbestos-containing insulation.
  Newly installed flooring, upholstery or carpet.
  Cabinetry or furniture made of certain pressed wood products.
- Products for household cleaning and maintenance, personal care, or hobbies.
- Central heating and cooling systems and humidification devices.
- Excess moisture.
- Outdoor sources such as radon, pesticides and outdoor air pollution.

15.3   Air Sampling and Storage

One of the most important steps in air analysis is the collection of the sample. We will describe a number of sample collection techniques. Once the sample has been collected, any number of standard measurement techniques may be employed.

The ideal method of measurement would involve the direct measurement of a pollutant in a stream of air drawn into the measuring apparatus. However, in all likelihood the number of substances that will be determined by direct measurement such as this will be rather limited for some time to come. Hence, samples are commonly collected by drawing the air into an appropriate adsorbing reagent or solution.

Many analytes of interest in air are rather reactive compounds, present in very low concentrations. They may be distributed between two or more phases, e.g., gases and solids or gases and liquids. Generally, the content of organic compounds in ambient air is very low. Sometimes there are higher concentrations inside and around certain industries. Thus, common types of air samples include indoor air, ambient (outdoor) air, and air from stacks or other kinds of emission exhausts (including automotive exhausts).

Sampling for volatile organics essentially means sampling for carbon-containing compounds that can get into the air. The term volatile usually means that the chemical gets into the air through a change of phase from liquid to gas. This phase change occurs when temperatures approach, equal, and exceed the boiling point and continue until equilibrium is established in the environment.

Various containers may be used to collect gases for later release into laboratory analytical chambers or sorbent beds. The remote collection devices include bags, canisters and evacuation chambers. Remote collection refers to the practice of collecting the gas sample, hopefully intact, at a site remote from the laboratory where analysis will occur.

This method of sample collection must always take into account the potential of the collecting vehicle reacting with the gaseous component collected during the time between collection and analysis. For this reason various plastic formulations and stainless steel compartments have been devised to minimize reactions with the collected gases. When bags are used, the fittings for the bags to the pumps must be relatively inert and are usually stainless steel.

Aerosol particles may be sampled by use of appropriate filters; however, various types of impactors for aerosol collection permit size discrete samples. These can be quite useful in transport and deposition studies. Particulate air sampling techniques include filtration, electrostatic precipitation, thermal precipitation, gravitational settling, centrifugal separation, and impingement. In sampling for particulates, the particulates must be filtered out or removed from the airstream by impaction. Particulates that are suspended in the airstream come in many sizes; therefore, the first question is whether exposure standards are based on the respirable fraction or the total particulate levels.

A variety of filtration options is available to collect particulates. Take care to avoid overloading the filter. Some examples of these options are as follows:

- Collect total dust on a preweighed, low-ash polyvinyl chloride (PVC) filter at a flow rate of about 2L/min, depending on the rate required to prevent overloading. Weigh PVC filters before and after taking the sample.

- Collect metal fumes on a 0.8μm mixed cellulose ester filter at approximately 1.5 L/min, not to exceed 2.0 L/min.
- When the gravimetric weight needs to be determined for welding fumes, collect these fumes on a low-ash PVC filter.

Personal sampling pumps must be calibrated before and after each day of sampling, using a bubble meter method (electronic or mechanical) or the precision rotameter (which has been calibrated against a bubble meter).

In pollution analysis, samples are generally collected for one of three important reasons: to establish hazardous levels in the environment, to evaluate the efficiency of pollution control measures, or to determine the source of a pollutant. Hence, the mode of sampling can be important.

15.3.1 Air Sampler

Many types of samplers have been used over the years, including liquid impingers, solid impactors, filters, electrostatic precipitators, and many others. The efficiencies of these samplers depend on a variety of environmental and methodological factors that can affect the integrity of the various structure.

An air sampler generally consists of an inlet to direct air into a collector, a filter to screen out larger particles that might interfere with an analysis, a collector where the sample is deposited, a flowmeter and valve to calibrate the air flow and a pump to pull air through the system.

15.3.2 Size of Sample

The volume of air sample is governed by the minimum pollutant concentration that must be measured, the sensitivity of the measurement, and the information desired. The concentration range of a pollutant may be unknown, and the sample size will have to be determined by trial and error.

15.3.3 Sampling Rate

The useful sampling rate will vary with the sampling device and should be determined experimentally. Most sampling devices for gaseous constituents have permissible flow rates of $0.003m^3/min$. The collection efficiency need not be 100% as long as it is reproducible and can be calibrated with known standards. The efficiency should be at least 90%, however. All gaseous samplers have threshold level below which their efficiency drops to near zero.

15.3.4 Duration of Sampling

The time of day and duration of sampling will be determined by the information that is desired. Remember that the sampling period will give an indication of only the average concentration during that period. It would be more meaningful to sample city air samples for lead content during rush hour, and between rush hours to obtain a realistic indication of the overall lead exposure of an individual in the city. It may be desirable in cases requiring many short interval samplings to employ instead automatic continuous monitoring using highly sensitive detection devices.

15.3.5 Sample Storage

Storage of air samples should be kept to a minimum. They should be protected from heat and light. Care should be taken that the desired test component does not react with other constituents or with the container. Gaseous samples are sometimes collected by adsorption onto a solid and the gases must not be lost by desorption prior to analysis.

15.4 Analyses of Air Pollutants

The World Health Organization reports on six major air pollutants, namely particle pollution, ground-level ozone, carbon monoxide, sulfur oxides, nitrogen oxides, and lead. China currently uses the air quality index (AQI) to describe air quality. The main evaluation factors include PM2.5, PM10, ozone, sulfur dioxide, nitrogen dioxide, and carbon monoxide. Air pollution can have a disastrous effect on all components of the environment, including groundwater, soil, and air. Additionally, it poses a serious threat to living organisms.

15.4.1 Nitrogen Dioxide

With the continuous development of industrialization and urbanization in China, current air pollution is becoming increasingly serious, and nitrogen dioxide as the main pollutant in the air, has been of urgent concern, and widely studied. The emission of nitrogen dioxide will lead to acid rain, photochemical smog and the formation of inhalable PM2.5. It will also damage the ozone layer of the atmosphere, causing serious harm to people's health while polluting the environment. Therefore, rapid and effective detection of nitrogen dioxide in the air is necessary. In recent years, the detection techniques for nitrogen dioxide in the air may be divided into two categories based on the detection principle: indirect detection technology and direct detection technology. Indirect detection techniques include spectrophotometry, ion chromatography, sensor method, fluorescence spectrometry and chemiluminescence. Direct detection techniques include differential optical absorption spectroscopy, laser induced fluorescence and cavity ring-down spectroscopy.

15.4.2 Particulate Matter (PM)

Examples of particles in the air include dust, smoke, aerosol, plant spores, bacteria and salt. Particulate matter may be a primary pollutant, such as smoke particles, or a secondary pollutant formed from the chemical reaction of gaseous pollutants. Particulate matter can be usefully classified by size. Large particles usually settle out of the air quickly while smaller particles may remain suspended for days and months. Particle pollution: PM10 inhalable particles, with aerodynamic diameters that are generally 10 micrometers and smaller; PM2.5 fine inhalable particles, with aerodynamic diameters that are generally 2.5 micrometers and smaller.

Dusts, silica, and other suspended particles in the air are measured by gravimetry. The filter in the cassette should be weighted before and after sampling for accurate determination of the mass of the deposited particles. For metal analysis, the metal dusts deposited on the filter must be acid-digested and analyzed by atomic absorption spectrophotometry or inductively coupled plasma spectrometry.

15.4.3 Identification of BTEX and Chlorobenzene Compounds by Gas Chromatography–Mass Spectrometry (GC–MS)

The volatile atmospheric contaminants, benzene, toluene, ethyl-benzene, and xylenes, shortly named BTEX, mainly originate from exhaust gases of internal combustion vehicles and are of particular concern in urban areas with intense road traffic; hence, the interest for monitoring their atmospheric concentrations.

GC is the most common analytical technique for the quantitative determination of organic pollutants in aqueous and nonaqueous samples. GC-MS is probably the best technique to identify a wide array of unknown organic substances in sample matrices. It is also the most effective method to determine the presence of pollutants in the sample.

The method is based on the principle of chromatographic separation of components of a mixture on a GC column, followed by their identification from their mass spectra. The compounds are separated on a suitable GC column, following which the components eluted from the column are subjected to electron-impact or chemical ionization (CI). The fragmented and molecular ions are identified from their characteristic mass spectra. Thus, the substances present in the sample are determined from their characteristic primary and secondary ions and from their retention times.

Experimental   Homemade calibration solutions of the BTEX analytes (benzene, toluene, ethyl benzene, m-, p-, and o-xylene) are prepared, with concentrations ranging between 40 and 500 pL/mL, in dichloromethane (DCM). The solvent elutes without interfering with the analytes. In each calibration solution, the internal standard, perdeuterated benzene from Supelco, is added in a constant concentration of 2 nL/mL. All the compounds used are of analytical grade purity. Of each calibration solution, 1microlitre is injected into the GC.

Sampling and Desorption of Analytes   Preconcentration of the atmospheric contaminants is performed in glass tubes filled with charcoal, using a portable, battery-operated pump set at 100 mL/min air flow, 45 minutes sampling time. A manually operated mechanical counter is used to determine the number of petrol-fueled vehicles passing the sampling site. The analytes are then desorbed in 0.5mL DCM, with 1-minute vortex and 2-minute ultrasonication. An internal standard (IS), deuterated benzene, is added to result in 2 nL/mL concentration in each sample extract, and 1microlitre of the supernatant is injected into the GC.

Equipment   The analytes are separated using a gas chromategraph equipped with a capillary column (30 m × 0.25 mm × 0.25 μm), with the GC oven temperature program: 30-150°C at 7°C/min, then to 270°C, at 20°C/min. The injector temperature is 270°C, with a split 10 : 1 and He carrier gas at 1.1 mL/min flow. The mass spectrometer is operated in the selected ion monitoring mode, under standard conditions, with 70 eV ionization energy, and the quadrupolar mass detector at 150°C.

Although GC-MS is the most confirmative technique to identify an analyte, it, however, has some limitations. First, the detection limit is relatively higher for any compound when compared to most other GC or HPLC detectors. In addition, the detection levels can be lowered using high-resolution MS. The cost and servicing of such instrument, however, for routine analysis could be expensive.

15.5   Air Monitoring for Occupational Health

Once substantial employee exposure is a potential concern, such exposure needs to be measured. The next step is to select a maximum-risk employee. When there are different processes where employees may be exposed to the chemical of concern, a maximum-risk employee should be selected for each work operation.

Selection of the maximum-risk employee requires professional judgment. The best procedure for selecting the maximum-risk employee is to observe employees and select the person closest to the chemical source. If measurement shows exposure to the chemical at or above the action level or the short-term exposure limit (STEL), all other employees who may be exposed at or above the action level or STEL need to be identified. Measurement or otherwise accurate characterization of their exposure must be accomplished.

Ammonia, with density of 0.771 g/L under standard conditions, is a colorless gas with a strong irritating odor. It is usually used as a refrigerant due to its low boiling point. Ammonia is also an important chemical raw material, widely used in industrial production of nitric acid, fertilizer, resin, plastics, synthetic fibers, etc. Its widespread usage makes it a common occupational hazard factor in the air of workplaces and creates a large potential for worker occupational exposure. Personal exposure to ammonia at a certain concentration could cause a strong stimulating and corrosive effect on human eyes, nose, throat, and skin. Exposure to ammonia at the concentration of about 20-95 mg/m^3 in the urea fertilizer factory could induce acute respiratory symptoms and acute decline in lung function. Chronic ammonia inhalation could also cause pulmonary fibrosis and interstitial lung disease.

The occupational exposure limits (OELs) of ammonia are 20 mg/m^3 (permissible concentration-time weighted average, PC-TWA) and 30 mg/m^3 (permissible concentration-short term exposure limit, PC-STEL) in the occupational health standard in China (GBZ 2.1-2007). The maximum workplace concentration of ammonia is established on the condition that the working week exceeds 40 hours, is 14 mg/m^3 in Germany. The common standard procedure for monitoring ammonia is performed by spectrophotometry with sampling using sulfuric acid (H_2SO_4) solution at different concentration, in the field of environmental protection and occupational health in China.

With the increasing requirement of the detection of occupational hazard factors in the air of workplaces, the current national standard method (0.5 mol/L H_2SO_4 solution collection-Nessler reagent spectrophotometry) for monitoring ammonia presents many defects and needs to be updated in China. For sampling, the decrease in absorbing solution (H_2SO_4 solution) concentration and the CH_4O_2S solution (15 mmol/L) as the alternate sampling solution were suggested. Although the improvement in the current method is investigated, some drawbacks still exists, such as only 1 day storage time for samples, inapplicability for long-distance shipment, and personal sampling. Alternate methods for sampling and analysis are considered. The method containing sampling conducted using acid-treated solid sorbent tubes and analysis performed by ion chromatography, were more suitable for the determination of ammonia in workplace air.

15.6   Air Pollution and Health

There are many pollutants that are major factors of diseases in humans. Among them, particulate matter, particles of variable but very small diameter, penetrate the respiratory system via inhalation, causing respiratory and cardiovascular diseases, reproductive and central nervous system dysfunctions, and cancer. Despite the fact that ozone in the stratosphere plays a protective role against ultraviolet irradiation, it is harmful when in high concentration at ground level, also affecting the respiratory and cardiovascular systems. Furthermore, nitrogen oxide, sulfur dioxide, volatile organic compounds (VOCs), dioxins, and polycyclic aromatic hydrocarbons (PAHs) are all considered air pollutants that are harmful to humans. Carbon monoxide can even provoke direct poisoning when breathed in at high levels. Heavy metals such as lead, when absorbed into the human body, can lead to direct poisoning or chronic intoxication, depending on exposure. Diseases occurring from the aforementioned substances include principally respiratory problems such as chronic obstructive pulmonary disease (COPD), asthma, bronchiolitis, and also lung cancer, cardiovascular events, central nervous system dysfunctions, and cutaneous diseases. Climate change resulting from environmental pollution affects the geographic distribution of many infectious diseases, as do natural disasters. The only way to tackle this problem is through public awareness coupled with a multidisciplinary approach by scientific experts. National and international organizations must address the emergence of this threat and propose sustainable solutions.

After the winter-long PM2.5 episode in eastern China in 2013, air pollution control policies have been experiencing significant changes on multiple fronts. For a long time we have known that reducing outdoor and indoor air pollution in cities or countries can have a significant effect on health almost immediately, and the benefits can far outweigh the costs. At this point, international cooperation in terms of research, development, administration policy, monitoring, and politics is vital for effective pollution control.

Glossary

magnesium *n.* 镁 a chemical element; a light, silver-white metal that burns with a bright white flame

carbon dioxide 二氧化碳 a gas breathed out by people and animals from the lungs or produced by burning carbon

hydrocarbon *n.* 烃; 碳氢化合物 an organic compound (such as acetylene or butane) containing only carbon and hydrogen and often occurring in petroleum, natural gas, coal, and bitumens

nitrogen oxide 氮氧化物 any of several oxides of nitrogen most of which are produced in combustion and are considered to be atmospheric pollutants

inorganic compound 无机化合物 any compound that does not contain carbon

pesticide *n.* 杀虫剂、农药 a chemical used to kill pests (such as rodents or insects)

volatile organic compounds 挥发性有机物 organic chemical compounds that evaporate easily at room temperature

aldehydes *n.* 乙醛、醛类 carbonyl-containing organic compounds in which the carbonyl function is at a terminal carbon

asbestos *n.* 石棉 a soft grey mineral that does not burn, used especially in the past in buildings as protection against fire or to prevent heat loss

aerosol particles 气溶胶颗粒 liquid or solid particles in the atmosphere whose sizes range from a fraction of a micron to several hundreds of microns (μm)

electrostatic precipitation 静电沉淀 a process that removes suspended dust particles from a gas by applying a high voltage electrostatic charge to the particles and collecting them on charged plates

polyvinyl chloride 聚氯乙烯 a polymer of vinyl chloride used especially for electrical insulation, films, and pipes

chemiluminescence *n.* 化学发光 luminescence resulting from a chemical reaction as the oxidation of luciferin in fireflies

chronic obstructive pulmonary disease 慢性阻塞性肺疾病 pulmonary disease (such as emphysema or chronic bronchitis) that is characterized by chronic typically irreversible airway obstruction resulting in a slowed rate of exhalation

（李敏）

新形态教材网·数字课程学习……

教学 PPT　　　自测题　　　推荐阅读

Chapter 16
Examination of Metals in Drinking Water

Learning objectives:

- Understand the sanitary significance of examination of metals in drinking water.
- Be familiar with the sampling and preservation of drinking water.
- Master the principles and pretreatment of metals in drinking water by different examination methods.

16.1   Introduction to Metals in Drinking Water

Drinking water refers to potable water and domestic water. Safe drinking water should follow epidemiological safety, prevent the occurrence and spread of water-borne infectious diseases, and ensure the microbiological safety of water quality. It is necessary to ensure that the sensitive properties of drinking water, such as the appearance, color, odor and taste, are good, and people's lifelong drinking will not cause acute poisoning, chronic poisoning, and potential long-term harm. Our government has always been very concerned and attaches great importance of drinking water. The national standard of drinking water has been issued and revised many times. The latest nation standard that is "Standards for Drinking Water Quality" (GB5749-2022) was implemented in April, 2023 to replace GB5749-2006. In the selection of water quality indices and their limitations in the national standard, China's actual situation has been fully considered, and "Guidelines for Drinking Water Quality" of the World Health Organization and the drinking water standards of the European Union, the United States, Russia and Japan are referred to. There are 97 water quality indices in "Standards for Drinking Water Quality" (GB5749-2022), including 5 microorganism indices, 21 inorganic compounds and 44 organic compounds in toxicological indices, 21 sensitive property and general chemical indices, 2 radioactive indices and 4 disinfectant indices.

With the development of industry, metal pollution in water has become increasingly obvious in recent years. Metal pollutants are derived from geological weathering, mineral smelting, production and use of metal, and the combustion of mineral fuels. Industrial waste water is the main source of metal pollution. Metal pollutants enter water and migrate in a cycle. In the process of migration, metal forms may change, but they are difficult to be degraded by microorganisms and can harm to human health when entering human body.

"Standards for Drinking Water Quality" (GB5749-2022) stipulates that arsenic, cadmium, chromium (Ⅵ), lead and mercury are the regular toxicological indices, and the expanded toxicological indices of metal include antimony, barium, beryllium, molybdenum, nickel, silver, thallium and selenium. Sensitive property and general chemical indices include four metal regular indices which are iron, manganese, copper and zinc, and one metal extended index which is sodium. Selenium is a regular toxicological index in GB5749-2006 and revised as an extended toxicological index in GB5749-2022. This chapter introduces the examinations of drinking water for metal indices including arsenic, cadmium, chromium (Ⅵ), lead, mercury, selenium, iron, manganese, copper and zinc. The examination methods are based on "Standard Examination Methods for Drinking Water–Part 6: Metal and Metalloid indices (GB/T 5750.6-2023)" .

Iron, manganese and copper are essential trace elements for human body. If the content of iron, manganese and copper exceeds the limitation in drinking water, it can cause sensitive property changes, such as colors and taste. When large amounts of iron, manganese and copper enter the body, a variety of diseases can be caused. A large amount of iron entering the human body can cause gastroenteritis. Too much manganese can damage mucosa, destroy red blood cells and proteins, and even damage the nervous system. Excessive intake of copper can cause liver and gallbladder function damage and brain nerve tissue lesions. Zinc is also an essential trace element for the human body which is less toxic. When the concentration of zinc in drinking water reaches 5 mg/L, the water will have an unpleasant metallic taste, and when the concentration reaches 10 mg/L, the water will become turbid. "Standards for Drinking Water Quality" (GB5749–2022) stipulates that the limitation of iron, manganese, copper and zinc in drinking water are 0.3 mg/L, 0.1 mg/L, 1.0 mg/L and 1.0 mg/L, respectively.

Lead entering the body and traveling throughout the body with the blood affects many systems and organs. It is mainly accumulated in nervous system, hematopoietic system, alimentary system, cardiovascular system and other systems. Cadmium is highly accumulative which can cause the symptoms such as renal dysfunction, emphysema, osteoporosis and bone deformation. Chromium mainly exists in the form of chromium (Ⅲ) and chromium (Ⅵ) in water. A moderate amount of chromium (Ⅲ) is beneficial to organisms, while chromium (Ⅵ) is toxic, which can cause vomiting, diarrhea and cancer. All forms of mercury are toxic mainly damaging the nervous system and kidneys. The toxicity of arsenic and its compounds decreases in the following order: arsenite > arsenic trioxide > arsenate > arsenic acid > metal arsenic. Arsenic has cardiovascular toxicity, neurotoxicity, hepatorenal toxicity, embryo development and reproductive toxicity and carcinogenicity. Selenium is an essential trace element for human body, but if ingested more than 10 times of the physiological requirement, the toxic threshold dose level can be reached, resulting in alopecia, fingernail shedding, skin itching and other symptoms. Severe excess can lead to liver cirrhosis and pulmonary edema. "Standards for Drinking Water Quality" (GB5749–2022) stipulates that the limitation of lead, cadmium, chromium (VI), mercury, arsenic and selenium are 0.01mg/L, 0.005 mg/L, 0.05 mg/L, 0.001 mg/L, 0.01 mg/L and 0.01 mg/L, respectively.

16.2   Sampling of Drinking Water and Storage of the Water Sample

16.2.1   Sampling of Drinking Water

Sampling is the first step of water quality analysis. Reasonable sampling is the basis to ensure the accuracy of analysis results. Drinking water samples include water sources, finished water, tap water, secondary water supply, and decentralized water supply.

Water sources for domestic drinking are divided into surface water (rivers, lakes, reservoirs, ditches and streams) and underground water (wells water and springs water). The sampling point is usually where the water is drawn.

Shallow Water

The appropriate container (bucket or sampling bottle) is placed directly into the water for sampling. Be careful not to mix with floating substances.

Water of a Certain Depth

For sampling water of a certain depth in lakes or reservoirs, an vertical water sampler can be used. Water flows through the water sampler during the sinking process, and when a predetermined depth is reached, the container closes automatically to sample water. When the water is deep and the current is rapid, the lead fish of corresponding quality should be tied up and the winch should be used.

Spring and Well Water

The self spraying spring water can be directly sampled at the water outlet. When sampling the spring water that does not spray, a water pump can be used. The water that is stagnant in the pumping pipe should be drawn. Do not sample until the pipe is filled with fresh water. To ensure the representativeness of water samples, water samples should be sampled from well water after fullly pumping.

Finished water refers to the centralized water supply treated by the water treatment process. The sampling point is located before the finished water entering the pipeline.

Tap water refers to the finished water that delivered to user tap through the pipe network. Attention should be paid to the sampling time. Sediments may be precipitated in water pipes at night, so when sampling the tap water should be released for several minutes to discharge sediments.

Secondary water supply refers to the water supply mode that the centralized water supply is stored, pressurized, disinfected again or advanced treated before entering the users, and then delivered to the users through pipelines or containers. Inlet, outlet and tap water should be sampled.

Decentralized water supply means that decentralized users directly fetch water from the water source without treatment by any facilities or just with simple facilities. Water is sampled according to the actual situation.

16.2.2　Storage of the Water Sample

For the determination of mercury, nitric acid (1+9, containing potassium dichromate 50 g/L) is added to the water sample to pH≤2, and the water sample can be stored for 30 days. For the determination of lead, cadmium, arsenic, selenium, iron, manganese, copper and zinc, the water sample can be stored for 14 days when added nitric acid to pH≤2.

16.3　Examination of Metals in Drinking Water

16.3.1　Examination of Iron, Manganese, Copper and Zinc in Drinking Water

The main examination methods for iron, manganese, copper and zinc in drinking water are ultraviolet-visible spectrophotometry, atomic absorption spectrophotometry, inductively coupled plasma-atomic emission spectrometry (ICP–AES), inductively coupled plasma-mass spectrometry (ICP–MS), among which flame atomic absorption spectrophotometry is convenient and widely used.

Principle

A sample solution is sprayed into flame, and the measuring element is transformed into ground state atoms. The characteristic spectral line radiated from the hollow cathode lamp (HCL) is absorbed to generate analysis signals. The measuring element is quantified compared with the standards substances.

Sample Pretreatment and Determination

The clarified water sample can be determined directly. For the determination of dissolved metals, the water sample should be filtered through a 0.45 μm microporous membrane during sampling and then acidified to pH≤2 by adding 1.5 mL nitric acid per liter of water sample. The water sample with more suspended substances needs acidification and digestion of organic compounds before analysis. The organic compounds in the water sample generally do not interfere with the determination. To ensure the metal ions can all enter the solution and promote the dissolution of particulate matter in favor of atomization, hydrochloric acid-nitric acid digestion method is often used. 5.0 mL of nitric acid is added to each liter of the acidified water sample, and then hydrochloric acid is added at the ratio of 5.0 mL hydrochloric acid to each 100 mL water sample. The sample solution is heated on an electric heating plate for 15 minutes, cooled to room temperature, filtered by a glass sand core filter, and diluted to a certain volume with pure water. The standard solutions, blank solution and the sample solution are sprayed into flame in turn, and the absorbance is measured. Then the standard curve is drawn and the concentration of the measuring element can be found.

See Table16-1 for reference operating conditions.

Table16–1   Reference operating conditions for determination of iron, manganese, copper and zinc by flame atomic absorption spectrophotometry

Elements	Fe	Mn	Cu	Zn
Analytical line (nm)	248.3	279.5	324.7	213.8
Spectral line passband (nm)	0.2	0.5	0.5	0.5
HCL electric current (mA)	10	5	5	5
Flame type	Air-acetylene flame	Air-acetylene flame	Air-acetylene flame	Air-acetylene flame
Burner height(mm)	7	7	7	7

16.3.2   Examination of Lead and Cadmium in Drinking Water

There are many methods for the determination of lead and cadmium in drinking water, such as flame atomic absorption spectrophotometry, graphite furnace atomic absorption spectrophotometry, atomic fluorescence spectrometry, ICP-AES and ICP-MS. The most commonly used method is graphite furnace atomic absorption spectrophotometry.

Principle

After proper pretreatment, the water sample is injected into the graphite furnace atomizer for atomization. The ground state atoms absorb the characteristic special line radiated by the hollow cathode lamp. Under certain conditions, the concentration of the measuring element is proportional to the absorbance and quantified accordingly.

Sample Pretreatment and Determination

1.0 mL of 120 g/L ammonium dihydrogen phosphate solution and 0.1 mL of 50 g/L magnesium nitrate solution are added into a 10.00 mL water sample and mixed well. At the same time, an equal volume of ammonium dihydrogen phosphate solution and magnesium nitrate solution are added into 10.00 mL nitric acid solution (1+99) as blank.

See Table16-2 for reference operating conditions.

Table16–2   Reference operating conditions for determination of lead and cadmium by graphite furnace atomic absorption spectrophotometry

Elements	Pb	Cd
Analytical line (nm)	283.3	228.8
Drying temperature and time	120℃, 30 s	120℃, 30 s
Ashing temperature and time	600℃, 30 s	900℃, 30 s
Atomization temperature and time	2 100℃, 3 s	1 800℃, 5 s
Purification temperature and time	2 600℃, 3 s	2 500℃, 3 s

16.3.3   Examination of Chromium (VI) in Drinking Water by Ultraviolet–Visible Spectrophotometry

Principle

Chromium (VI) reacts with diphenylcarbazide in acidic environment to form a purple water-soluble complex. Then the absorbance of the solution is measured at 540 nm, and chromium (VI) is quantified by standard curve.

Drawing Standard Curve and Determination

0, 0.20, 0.50, 1.00, 2.00, 4.00, 6.00, 8.00 and 10.00 mL of 1.00 μg/mL chromium (VI) standard application solutions are added into nine 50 mL colorimetric tubes, respectively, then the volumes are diluted to 50 mL with pure water. 50 mL of the clarified or pretreated water sample is added into a 50 mL colorimetric tube. 2.5 mL of sulfuric acid solution (1+7) and 2.5 mL of diphenylcarbazide solution are added to the water sample and the standard solutions, mixed and left for 10 minutes. The absorbance of standard solutions and the sample solution are measured at 540 nm with water as the reference. The absorbance - concentration curve is drawn, the regression equation is obtained, and the concentration of chromium (VI) in the water sample is calculated according to the regression equation.

16.3.4   Examination of Arsenic, Selenium and Mercury in Drinking Water

Arsenic in drinking water can be determined by hydride generation-atomic fluorescence spectrometry, ultraviolet-visible spectrophotometry, ICP-AES and ICP-MS, etc. The methods for the determination of selenium mainly include atomic fluorescence spectrometry, hydride generation atomic absorption spectrophotometry, ICP-AES and ICP-MS, etc. The analysis methods for detecting total mercury include atomic fluorescence spectrometry, cold atomic absorption spectrometry, dithizone spectrophotometry and ICP-MS, etc.

Atomic fluorescence spectrometry has been widely used in the detection of arsenic, selenium and mercury due to its high sensitivity, low detection limit, high accuracy and selectivity. Stannous chloride reduction-cold atomic absorption spectrometry is a special method for mercury analysis, which has the advantages of less interference and simple operation. Hydride generation atomic absorption spectrophotometry is an important method for the determination of selenium in water due to its advantages of low interference and high sensitivity.

16.3.4.1   Examination of Arsenic, Selenium and Mercury in Drinking Water by Atomic Fluorescence Spectrometry

Principle

After appropriate pretreatment, the various forms of arsenic, selenium and mercury in the drinking water are converted to arsenic (III), selenium (IV), mercury (II), respectively. in acidic environment, arsenic (III), selenium (IV), mercury (II) can be reduced by sodium borohydride (or potassium borohydride) to arsenic hydride (H_3As), selenium hydride (H_2Se) and elemental mercury, respectively, which are carried into electrically heated quartz atomizer by the carrier gas (argon) for atomization. The ground state atoms are excited to the excited-state by the emission line of the corresponding high-performance hollow cathode lamp, then the atomic fluorescence is emitted when excited state atoms return to the ground state. The concentrations of arsenic, selenium and mercury in the solution are proportional to their fluorescence intensity and are quantified by the calibration curve. The method detection limits of arsenic, selenium and mercury are 1.0 μg/L, 0.4 μg/L and 0.1 μg/L, respectively.

Sample Pretreatment and Determination

For the analysis of arsenic, 10.00 mL of water sample is added into colorimetric tube, then 1.0 mL of hydrochloric acid and 1.0 mL of solution (10% thiourea + 10% ascorbic acid) are added to the sample. Arsenic (V) in the sample is transformed to arsenic (III) for determination. For selenium analysis, 25.00 mL of water sample is added with 2.5 mL of nitric acid and perchloric acid mixture (1 : 1) in a conical flask. Then the conical flask is heated on an electric heating plate for digestion. When white fog appears in the conical flask, the conical flask should be removed and cooled. 2.5 mL of hydrochloric acid solution (1+1) is added in the solution. In order to reduce selenium (VI) to selenium (IV) completely, the solution is heated again until white fog appears. After cooled again, the solution is transferred to a colorimetric tube, and the volume is fixed to 10.00 mL with pure water. To analyze mercury, 1.0 mL of hydrochloric acid and 0.5 mL of potassium bromate - potassium bromide mixed solution are added to 10.00 mL water sample, blank solution and standard solutions. After being mixed well, the solutions are placed for 20 minutes, and all mercury is transformed to mercury (II). Finally, 1–2 drops of hydroxylamine hydrochloride solution are added to the water sample, blank solution and standard solutions to the yellow faded. The atomic fluorescence spectrometer is used for measuring. The reducing agent is 2% NaBH₄ solution and the carrier is 5% HCl solution.

See Table 16-3 for reference operating conditions.

Table16-3   Reference operating conditions for the determination of arsenic, selenium and mercury by atomic fluorescence spectrometry

Elements	As	Se	Hg
HCL electric current (mA)	45	70	30
Negative high voltage (V)	305	340	260
Furnace height (mm)	8.5	8	8.5
Carrier gas flow rate (mL/min)	500	500	500
Shield gas flow rate (mL/min)	1000	1000	1000

16.3.4.2   Examination of Total Selenium in Drinking Water by Hydride Generation Atomic Absorption Spectrophotometry

Principle

The drinking water sample is digested by nitric acid-perchloric acid (4:1), and then selenium (VI) is reduced to selenium (IV) by hydrochloric acid. In acidic environment, selenium (IV) is reduced to hydrogen selenide (H_2Se) by sodium borohydride (or potassium borohydride). H_2Se is carried by the carrier gas (argon) into an electrically heated quartz atomizer to atomization. The ground state selenium atoms absorb characteristic spectral line (196.0 nm) emitted by selenium hollow cathode lamp. Under certain conditions, the absorbance value is proportional to the concentration of selenium in the sample solution. The detection limit of selenium is 0.2 μg/L.

Sample Pretreatment and Determination

50.00 mL of water sample is added into a 100 mL conical flask. 2.0 mL of nitric acid-perchloric acid mixed solution (4 ∶ 1) is added to the sample. The sample solution is heated on an electric heating plate until perchloric acid fogs. After cooled, 4.0 mL of hydrochloric acid solution (1+1) is added to the sample solution, and it is heated for 10 minutes in water bath at 100°C. After cooled again, the solution is transferred into a 10 mL colorimetric tube where 1.0 mL of potassium ferricyanide solution (100 g/L) has been added before. Finally, the solution is diluted to 10.00 mL with pure water and mixed well being ready for atomic absorption spectrophotometer determination.

The reference operating conditions are as follows: Analysis line: 196 nm; current: 8 mA; slit width: 0.5 nm; carrier gas (argon) flow rate: 1.2 L/min; atomization temperature: 800 ℃.

16.3.4.3   Examination of Mercury in Drinking Water by Cold Atomic Absorption Spectrometry

Principle

After digestion of the water sample, the bond mercury is transformed to mercury ions, and then the mercury ions are reduced to elemental mercury vapor by stannous chloride($SnCl_2$). Mercury vapor is carried to the lightpath by the carrier gas and absorbs 253.7 nm characteristic spectral line. Within a certain range of mercury concentration, the concentration of mercury is proportional to the absorbance and is quantified by the work curve.

Sample Pretreatment and Determination

The polluted water sample is digested by sulfuric acid-potassium permanganate, and the clarified water sample is digested by potassium bromate-potassium bromide. The standard solutions are pretreated in the same way as the sample solution.

Sulfuric acid-potassium permanganate digestion method is as follows. 2.0 mL of 50 g/L potassium permanganate solution and 50.00 mL of water sample are added into a 100 mL conical flask, then 2.0 mL of sulfuric acid is dropped into the sample. The sample solution is heated to boiling for 5 minutes on the electric stove, and then cooled. Next, 100 g/L hydroxylamine hydrochloride solution is added drop by drop until the purple color of potassium permanganate fades. And then the solution is placed for 30 min. Finally, the solution is transferred to a 100 mL volumetric flask and diluted with pure water to 100 mL for determination.

The potassium bromate-potassium bromide method is shown below. The 50.00 mL of water sample is added into a 100 mL volumetric flask, and 2.0 mL of sulfuric acid and 4.0 mL potassium bromate-potassium bromate solution are successively added to the sample, which is mixed and laid up for 10 min. Several drops of hydroxylamine hydrochloride solution are added until the yellow color disappears to terminate bromination. Then the solution volume is diluted to100 mL with pure water. It is determined by the cold atomic absorption mercury meter.

The reference operating conditions are as follows: The connection between the mercury meter and the mercury bottle is checked for no air leakage. The cold atomic absorption mercury meter is adjusted according to the instructions.

16.3.5   Simultaneous Examination of Metals in Drinking Water

16.3.5.1   ICP-AES

ICP-AES is suitable for simultaneous determination of several metals in drinking water, including silver, aluminum, arsenic, barium, beryllium, calcium, cadmium, cobalt, chromium, copper, iron, potassium, lithium, magnesium, manganese, molybdenum, sodium, nickel, lead, antimony, selenium, strontium, thallium, vanadium and zinc.

Principle

A water sample is carried into the atomization system of the inductively coupled plasma-atomic emission spectrometer by high-purity argon to form aerosol which enters the axial channel of plasma. The water sample is fully evaporated, atomized, ionized and excited in a plasma torch in inert atmosphere at high temperature. The characteristic spectral line of the mesauring elements is emitted. After splitting, each element is qualitatively analyzed according to characteristic emission spectral line and quantitatively analyzed according to characteristic emission spectral line intensity using the standard curve method.

Sample Pretreatment and Determination

100.00 mL of drinking water sample is filtered by 0.45 μm microporous membrane. 2.00 mL of concentrated nitric acid is added into a 100 mL volumetric flask and diluted to 100 mL with the filtered water sample. The solution is mixed well for measuring. The reagent blank solution is prepared at the same time. The mixed metals standard series solutions, blank solution and sample solution are determined successively. The standard curves of multiple metal elements are drawn and the concentrations of multiple metals are determined.

The reference operating conditions are as follows: Incident power:1200 W; working gas: argon; cooling gas flow rate:15 L/min; carrier gas flow rate: 0.80 L/min; auxiliary flow rate: 1.50 L/min: injection time:30s; integral time:3s. The recommended analysis lines are as follows: lead: 220.35 nm, cadmium: 226.50 nm, chromium: 267.72, arsenic: 193.70 nm, selenium: 196.03 nm, iron: 259.94 nm, manganese: 257.61 nm, copper: 324.75 nm. The analysis lines of other metal elements can be found in "Standard Examination Methods for Drinking Water—Metal Parameters" (GB 5750.6-2023).

16.3.5.2   ICP-MS

ICP-MS is suitable for the simultaneous determination of various metals in drinking water including silver, aluminum, arsenic, barium, beryllium, calcium, cadmium, cobalt, chromium, copper, iron, lithium, magnesium, manganese, molybdenum, sodium, nickel, lead, antimony, selenium, strontium, tin, thorium, thallium, titanium, uranium, vanadium, zinc and mercury.

Principle

A water sample is pumped through a peristaltic pump into a ncbulizer to produce a fine aerosol spray. The smallest droplets filtered by the spray chamber are injected at a high speed into the ICP torch, where the inductively coupled plasma is formed from ionization of argon gas. The hot plasma heated to a temperature of 6 000 K to 10 000 K dries the aerosol, dissociates the molecules, and forms singly charged positive ions by stripping off an electron from the metal atoms. The positive ions pass through the interface cones into the mass spectrometer, which separates the positive ions according to the mass-to-charge ratio(m/z). The positive ions with a specific m/z are allowed to pass and hit the ion detector, thereby translating the signal into analyte concentration.

Determination

The water samples are directly injected for determination. When the vacuum degree of the instrument reaches the requirement, the instrument indicators are adjusted well using 10 ng/L of lithium, yttrium, cerium, thallium and cobalt mixed mass spectrometry tuning solution. After the sensitivity, oxide, double charge and resolution reach the determination requirements, the internal standard solution (1 μg/mL mixed solution of lithium, scandium, germanium, yttrium, thallium and cobalt) is used to adjust the sensitivity. After the sensitivity of internal standard and P/A adjustment index reach the requirements, the reagent blank solution, standard series solutions and sample solution are determined, respectively.

The reference operating conditions are as follows: Radio frequency (RF) power: 1 200 W~ 1550 W; carrier gas flow: 1.10 L/min; sampling depth: 7 mm; atomizer: barbinton type; sampling cone: nickel cone.

Glossary

drinking water 生活饮用水 potable water and domestic water

centralized water supply 集中式供水 water catchment is concentrated in the water source and the water is delivered to the users or the public watering points through water distribution network

regular indices 常规指标 indicators reflecting the basic condition of drinking water quality

expanded indices 扩展指标 indicators reflecting the characteristics of drinking water quality and water quality in a certain period of time or under special circumstances

iron *n.* 铁 a metallic element with atomic number 26 in the periodic table of elements and relative atomic mass 55.85

manganese *n.* 锰 a metallic element with atomic number 25 in the periodic table of elements and relative atomic mass 54.94

copper *n.* 铜 a metallic element with atomic number 29 in the periodic table of elements and relative atomic mass 63.55

zinc *n.* 锌 a metallic element with atomic number 30 in the periodic table of elements and relative atomic mass 65.38

lead *n*. 铅 a metallic element with atomic number 82 in the periodic table of elements and relative atomic mass 207.2

cadmium *n*. 镉 a metallic element with atomic number 48 in the periodic table of elements and relative atomic mass 112.41

chromium *n*. 铬 a metallic element with atomic number 24 in the periodic table of elements and relative atomic mass 51.996

arsenic *n*. 砷 a metalloid element with atomic number 33 in the periodic table of elements and relative atomic mass 74.92

selenium *n*. 硒 a metalloid element with atomic number 34 in the periodic table of elements and relative atomic mass 78.96

mercury *n*. 汞 a metallic element with atomic number 80 in the periodic table of elements and relative atomic mass 200.59

ground state 基态 a state when an atom or molecule is in the lowest of all possible energy levels

excited state 激发态 a state when the ground state electrons jump to higher energy states after atoms or molecules absorb energy equivalent to the energy level difference

standard curve 标准曲线 a curve describing the quantitative relationship between the standard substance content and the instrument response value

characteristic spectral line 特征谱线 the radiation absorbed (or emitted) by elements atoms when they are excited from the ground state to the first excited state (or jump back from the first excited state to the ground state)

digestion *n*. 消化 the decomposition of a solid sample by a liquid reagent into a homogeneous system

analytical line 分析线 spectral lines used for qualitative identification and quantitative analysis by atomic spectrometry

sensitivity *n*. 灵敏度 the amount of changes in the analysis signals when the quantity or concentration of the measured component changes by one unit

detection limit 检出限 the minimum mass or concentration of a component can be detected by the analytical method with an appropriate confidence probability (typically 95%)

absorbance *n*. 吸光度 the logarithm of the ratio of the incident light intensity to the transmitted light intensity

（李淑荣）

新形态教材网·数字课程学习……

📺教学 PPT   📝自测题   💬推荐阅读

Chapter 17
Determination of Hippuric Acid and Methylhippuric Acid in Urine by HPLC

Learning objectives:

- Know the collection and pretreatment methods of urine samples.
- Understand the value of hippuric acid determination.
- Master the analytical method of HPLC.

17.1 The Significance of Determination of Hippuric Acid and Methylhippuric Acid in Urine

Toluene and xylene are frequently utilized in the production of dyes, plastics, artificial flavors, and synthetic fibers. Additionally, they serve as solvents or diluents and are widely employed in industrial processes such as paint, rubber, and leather production. Both toluene and xylene are clear, transparent, and volatile liquids with an aromatic scent. At room temperature and under constant pressure, they exist in the air as vapors and are primarily absorbed into the human body through the respiratory tract. In their liquid state, they can also be absorbed through the digestive tract and skin.

Both toluene and xylene are organic compounds that are considered to be low-toxic. However, in large doses, they can have adverse effects on the central nervous system and cause irritation to the skin and mucous membranes. When toluenc enters the human body, approximately 15% to 20% of it is excreted through the respiratory tract in its original form, which is a specific indicator used in toluene biological monitoring. Only about 1% of the toluene is excreted in the urine, while the rest is primarily metabolized in the body. During metabolism, the liver microsome monoamine oxidase enzyme, in the presence of the coenzyme II, oxidizes about 80% of the toluene to benzyl methanol. This is then further oxidized to benzaldehyde in the presence of the coenzyme I, and finally oxidized to benzoic acid.

In the presence of coenzyme A and adenosine triphosphate, benzoic acid readily combines with glycine to form hippuric acid (HA), which is subsequently excreted in the urine. Additionally, small amounts of benzoic acid, sulfuric acid, and glucuronic acid are also excreted in the urine. When toluene is present, it is oxidized to methyl hydroxybenzene and then combined with sulfuric acid and glucuronic acid. The concentration of HA in urine increases rapidly 2 hours after exposure to toluene and reaches its peak after 16 to 18 hours following the cessation of exposure. Therefore, HA can serve as a reliable biomarker for toluene exposure.

It is important to acknowledge that HA is present in normal urine and exposure to organic compounds like ethylene benzene, benzene, styrene, benzene formaldehyde, benzyl methanol, and benzoic acid can elevate the HA levels in human urine. As a result, urinary HA cannot be considered a specific biomonitoring indicator of toluene exposure. Nevertheless, due to its straightforward measurement process and ease of use, it still holds some value in assessing human toluene exposure in studies involving the exposed population.

Approximately 5% of xylene in the body is expelled through the lungs, while 60% to 80% is metabolized in the liver to form methyl benzoic acid, diphenol, and hydroxybenzoic acid. The majority of methyl benzoic acid binds with glycine to produce methylhippuric acid (MHA), with 15% to 20% of MHA being excreted in the urine after binding with glucuronic acid or sulfuric acid. The concentration of free methyl benzoic acid in urine is typically low in healthy individuals, but exposure to xylene can increase MHA levels in urine, which is a specific and widely used biological monitoring indicator of xylene exposure. The National Health Commission of the People's Republic of China has set occupational exposure limits for hazardous agents in the workplace, with a limit of 1.5 g/g Cr or 2.0 g/L for toluene in the urine of occupational workers after work, and a limit of 0.3 g/g Cr or 0.4 g/L for MHA in workers exposed to xylene after work.

17.2 Collection and Preservation of Urine Samples

17.2.1 Characteristics of Urine Samples

Urine is a widely used biological material for testing, owing to its ease of collection. It is particularly suitable for monitoring water-soluble chemicals, such as metabolites and metals. When the body absorbs and metabolizes various chemicals, their original form or metabolites are excreted in the urine. The concentration of these substances in urine is positively correlated with their concentration in the blood, making urine an effective indicator of chemical exposure and body homeostasis. The amount of chemicals excreted through urine is influenced by renal function, including the degree of water reabsorption. Additionally, the content of foreign chemicals in urine is affected by factors such as water intake, diet, physical activity, and metabolic characteristics.

Urine samples come in various types, including whole day's urine (also known as 24-hour urine), first-time urine, random urine, and timed urine. Timed urine refers to samples collected at specific times, such as pre-shift, during-shift, and post-shift. Pre-shift samples are collected at 16 hours after occupational exposure, within 30 minutes before the start of the next shift. During-shift samples are collected from 2 hours after occupational contact until before work. Post-shift samples are collected within 30 minutes after stopping occupational contact. Whole day's urine is the best option for reflecting the excretion of chemicals and their metabolites, as well as the dose in vivo, as it is less affected by the amount of drinking water and sweating. However, it is difficult to collect, transport, and save total urine. Morning urine, random urine, and regular urine are easier to collect, but the measurement results may deviate due to changes in urine sample gravity. Therefore, the concentration of measured objects should be corrected using the urine specific gravity method or urine creatinine method. During biological monitoring of workers, the appropriate urine sample type should be selected based on the biological half-reduction period of the chemicals, inspection requirements, and biomarker characteristics.

17.2.2   The Collection of Urine Samples

The sampling time plays a crucial role in determining the accuracy of biomaterial test results and their evaluation. It is imperative to strictly control the sampling time due to the short half-reduction period of HA. Typically, 100 mL urine samples are collected in either plastic or glass bottles, and the urine specific gravity or creatinine content should be determined promptly before adding any preservatives. When determining HA in urine using the photometric method, trichloromethane should be added in a volume ratio of 100 + 1 and thoroughly shaken. The bottle should be sealed and stored in a 4℃ refrigerator for two weeks or in a -20℃ refrigerator for more than a month. If determined by liquid chromatography, concentrated hydrochloric acid should be added to 0.1% of the urine, which can be stored for up to two weeks. It is essential to be mindful of any factors that can affect the HA content during sampling, such as drinking, medication, and other poisons.

17.2.3   Preservation and Transport of Urine Samples

At room temperature, urine can degrade, leading to precipitation or bacterial growth, which can damage the chemicals being measured. Therefore, it is crucial to seal collected samples promptly, cryopreserve them, and transport them as soon as possible for analysis. If immediate analysis is not possible, samples should be stored at either 4℃ or -20℃. It is important to note that cryopreserved samples should not be packed in glass containers to prevent freezing and cracking.

17.3   Determination of Urine Specific Gravity and Urinary Creatinine

To mitigate the impact of drinking water and perspiration, and to accurately compare urine samples collected at different times, it is crucial to determine the specific proportion of urine or creatinine content immediately after sampling. This correction helps to ensure the accuracy of measurement results.

17.3.1   Determination of Urine Specific Gravity

The specific gravity of urine is a measure of its weight in relation to the weight of an equal amount of pure water at 4℃, as determined by a specialized hydrometer. The specific gravity of urine can vary significantly among individuals due to differences in diet, hydration, sweating, and urination. Typically, the specific gravity of urine should fall between 1.010 and 1.025, but it can fluctuate between 1.003 and 1.030 depending on various factors. For instance, drinking ample water can lower the specific gravity of urine to 1.003, while drinking less water and sweating more can increase it to over 1.030. Urine samples with a specific gravity below 1.010 or above 1.030 should be discarded and resampled for accurate determination, as they indicate high or low concentration after gravity correction

17.3.2   Determination of Urinary Creatinine

Urinary creatinine levels are measured using spectrophotometry (WS/T 97-1996) or high-performance liquid chromatography (WS/T 97-1996), in accordance with the current health industry standards set forth by the Ministry of Health of the People's Republic of China.

17.3.2.1   Spectrophotometry

Reagent

To prepare the alkaline saturated bitter acid solution, mix 1 portion of 100 g/L sodium hydroxide solution with 10 parts of saturated bitter acid solution (approximately 15 g/L) and ensure thorough mixing before use. For the creatinine standard solution, dry 100 mg of creatinine at 110°C for 2 hours, dissolve it in hydrochloric solution, and dilute with water to obtain a 0.1 mg/mL standard solution.

Analytical Procedure

0.1 mL of urine sample is transfered into a 10 mL test tube, which is then diluted with water to a volume of 3 mL. A reagent blank is prepared by adding 3 mL of pure water to a 10 mL test tube. To prepare the standard tubes, six test tubes are used and the contents are prepared according to the specifications outlined in Table 17-1:

Table 17–1   Preparation of creatinine standard tubes

Tube number	0	1	2	3	4	5
Creatinine standard solution (0.1mg/mL), mL	0	0.2	0.4	0.6	0.8	1.0
Deionized water ,mL	3.0	2.8	2.6	2.4	2.2	2.0
The concentration of creatinine,g/L	0	0.2	0.4	0.6	0.8	1.0

To begin the analysis, 2.0 mL of basic picric acid solution is added to each standard tube and allowed to react for 20-30 minutes at room temperature. The resulting mixture is then mixed with 5 mL of pure water. Using the zero tube as a reference, the absorbance of the mixture is measured at 490 nm within 0.5 hours. Each concentration solution is measured three times to obtain the mean absorbance value, which is then used to create a calibration curve with creatinine concentration (g/L) as the x-coordinate and the mean absorbance as the y-coordinate. The sensitivity parameters of the reagent blank are analyzed using calibration curves under the same conditions. Finally, the absorbance of the sample is measured with the reagent blank as a reference under the same conditions as the calibration curve.

Results Calculated

Concentration of creatinine are calculated based on the calibration curve. To calculate the concentration of creatinine in urine, the following formula is used (17-1)

$$C = c \times f \qquad\qquad 17\text{--}1$$

Here, C represents the concentration of creatinine (g/L) in urine, c is the concentration of creatinine (g/L) obtained from the standard curve, and f denotes the urine dilution factor.

17.3.2.2   High performance liquid chromatography

High performance liquid chromatography (HPLC) is a crucial branch of chromatography that utilizes liquid as the mobile phase. It employs a high-pressure infusion system to pump a single solvent with varying polarities or mixed solvents, buffers, and other mobile phases with different polarities into a stationary phase. In the chromatographic column, each component is separated, and then it enters the detector for detection, enabling the analysis of the sample. HPLC boasts high separation efficiency, sensitivity, fast analysis speed, and a wide range of applications, making it a popular choice for analyzing biological materials.

Chromatographic Conditions

The column: C18, 4 mm × 300 mm, 5 μm; Mobile phase: a mixture of 95%:5% v/v 0.05 mol/L sodiumacetate methanol; Flflow rate: 0.9 mL/min; Column temperature: room temperature; UV detector: λ = 254 nm.

Creatinine Calibration Curves

250 mg of creatinine is first dissolved and diluted with methanol to create a 25 mL creatinine standard stock solution with a concentration of 10 mg/mL. This stock solution is then further diluted with methanol to create a 100 μg/mL creatinine standard solution, which is subsequently used to prepare a series of creatinine standard solutions with concentrations ranging of 0, 2.0, 4.0, 6.0, 8.0, 10.0 μg/mL. For each concentration in the standard series, 10 μL of the solution is analyzed to determine the corresponding peak height or peak area. To ensure accuracy, each concentration solution is injected six times and the average is calculated. The resulting calibration curve is plotted using the creatinine concentration (μg/mL) as the x-coordinate and the mean peak height or peak area as the y-coordinate.

Sample Analysis

0.05 mL urine samples is diluted 200-500 times in the mobile phase and mix on a vortex mixer for 1min to determine the peak height or peak area under the same conditions. The concentration of creatinine (μg/mL) is then checked using the calibration curve.

Results Calculated

Urine creatinine concentration is calculated by the equation (17-2)

$$C = \frac{c \times v}{V} \qquad\qquad 17\text{--}2$$

C is the urinary creatinine concentration, μg/mL; c is the creatinine concentration obtained from the calibration curve, μg/mL; v is the volume of the urine sample dilution , mL, and V is the volume of the urine sample , mL.

The urine samples should be discarded and resanpled for determination, while it with a creatinine concentration of less than 0.3 g/L or greater than 3.0 g/L.

17.4   Determination of Urinary HA and MHA

The determination of urinary HA can be carried out using various methods, including spectrophotometry, gas chromatography, and HPLC.

Spectrophotometry techniques such as pyridine-phenylsulfonyl chlorophotometry, subbromine photometry, and fluorescence photometry are commonly used. Pyridine-phenylsulfonyl chlorophotometry is preferred for large sample analysis due to its simplicity and no sample preparation requirement. However, this method can be affected by MHA and creatinine, and the pyridine used has an unpleasant odor. Hypobromine photometry is not recommended due to the interference of urea. Fluorescent photometry is highly sensitive and requires minimal sample size and processing, but it can be affected by benzoyl derivatives.

Urinary HA and MHA can be accurately determined through gas chromatography after esterification. Although this method can effectively separate HA and MHA from other interfering components in urine, it is a complex process. Alternatively, the most widely used analytical method is HPLC, which can easily separate HA and MHA from other coexisting components in urine. This method is highly sensitive, simple, and rapid, making it an ideal choice for determining HA and MHA in urine. Therefore, the following will mainly focus on the HPLC method for determining HA and MHA in urine.

Principle

The principle urine is acidified and then HA and MHA are extracted using ethyl acetate. The two compounds are then separated using a Cl8 column and quantified using a UV detector and peak area. The lowest detectable concentrations of HA and MHA are 0.015 mg/L and 0.03 mg/L (per 1 ml urine sample), respectively.

Standard Curve

50.00 mg of HA and MHA are dissolved in pure water and transferred to a 50 mL volumetric flask, which is then diluted to volume. The concentration of the stock standard solution for HA and MHA is 1 mg/mL, respectively. A series of multicomponent working standard solutions are prepared according to table 17-2. The calibration curve is generated using either HA or MHA as the x-coordinate and the peak area of HA or MHA as the y-coordinate.

Table 17-2　Preparation of working standard for the HA and MHA

Tube number	0	1	2	3
Stock standard solution, mL	0	0.10	0.20	0.5
Deionized water, mL	1.0	0.90	0.80	0.5
The mass of HA, mg	0	0.10	0.20	0.5
The mass of MHA, mg	0	0.10	0.20	0.5

The working standard tube can be increased to 5 units. For example, in the fourth tube, the mass of HA and MHA is 0.8 mg, while in the fifth tube, the mass of HA and MHA is 1.0 mg.

Sample Treatment

1.0 mL of the sample is transferred to a 10 mL centrifuge tube. Next, 0.10 mL of hydrochloric acid solution (1:1) is added to the tube and mixed thoroughly. To this mixture, 0.3 g of sodium chloride and 4 mL of ethyl acetate are added. The tube is then vortexed for 1 minute and centrifuged at 1,000 r/min for 5 minutes. After centrifugation, 0.40 mL of the supernatant is carefully transferred to a test tube and either bathed at 70℃ or dried using nitrogen flow. The residue is then dissolved in 1.0 mL of pure water to create the final test solution.

Instrument Reference Condition

Chromatcolumn: C18 column (15 cm × 4.6 mm × 5 μm); Column temperature: 35℃; Mobile phase: a mixture of 20% methanol: 80% deionized water:0.01% glacial acetic acid (v/v); Flflow rate: 1 mL/min; UV detection wavelength: 254 nm.

HPLC Determination

A 10 mL test solution and a mixture of working standard solution of HA and MHA are separately injected into the HPLC instrument. The operating conditions of the instrument are followed to obtain qualitative information on the retention time and quantified information on the peak area. Each solution is injected three times, and the mean peak area is calculated. The concentration of HA or MHA in the urine sample is determined using equation (17-3)

$$c = \frac{m \times 1000}{V} \qquad 17\text{-}3$$

Where c represents the concentration of HA or MHA, mg/L; m is the content of HA or MHA checked on the calibration curve, μg, V is the sample volume, μL.

Result Representation

To represent the results of urine sample determination accurately, it is necessary to correct the urine specific gravity to a standard specific gravity of 1.020. Alternatively, the results can be indicated by the total 24-hour discharge or content in creatinine per gram.

The corrected urine concentration can be calculated using the following equation:

$$c_{\text{correction}} = \frac{1.020 - 1.000}{d - 1.000} \times c \qquad 17\text{-}4$$

Where $c_{\text{correction}}$ is the concentration of the corrected urine (mg/L); c is the concentration (mg/L) of the measured urine (mg/L); 1.020 is the standard gravity of urine; d is the actual urine gravity.

It is generally observed that diet, drinking volume, and diuretics have minimal impact on creatinine discharge rates. Healthy individuals typically excrete around 1.8 g of creatinine in their urine per day. Therefore, the amount of the components to be measured corresponding to 1 g of creatinine excreted in the urine can be used to determine the concentration of the components in the urine. The conversion equation for this purpose is:

$$C\ (mg/gCr) = \frac{c_{HA/MHA}}{c_{Cr}} \qquad 17\text{-}5$$

Where $C\ (mg/gCr)$ is the concentration (mg/g) of HA or MHA that has been adjusted for urinary creatinine. $c_{HA/MHA}$, is the concentration of HA or MHA that has been directly measured in urine, while c_{Cr} is the concentration of creatinine in urine. By multiplying the C value by 1.8, we can determine the content of the components being tested in 24-hour urine (mg/24 h).

Precautions

1. To stabilize a urine sample for at least 15 days, HCL can be added at a concentration of 0.1%, or thymol can be added at the same concentration and stored at 4℃. Alternatively, the sample can be acidified, extracted with ethyl acetate, steamed in the extraction water bath, or stored in a 4℃ refrigerator, which will maintain stability for at least six months.

2. The presence of urinary creatinine, zoic acid, phenol, nitrophenol and other cophorents will not affect the determination of HA and MHA.

Glossary

biological monitoring 生物监测 the systematic collection of human biological material samples, and the regular detection of the content of toxicants or their metabolites, to evaluate the degree of human exposure to chemical substances and their impact on health

indicator(s) of biological monitoring 生物监测指标 the harmful substances and their metabolites in the body, which can be used for biological monitoring after occupational exposure to harmful substances

metabolism *in vivo* 体内代谢 the general term for a series of ordered chemical reactions in the body to maintain life

biomarker *n*. 生物标志物 a change that occurs after the biological system is exposed to exogenous substances, mainly the metabolites formed by chemical substances in the organism and measurable biochemical, physiological, immune, cellular or molecular changes

biological material 生物材料 a general term for human body fluids (such as blood), excrement (such as exhaled breath, urine), hair, nails, and tissue organs

occupational exposure biological limit 职业接触限值 the allowable exposure level of workers who have been exposed repeatedly for a long time in the process of occupational activities without harmful effects on the health of most contacts

urinary creatinine 尿肌酐 the amount of creatinine excreted in the urine

specific gravity of urine 尿比重 the weight ratio of urine to the same volume of pure water at 4℃

whole day's urine 全日尿 all urine within 24 hours

first morning urine 晨尿 the urine discharged for the first time after getting up in the morning without having breakfast and exercise

random urine 随机尿 urine samples taken at random

timed urine 定时尿 urine samples collected at a specific time, such as pre-shift, during-shift, post-shift, etc.

pre-shift *n*. 班前 16 hours after occupational exposure (within 30 minutes before the start of the next shift)

during-shift *n*. 班中 the period from 2 h after occupational contact to before work

post-shift *n*. 班末 the shortest time (30 minutes) after stopping occupational contact

（黄东萍）

新形态教材网·数字课程学习……

🖥教学 PPT　　📝自测题　　💬推荐阅读

Chapter 18
Physicochemical Determinantion of Cosmetics

Learning objectives:

- Know the detection of the special chemical components of cosmetics.
- Understand the testing basis of cosmetics.
- Be familiar with the sample collection method for cosmetics.
- Master the sensory test and general physical and chemical indicators test of cosmetics.

18.1   Overview of Cosmetics Testing

Cosmetics are daily chemical products that are applied to various parts of the human body, including the skin, hair, nails, and lips, through methods such as embrocation, spraying, or other similar techniques. Their primary purpose is to clean, eliminate bad odors, provide skin care, enhance beauty, and modify appearance. With a wide range of functions, shapes, and appearances, cosmetics can be categorized into two main types: general-purpose cosmetics and special-purpose cosmetics. General-purpose cosmetics include skin care, hair care, aroma, and beauty products, while special-purpose cosmetics are designed for specific uses such as hair growth, hair coloring, perm, hair removal, breast beauty, bodybuilding, deodorant, freckle removal, and sun protection.

Cosmetics play a significant role in people's daily lives, and ensuring their safety is of utmost importance. To achieve this, it is crucial to strengthen the quality inspection of cosmetics. In our country, current regulations for cosmetics quality management include "Safety and Technical Standards for Cosmetics" (2015 Edition) promulgated by the former State Food and Drug Administration, and "Inspection Rules for Cosmetics" (GB/T 37625-2019) jointly promulgated by the State Administration for Market Regulation and the China National Standardization Administration. "Safety and Technical Standards for Cosmetics" is a revised version of "Cosmetics Hygiene Specifications" (2007 Edition) issued by the former Ministry of Health. These standards outline the requirements for permitted components and inspection and evaluation methods, which are crucial for cosmetic production and supervision in China. "Inspection Rules for Cosmetics (GB/T 37625-2019)" stipulates the terms and definitions of cosmetic inspection,

inspection classification, batching rules and sampling plans, sampling methods, judgment and re-inspection rules, transfer rules, suspension and resumption, and selection of inspection methods. By adhering to these regulations, we can ensure the safe use of cosmetics and protect the health of consumers.

Cosmetics testing items are categorized into routine inspection items and non-routine inspection items based on the type of inspection required. Routine inspection items are designed to evaluate the sensory, physical, and chemical performance indicators (excluding heat and cold resistance), net content, packaging appearance requirements, and the total number of colonies, molds, and yeasts in the hygienic indicators for each batch of cosmetics. On the other hand, non-routine inspection items are intended to assess the heat resistance and cold resistance in the physical and chemical properties of each batch of cosmetics, as well as other hygienic indicators, except for the total number of bacterial colonies, mold, and yeast.

Cosmetics must undergo rigorous testing before they are made available to consumers. These tests include physical and chemical tests, microbiological tests, toxicological tests, and human safety tests. Additionally, cosmetics must undergo a safety risk assessment to ensure that they do not pose any harm to human health when used normally and reasonably. The production of cosmetics must adhere to strict cosmetic production specifications, and the production process must be scientifically designed and executed to guarantee product safety.

18.2　Sampling Method of Cosmetics

18.2.1　Sampling of cosmetics

The importance of using the correct sampling method cannot be overstated when it comes to cosmetic detection. To ensure accurate inspection of sensory, physical, and chemical performance indicators, net content, and hygienic indicators, samples must be randomly selected from the batch and sufficient in quantity to cover all necessary indicators and reserve samples. The samples should be labeled with the production date, shelf life or production batch number, expiration date, date of sampling, and the name of the person who took the sample. For inspecting the appearance of the package, a representative sampling method should be used to ensure the quality of the entire batch. If the inspection batch consists of several layers of pumping unit products, a hierarchical method should be used. Any intact units of product after inspection can be returned to the original lot. During type inspection, unconventional inspection items can be randomly selected from 2 to 4 units of products from any batch of products and inspected according to the methods specified in the product standards. It is important to note that routine inspection items are subject to the results of the factory inspection during type inspection, and the type inspection of the reserved samples will be carried out, and the samples will not be repeated.

18.2.2 Sampling Principles for Cosmetic Inspection

(1) During the sampling process of cosmetic products, it is crucial to consider the representativeness and uniformity of the samples. Sampling should be carried out in accordance with the use method of cosmetic samples to ensure that the result analysis accurately reflects the quality of cosmetics.

(2) Upon receipt of the sample, the laboratory worker must register and verify the integrity of the seal.

(3) Prior to analysis, it is imperative to observe the properties and characteristics of the sample, ensuring it is mixed thoroughly.

(4) After opening the package, it is important to analyze the samples promptly. If storage is necessary (excluding easily oxidized products), the container should be tightly sealed to maintain the product's quality. In cases where the product is sold in bulk or subpackaged, existing regulations may not provide a sampling method. In such instances, it is essential to develop a reasonable sampling method and document the actual sampling steps, attaching them to the original record.

18.2.3 Sampling Requirements for Different Types of Cosmetic Inspection

Liquid Samples

Liquid samples, including oil solutions, alcohol solutions, aqueous solutions, floral water, and skin lotions, should possess good fluidity. It is important to read the instructions for using the product before sampling to ensure the uniformity of the sample. After removing the sample to be analyzed, the container should be closed promptly.

Semi-fluid Samples and Semi-solid Samples

Semi-fluid and semi-solid cosmetic products, such as creams, honey, and gels, require specific sampling techniques. For narrow-necked containers, it is recommended to discard at least 1 cm of the cosmetic initially before squeezing out the required sample size. The container should be closed immediately after sampling. For wide-mouth containers, the surface layer should be scraped off before taking out the sample, and the container should be closed immediately after sampling.

Solid Samples

Solid samples, including loose powder, powder, and lipstick, require specific sampling techniques. Prior to opening, the loose powder sample should be shaken vigorously to ensure uniformity, and then a test portion should be removed. For powder cake and lipstick samples, the surface layer should be scraped off before sampling.

Other dosage forms can be sampled using appropriate methods based on the sampling principle or product standard.

18.3 Sensory Inspection of Cosmetics

The primary factors that are assessed during cosmetic sensory inspection are color, aroma, texture, appearance, clarity, powder, block shape, and structure. The sensory evaluation process involves various methods, including:

Visual Inspection

Visual inspection is a crucial sensory evaluation method for assessing the quality of cosmetics. This method involves evaluating cosmetics based on their reaction on the visual organ. The primary indicators for visual inspection include appearance, gloss, color, powder, transparency, block type, and uniformity. It is essential to conduct visual inspection under natural light or similar lighting conditions to ensure accurate assessment.

Olfactory Test

Olfactory testing is a reliable method for assessing the response of cosmetic products to the sense of smell. This test evaluates the product's ability to stimulate the olfactory organs and elicit a positive sensory experience.

Odors Test

This test is used to detect the volatile substances, such as fragrances, that are emitted by cosmetic products. This test involves rubbing the product on a clean palm and identifying the scent through olfactory identification.

Taste Test

Taste tests are typically conducted when visual and olfactory tests yield normal results. For instance, toothpaste aroma is evaluated through the taste method.

Tactile Test

The tactile test relies on the sensory nerves in the hands, skin, and other organs to assess the softness, hardness, stickiness, packing, adhesion, caking, and doughiness of cosmetics. This is achieved through actions such as touching, stroking, pinching, kneading, rubbing, and pressing, and the quality of the product is determined through judgment.

18.4 Detection of General Physical and Chemical Test Indicators of Cosmetics

The detection of general physical and chemical test indicators is a crucial aspect of cosmetic inspection quality. This routine test item encompasses a range of factors, such as pH value, turbidity, relative density, color stability, heat/cold resistance, centrifugal strength, leakage, and drying time. By assessing these indicators, the quality and effectiveness of cosmetics can be evaluated and improved.

pH

pH is a crucial performance indicator for cosmetics. The pH range of human skin typically falls between 4.5 to 6.5. Therefore, creams and lotions applied to the skin must have an

221

appropriate pH value. Products that are too acidic or too alkaline can lead to skin irritation. The "Safety and Technical Standards for Cosmetics" mandates the potentiometric method as the standard approach for measuring the pH value of cosmetics.

Turbidity

Turbidity refers to the cloudy or hazy state of certain substances or their aqueous solutions, which results in the absorption or obstruction of light passing through the sample. This property reflects the water solubility of the substance and is closely related to its chemical composition. In the context of water-based cosmetics, such as perfumes, turbidity is considered a key indicator of their physical and chemical quality. Cosmetic turbidity is typically assessed through visual inspection, which involves observing the clarity of the sample in a water bath or other refrigerants.

Relative Density

Relative density refers to the mass ratio of a given volume of a cosmetic sample to pure water at a specific temperature, denoted as d. The temperature of the water used should be indicated in the lower right corner of d, while the temperature of the object being tested should be indicated in the upper right corner. For instance, d? represents the relative density of a liquid at 25℃ compared to pure water at 4℃. There are three methods for determining the relative density of cosmetics: the density bottle method, densitometer method, and instrument method. The density bottle and densitometer methods are used for liquid cosmetics, while the instrument method is used for semi-solid cosmetics.

Color Stability

Color stability refers to the process of observing the color of cosmetics and testing its resistance to high temperatures. This is achieved by placing two samples in different environments, one in a 48-hour incubator and the other at room temperature. After 24 hours, a visual comparison is made to determine whether the color of the incubator sample has changed.

Heat/cold Resistance Test

Heat/cold resistance testing involves placing a specific amount of cosmetic product in a constant temperature incubator at a predetermined temperature. After a specified amount of time, the sample is removed from the incubator and returned to room temperature. The properties and performance of the sample are then observed, or it is compared to the original product.

Centrifugation Test

Centrifugation test is a method used to determine the stability of cosmetics. This involves placing the cosmetics in a constant temperature incubator for a specific duration, followed by immediate centrifugation. After a certain period, the samples are taken out and observed for any signs of stratification.

Leak Test

The leak test involves adjusting the temperature of the constant temperature water bath to (50 ± 2)℃ beforehand. Next, three bottles of samples are added and shaken thoroughly before placing them upright in the water bath with the plastic caps removed. A maximum of five test bubbles per bottle within five minutes is considered acceptable for qualification.

Drying Time

Drying time is a crucial factor in determining the effectiveness of cosmetics. It refers to the duration required for the product to dry at room temperature $(20 \pm 5)°C$ and relative humidity of less than or equal to 80%. To test the drying time, we first wash the slide plant with ethyl acetate and dry it. Then, we use a brush to fill the sample and apply it to the slide in one go. Next, we start the stopwatch and wait for 8 minutes before touching the sample to check if it is dry. If the sample is dry, it is considered qualified.

18.5 Detection of Special Chemical Components of Cosmetics

The detection of special chemical components in cosmetics is a crucial process that involves identifying harmful substances, prohibited and restricted components, preservatives, sunscreens, coloring agents, hair dyes, and other ingredients. It is essential to ensure that cosmetics are safe for use and do not pose any health risks to consumers. By detecting these special components, manufacturers can ensure that their products comply with regulatory standards and are safe for use by the general public. Therefore, the detection of special chemical components in cosmetics is a critical step in the production process that should not be overlooked.

18.5.1 Detection of Hazardous Substances

The "Safety and Technical Standards for Cosmetics" outlines the maximum allowable levels of heavy metals, including mercury, lead, arsenic, and cadmium, as well as harmful substances such as methanol, dioxane, and asbestos, as detailed in Table 18-1. These harmful substances may contaminate cosmetics during production, packaging, or transportation, and can be absorbed through the skin, leading to toxic reactions and posing a threat to human health.

Table 18–1　Limits of hazardous substances in cosmetics and their detection methods

Hazardous substance	Limit (mg/kg)	Detection methods
Mercury	1	HAFS,CAA, mercury analyzer method
Lead	10	GFAAS, FAAS
Arsenic	2	HAFS, HGAAS
Cadmium	5	FAAS
Methanol	2000	GC
Dioxane	30	GC-MS
Asbestos	Shall not be detected	X-ray diffractometer and polarizing microscope

Abbreviation: HAFS: Hydride atomic fluorescence spectrometry; CAA: Cold atomic absorption; GFAAS:Graphite furnace atomic absorption spectrophotometry; FAAS: Flame atomic absorption spectrophotometry; HAFS:Hydride atomic fluorescence spectrometry; HGAAS:Hydride generation atomic absorption spectrometry; GC:Gas Chromatography:GC-MS:Gas Chromatography-Mass Spectrometry

18.5.2 Forbidden Component

Forbidden components are substances that are not allowed to be used as raw materials in cosmetics. The "Safety and Technical Standards for Cosmetics" lists a total of 1388 forbidden components. Table 18-2 highlights some of the most commonly found forbidden components and their respective detection methods.

Table 18–2   Some forbidden components in cosmetics and their detection methods

Forbidden components	Detection methods
9 components in cosmetics include fluconazole, ketoconazole, naftifine, bibenbenzazole, clotrimazole, econazole, griseofulvin, miconazole, ciclopirox olamine ciclopiroxamine	LC-MS/MS
10 components in cosmetics include enoxacin, fleroxacin, ofloxacin, norfloxacin, pefloxacin, ciprofloxacin, enrofloxacin, sarafloxacin, difloxacin and moxifloxacin component	
7 components in cosmetics include minoxidil, hydrocortisone, spironolactone, estrone, canrenone, triamcinolone acetonide acetate, progesterone and others	
4-Aminobiphenyl and its salts in cosmetics	
15 components in liquid water-based, cream emulsion and gel cosmetics which include desloratadine, chlorpheniramine, astemizole, tripinamine, brompheniramine, diphenhydramine, promethazine, hydroxyzine, perphenazine, cetirizine, fluphenazine, chlorpromazine, loratadine, terfenadine, cyproheptadine and others	
7 components in cosmetics include minocycline hydrochloride, metronidazole, oxytetracycline dihydrate, tetracycline hydrochloride, chlortetracycline hydrochloride, doxycycline hydrochloride and chloramphenicol	HPLC-DAD
7 sex hormones in cosmetics include estriol, estrone, diethylstilbestrol, estradiol, testosterone, methyl testosterone and progesterone	1. HPLC-DAD
Hydroquinone and phenol in freckle cosmetics and shampoos	2. HPLC-UV/FLD 3. GC-MS
6-Methylcoumarin in liquid water-based, cream emulsion and powder cosmetics	1. HPLC 2. GC Confirmatory method: GC-MS
4 components in cosmetics including 8-methoxypsoralen, 5-methoxypsoralen, Trioxysalen and imperatorin	HPLC, confirmed method: LC-MS
5 components in lipstick, loose powder and nail polish cosmetics which including acid Yellow 36 (CI 13065), Pigment Red 53:1 (CI 15585:1), Pigment Orange 5 (CI 12075), Sudan Red Ⅱ (CI 12140) and Sudan Red Ⅳ (CI 26105)	
Aminocaproic acid in cream, lotion and powder cosmetics	
7 components in liquid water-based, liquid oil-based, cream lotion, gel which include procainamide, procaine, chloroprocaine, benzocaine, lidocaine, tetracaine, Cincocaine	
Retinoic acid and isotretinoin in creams, lotions and liquid water-based cosmetics	
4 components in cosmetics including psoralen, isopsoralen, new psoralen isoflavone and psoralen dihydroflavonoid	HPLC
Vitamin D$_2$ and Vitamin D$_3$ in Cosmetics	

(*Continued*)

Table 18-2 (*Continued*)

Forbidden components	Detection methods
5-aminoazobenzene and benzidine in liquid water-based, liquid oil-based, cream emulsions, powder cosmetics	GC-MS
Dioxane in liquid water-based, cream emulsion and gel cosmetics	
8 components in cosmetics including dibutyl phthalate (DBP), di(2-methoxyethyl) phthalate (DMEP), diisoamyl phthalate (DIPP),amyl isoamyl phthalate (DnIPP), di-n-pentyl phthalate (DnPP), butyl benzyl phthalate (BBP), di(2-ethylhexyl) phthalate (DEHP) and 1,2-Phenyldicarboxylic acid branched and linear dipentyl ester	
37 volatile organic solvents in cosmetics include ethanol, ether, acetone, ethyl formate, isopropanol, acetonitrile, methyl acetate, dichloromethane, methyl tert-butyl ether, N-propanol, 2-butanone, ethyl acetate, tetrahydrofuran, sec-butyl alcohol, chloroform, cyclohexane, carbon tetrachloride, benzene, 1,2-dichloroethane, isobutanol, isopropyl acetate, trichloroethylene, n-butanol, dioxane, propyl acetate, 4-Methyl-2-pentanone, toluene, isoamyl alcohol, isobutyl acetate, tetrachloroethylene, N-amyl alcohol, butyl acetate, ethylbenzene, para/meta-xylene, isoamyl acetate and O-xylene	
α-Chlorotoluene in creams, emulsions and liquid water-based cosmetics	GC
Diethylene glycol in propylene glycol,cosmetic raw material	Confirmatory
Ethylene oxide and methyl ethylene oxide in cleaning and liquid water-based cosmetics with polyethylene glycol and polypropylene glycol as raw materials	method: GC-MS
15 components in cosmetics include dichloromethane, 1,1-dichloroethane, 1,2-dichloroethylene, chloroform, 1,2-dichloroethane, benzene, trichloroethylene, toluene, tetrachloroethylene, ethylbenzene , m-, p-xylene, styrene, o-xylene and cumene	
Cantharidin in hair cosmetics	GC
Chlormethine in hair cosmetics	
Benzo[a] pyrene in liquid water-based, liquid oil-based and cream emulsion cosmetics	HPLC, confirmed
10 components in cosmetics include dimethyl phthalate (DMP), diethyl phthalate (DEP), di-n-propyl phthalate (DPP), butyl benzyl phthalate (BBP), di-n-butyl phthalate (DBP), di-n-pentyl phthalate ester (DAP), dicyclohexyl phthalate (DCHP), di-n-hexyl phthalate (DHP), diisooctyl phthalate (DEHP) and di-n-octyl phthalate (DOP)	method: GC-MS
Acrylamide in cosmetics	LC-MS
Diethyl maleate in cream emulsions, liquid oil-based and liquid water-based cosmetics	HPLC, confirmed
Minoxidil in liquid water-based cosmetics for hair	method: LC-MS/MS

Abbreviation: HPLC: high performance liquid chromatography; GC: gas chromatography; GC-MS: Gas chromatography- mass spectrometry; LC-MS: liquid chromatography-mass spectrography; LC-MS/MS:liquid chromatography-tandem mass spectrometry; DAD: diode array detector; FLD: Fluorescence Detector

18.5.3 Restricted Components

Restricted components are substances that can be utilized as cosmetic raw materials, but only under specific conditions. The "Safety and Technical Standards for Cosmetics" outlines 47 requirements for their use. Table 18-3 highlights some of the most commonly used detection methods for restricted components.

Table 18-3　Common restricted component in cosmetics and their detection methods

Restricted components	Maximum allowable concentration for cosmetic use	Detection methods
α-hydroxy acids (tartaric acid, glycolic acid, malic acid, lactic acid, citric acid) in cosmetics for washing, hair care and skin care	6% of total (calculated as acid)	1. HPLC 2. IC 3. GC
Selenium (IV) in selenium disulfide in anti-dandruff shampoo cosmetics	1%	FS
Hydrogen peroxide in hair dye and cream mask cosmetics	A. Hair products: 12% of total (calculated as H_2O_2 present or released) B. Skin products: 4% of total (by presence or release of H_2O_2 meter) C. Finger (toe) nail hardening products: 2% of total (calculated as H_2O_2 present or released)	HPLC
Catechol for non-colored hair cosmetics	0.5%	HPLC
Soluble zinc salts in deodorant cosmetics	1% of total(calculated as zinc)	FAAS
Quinine in shampoo and resident hair care cosmetics	A. Rinse hair products: 0.5% of total (calculated as quinine) B. Leave-on hair products: 0.2% of total (calculated as quinine)	HPLC
Boric acid and borates in cosmetics	A. Talcum powder；5% of total (calculated as boric acid) B. Other products (except bath and perm products): 3% of total (calculated as boric acid)	Methimine-H spectrophotometry
Hydroxyquinoline in hair cosmetics	A. Used as a stabilizer for hydrogen peroxide in rinse-off hair products: 0.3% of total (calculated as base) B. Used as a stabilizer for hydrogen peroxide in leave-on hair products: 0.03% of total (calculated as base)	HPLC
Thioglycolic acid in hair curling agent or straightening agent, hair removal cream cosmetics	A. Perm products (a) General use: 8% of total (calculated as thioglycolic acid), pH7-9.5 (b) Professional use: 11% of total (calculated as thioglycolic acid), pH7-9.5 B. Depilatory products: 5% of total (as thioglycolic acid), pH 7-12.7	HPLC
Thioglycolic acid and its salts in cosmetics	Other rinse-off hair products: 2% of Total (calculated as thioglycolic acid), pH7-9.5	IC
Thioglycolic acid and its salts and esters in hair removal, perm and other hair cosmetic products	Perm products (a) General use: 8% of total (calculated as thioglycolic acid), pH6-9.5 (b) Professional use: 11% of total (calculated as thioglycolic acid), pH6-9.5	Chemical titration

(Continued)

Table 18–3 (*Continued*)

Restricted components	Maximum allowable concentration for cosmetic use	Detection methods
Salicylic acid in skin and rinse-off hair cosmetics	A. Leave-in products and rinse-off skin products: 2.0% B. Rinse hair products: 3.0%	HPLC
Keto musk in perfume and cream emulsion cosmetics	A. Perfume:1.4% B. Weak perfume: 0.56% C. Other products: 0.042%	HPLC
Free hydroxide in various types of hair straightening products	A. Finger (toe) nail protective film solvent: 5% (by weight) B. Finger (toe) nail protective film solvent: 5% (by weight)	PT

Abbreviation: HPLC: high performance liquid chromatography; GC: gas chromatography; FAAS: Flame atomic absorption spectrophotometry; IC: ion chromatography; PT: potentiometric titration; FS: fluorescence spectrophotometry

18.5.4   Preservatives

Preservatives are substances added to cosmetics to prevent the growth of microorganisms. The "Safety and Technical Standards for Cosmetics" lists 51 permitted preservatives. Table 18-4 outlines some of the commonly used methods for detecting preservatives.

Table 18–4   Common preservatives in cosmetics and their detection methods

Preservatives	Maximum permissible concentration for cosmetic use	Detection methods
Benzyl alcohol in liquid water-based, cream emulsion, powder cosmetics	1.0%	1.GC 2. HPLC Confirmation method: GC-MS
Benzoic acid and its sodium salt in liquid water-based, cream emulsion, powder cosmetics	2.5% of total (calculated as acid)	1. HPLC 2. GC Confirmation method: GC-MS
Phenoxyisopropanol in rinse-off cosmetics (including liquid water-based and creams and lotions, excluding oral hygiene products)	1.0%	HPLC
Benzalkonium chloride (sum of dodecyl dimethyl benzyl ammonium chloride, tetradecyl dimethyl benzyl ammonium chloride and hexadecyl dimethyl benzyl ammonium chloride) in washing hair products or liquid water based products, cream cream emulsion cosmetics	0.1% of total (calculated as benzalkonium chloride)	HPLC

(*Continued*)

Table 18–4 (*Continued*)

Preservatives	Maximum permissible concentration for cosmetic use	Detection methods
Lauralkonium chloride, benzethonium chloride and sitalkonium chloride in liquid Water-Based, cream-emulsion cosmetics	Benzethonium chloride: 0.1%	HPLC
Determination of formaldehyde content in cosmetics, not applicable to the determination of formaldehyde content in nail polish containing toluene sulfonamide resin	0.2% of total(calculated as free formaldehyde)	(a) Acetylacetone spectrophotometry (b) Precolumn-derived- HPLC
12 components in cosmetics include methylchloroisothiazolinone, 2-bromo-2-nitropropane-1,3-diol, methylisothiazolinone, benzyl alcohol, phenoxyethanol, methyl 4-hydroxybenzoate, benzene formic acid, ethyl 4-hydroxybenzoate, isopropyl 4-hydroxybenzoate, propyl 4-hydroxybenzoate, isobutyl 4-hydroxybenzoate and butyl 4-hydroxybenzoate	A. Mixture of methylchloroisothiazolinone and methylisothiazolinone with magnesium chloride and magnesium nitrate: 0.0015% B. Benzyl alcohol: 1.0% C. Methylisothiazolinone: 0.01% D. Phenoxyethanol: 1.0% E. Benzoic acid: 0.5% of total (calculated as acid)	HPLC
Chlorphenesin in liquid water-based, cream emulsion and powder cosmetics	0.3%	HPLC
Triclocarban in cosmetics such as liquid water-based, creams, lotions, and solid soaps	0.2%	HPLC
Sorbic acid and dehydroacetic acid and their salts in creams, emulsions, liquid water-based and gel cosmetics	0.6% of total (calculated as acid)	HPLC
5 components in hair cosmetics include salicylic acid, zinc pyrithione, ketoconazole, climbazole and piroctone ethanolamine salt	A. Salicylic acid and its salts: 0.5% of total (calculated as acid) B. Zinc pyrithione:0.5% C. Climbazole: 0.5% D. Piroctone and piroctone ethanolamine salts: (a) Rinse products: 1.0% of total (b) Other products: 0.5% of total	HPLC

Abbreviation: HPLC: high performance liquid chromatography; GC: gas chromatography; GC-MS:Gas chromatography-mass spectrometry

18.5.5 Sunscreens

Sunscreens are cosmetic additives that utilize the absorption, reflection, or scattering of light to safeguard the skin from specific ultraviolet rays or to preserve the product. The "Safety and Technical Standards for Cosmetics" specifies 27 authorized sunscreen agents. Table 18-5 outlines various commonly used methods for detecting sunscreens.

Table 18–5   Common sunscreens in cosmetics and their detection method

Sunscreens	Maximum permissible concentration for cosmetic use	Detection methods
15 components in cosmetics,including phenylbenzimidazole sulfonic acid, benzophenone-4 and benzophenone-5, p-aminobenzoic acid, benzophenone-3, isoamyl p-methoxycinnamate, 4-methylbenzylidene in cosmetics camphor, PABA ethylhexyl, butylmethoxydibenzoylmethane, octocrylene, ethylhexyl methoxycinnamate, ethylhexyl salicylate, homosalate, ethylhexyltriazine, ketones, methylenebis-benzotriazolyl tetramethylbutylphenol and bis-ethylhexyloxyphenol methoxyphenyltriazine	Phenylbenzimidazole sulfonic acid and its potassium, sodium and triethanolamine salts: 8% of total (calculated as acid) Benzophenone-4 and Benzophenone-5: 5% of total (calculated as acid) Benzophenone-3: 10% Isoamyl p-methoxycinnamate: 10% 4-methylbenzylidene camphor: 4% Dimethyl PABA ethylhexyl ester: 8% Butylmethoxydibenzoylmethane: 5% Octrelin: 10% of total (calculated as acid) Ethylhexyl methoxycinnamate: 10% Ethylhexyl salicylate: 5% Homosalate: 10% Ethylhexyltriazinone: 5% Methylenebis-benzotriazolyltetramethylbutylphenol: 10% Bis-ethylhexyloxyphenol methoxyphenyl triazine: 10%	1. HPLC-DAD 2. HPLC-UV
Total titanium (calculated as titanium dioxide) in cream, lotion, liquid and other cosmetics	25%	Spectrophotometry
Diethylaminohydroxybenzoylhexylbenzoate in liquid water-based, cream and lotion cosmetics	10%	HPLC
Diethylhexylbutyramidotriazinone in liquid water-based, cream and lotion products	10%	HPLC
Benzylidene camphorsulfonic acid in liquid water-based, cream emulsion cosmetics	6% of total (calculated as acid)	HPLC
Total zinc content (calculated as zinc oxide) in creams, lotions, liquids and other cosmetics	25%	FAA

Abbreviation: HPLC: high performance liquid chromatography; FAA: Flame atomic absorption

18.5.6   Colouring Agents

Colouring agents are substances that are added to cosmetic products to provide color to the product or the area where it is applied by absorbing or reflecting visible light. It is important to note that hair dyes are not included in this definition. According to the Safety and Technical Standards for Cosmetics, there are 157 permitted colouring agents. Table 18-6 provides information on several commonly used colouring agents and their detection methods.

Table 18-6   Common colouring agent in cosmetics and their detection methods

Colouring agents	Detection methods
Seven components of hair color and perm cosmetics include basic orange 31, basic yellow 87, basic red 51, basic purple 14 (CI 42510), acid orange 3 (CI 10385), acid purple 43 (CI 60730), basic blue 26 (CI 44045)	HPLC
10 components in rouge, lipstick, foundation, nail polish, mascara, eye shadow and other cosmetic products, including CI 59040, CI 16185, CI 16255, CI 10316, CI 15985, CI 16035, CI 14700, Orange yellow I, CI 45380, CI 15510	HPLC;Confirmation method: LC-MS

Abbreviation: HPLC: high performance liquid chromatography; LC-MS: liquid chromatography-mass spectrography

18.5.7   Hair Dye

Hair dye is a cosmetic substance used to alter the color of hair. According to the "Safety and Technical Standards for Cosmetics," there are 75 permitted hair dyes. Table 18-7 outlines several commonly used methods for detecting hair dye.

Table 18-7   Common hair dye in cosmetics and their detection methods

Hair dye	Maximum permissible concentration for cosmetic use	Detection methods
Eight kinds of oxidative dyes include p-phenylenediamine, p-aminophenol, hydroquinone, toluene 2,5-diamine, m-aminophenol, o-phenylenediamine, resorcinol and p-methylaminophenol in hair color cosmetics	(a) p-phenylenediamine: 2.0% (b) p-aminophenol: 0.5% (c) Toluene 2,5-diamine: 4.0% (d) m-aminophenol: 1.0% (e) 4-Nitro-o-phenylenediamine: 0.5% (f) Resorcinol: 1.25% (g) p-methylaminophenol: 0.68% (calculated as sulfate)	HPLC
32 dyes in hair color cosmetics include P-phenylenediamine, p-aminophenol, toluene-2,5-diamine sulfate, m-aminophenol, o-phenylenediamine, 2-chloro-p-phenylenediamine sulfate, o-aminophenol, Resorcinol, 2-nitro-p-phenylenediamine, toluene-3,4-diamine, 4-amino-2-hydroxytoluene, 2-methylresorcinol, 6-amino-m-cresol, phenylmethylpyrazolone, *N,N*-diethyltoluene-2,5-diamine hydrochloride, 4-amino-3-nitrophenol, m-phenylenediamine, 2,4-diaminophenoxyethanol hydrochloride salt, hydroquinone,4-amino-m-cresol,2-amino-3-	(a) p-methylaminophenol sulfate: 0.68% (b) p-phenylenediamine hydrochloride: 2.0% (c) m-aminophenol hydrochloride, m-aminophenol sulfate: 1.0% (based on free radicals) (d) Toluene-2,5-diamine sulfate: 4.0% (calculated as free radicals) (e) 4-Nitro-o-phenylenediamine sulfate: 0.5% (calculated as free radicals) (f) 2-Chloro-p-phenylenediamine sulfate: 0.5% (oxidative hair coloring products); 1.0% (non-oxidative hair coloring products) (g) 4-Amino-2-hydroxytoluene: 1.5% (h) 2-Methylresorcinol: 1.0% (oxidative hair coloring products); 1.8% (non-oxidative hair coloring products) (i) 6-Amino-m-cresol: 1.2% (oxidative hair coloring products); 2.4% (non-oxidative hair coloring products) (j) Phenylmethylpyrazolone: 0.25%	HPLC

(Continued)

Table 18–7 (*Continued*)

Hair dye	Maximum permissible concentration for cosmetic use	Detection methods
hydroxypyridine, N,N-bis(2-hydroxyethyl)-p-phenylenediamine sulfate, p-methylaminophenol sulfate, 4- Nitro-o-phenylenediamine, 2,6-diaminopyridine, N,N-diethyl-p-phenylenediamine sulfate, 6-hydroxyindole, 4-chlororesorcinol, 2,7-naphthalenediol , N-phenyl-p-phenylenediamine, 1,5-naphthalenediol and 1-naphthol	(k) 4-Amino-3-nitrophenol: 1.5% (oxidative hair coloring products); 1.0% (non-oxidative hair coloring products) (l) 2,4-Diaminophenoxyethanol hydrochloride: 2.0% (m) 4-Amino-m-cresol: 1.5% (n) 2-amino-3-hydroxypyridine: 0.3% (o) *N,N*-bis(2-hydroxyethyl)-p-phenylenediamine sulfate: 2.5% (calculated as sulfate) (p) 2,6-diaminopyridine: 0.15% (q) 6-hydroxyindole: 0.5% (r) 4-chlororesorcinol: 0.5% (s) 2,7-Naphthalenediol: 0.5% (oxidative hair coloring products); 1.0% (non-oxidative hair coloring products) (t) N-phenyl-p-phenylenediamine: 3.0% (u) 1,5-Naphthalenediol: 0.5% (oxidative hair coloring products); 1.0% (non-oxidative hair coloring products) (v) 1-Naphthol: 1.0%	

Abbreviation: HPLC: high performance liquid chromatography

In addition to the physical and chemical indicators mentioned earlier, the "Technical Specifications for Cosmetics" also outlines microbial indicators that must be met. These include total bacterial counts, mold and yeast counts, coliforms, fecal coliforms, Escherichia coli, Staphylococcus aureus, hemolytic streptococcus, Salmonella, Pseudomonas aeruginosa, Legionella, and more. Enzyme activity detection is also required for certain cosmetics, such as cellulase, saccharification enzyme, amylase, protease, thermostable amylase, and superoxide dismutase (SOD). Cosmetic additives must meet the relevant requirements for product quality and safety. Once the products pass inspection, they can be released into the market.

Glossary

cosmetic *n.* 化妆品 the daily chemical industrial products spread on any part of the human body (skin, hair, nails, lips, etc.) by embrocating, spraying or other similar methods for cleaning, eliminating bad odor, skin care, beauty and modification

routine inspection items 常规检验项目 the items for each batch of cosmetics to inspect its sensory, physical and chemical performance indicators (except heat and cold resistance), net content, packaging appearance requirements and the total number of colonies, molds and yeasts in the hygienic indicators

the non-routine inspection items 非常规检验项目 the items for each batch of cosmetics to inspect the heat resistance and cold resistance in its physical and chemical properties, as well as other hygienic indicators except the total number of bacterial colonies, mold and yeast

forbidden components 禁用成分 the substances that cannot be used as cosmetic raw materials

restricted components 限用成分 the substances that can be used as cosmetic raw materials under limited conditions

preservatives *n.* 防腐剂 the substances added to cosmetics for the purpose of inhibiting the growth of microorganisms in cosmetics

sunscreens *n.* 防晒剂 the substances added to cosmetics for absorption, reflection or scattering of light to protect the skin from specific UV rays

colouring agents 着色剂 the substances added to cosmetic products by absorbing or reflecting visible light to give color to the cosmetic product or its application site, excluding hair dyes

hair dye 染发剂 the substance added to cosmetics to change hair color

（黄东萍）

新形态教材网 · 数字课程学习……

教学 PPT   自测题   推荐阅读

PART V
Sanitary Quarantine

Chapter 19
Epidemiology in Sanitary Inspection

Learning objectives:

- Know the concepts and characteristics of epidemiology in sanitary inspection.
- Be able to calculate disease-related measures.
- Learn how to choose the right research method.
- Master the epidemiological methods in sanitary inspection, from the exploration of causes to the verification of causes.

19.1　Introduction

Epidemiology in sanitary inspection is a combination of traditional epidemiology and health technology to generate a new branch of epidemiology, which utilizes modern medical theory and science and technology to supervise, monitor and identify potential health hazards existing in environment, food, cosmetics, workplace, and provides basis and measures for prevention and treatment of disease. The application of epidemiology methods in sanitary inspection makes disease prevention and intervention measures more effective and targeted. For example, epidemiology is applied to study the influencing factors of food hygiene and quality, to study the impact of environmental and biological factors on human beings, and to evaluate the scientificity of sanitary inspection systems.

Descriptive epidemiology in sanitary inspection mainly describes the distribution of biological or environmental factors that cause diseases or affect health status, and makes a preliminary analysis of distribution to provide clues for specific etiology research. Analytical epidemiology in sanitary inspection mainly starts from analyzing the different distribution of influence factors and health status among groups to find out the law and reason of epidemic and distribution, and to test or verify the hypothesis of etiology. Experimental epidemiology in sanitary inspection is to identify strategies and measures for disease prevention and control, and to confirm the hypothesis of cause through the rational application of the results of the first two stages.

19.1.1   Measures of the Disease Frequency

In epidemiology, there are many kinds of frequency indicators of disease or health effects, such as incidence rate, prevalence, prevalence of infection, mortality rate, and case fatality rate, and so on.

19.1.1.1   Incidence Rate

Incidence rate refers to the frequency of new cases of a disease in a certain range of people within a certain period of time. Incidence rate is a common indicator of disease epidemic intensity, reflecting the degree of impact of a disease on the health of the population. A high incidence rate of a disease represents the great harm of the disease to the population.

$$Incidence\ rate = \frac{the\ number\ of\ new\ cases\ of\ a\ disease\ in\ a\ population\ during\ a\ certain\ period}{number\ of\ person\text{-}time\ at\ risk\ in\ that\ population\ during\ the\ same\ period}$$
$$\times K$$

K=100%, 1 000‰, 10 000/ ten thousand, 1 000 000/ hundred thousand…

19.1.1.2   Attack Rate

The attack rate refers to the incidence rate within a limited period of time. It is also an indicator to measure the frequency of new cases of a disease in a population, but it is observed over a shorter period of time. Attack rates are often used in outbreak investigations to describe the intensity of an outbreak and to explore the relationship between exposure factors and disease, such as food poisoning or infectious disease outbreak investigations.

$$Attack\ rate = \frac{The\ number\ of\ new\ cases\ of\ a\ disease\ during\ the\ observation\ period}{Population\ exposed\ during\ the\ same\ period} \times K$$

K = 100%, 1 000‰…

19.1.1.3   Prevalence

Prevalence refers to the proportion of new and old cases of disease in the total population at a certain time. It is usually used to reflect the disease status of a certain disease, and can also be used to estimate the severity of a certain disease on the health of the population. For chronic diseases with a long course, prevalence can reflect the epidemic status of these diseases.

$$Prevalence = \frac{New\ and\ old\ cases\ of\ a\ disease\ in\ a\ population\ during\ a\ certain\ observation\ period}{The\ average\ population\ over\ the\ same\ period}$$
$$\times K$$

K=100%, 1 000‰, 10 000/ten thousand, 1 000 000/ hundred thousand…

19.1.1.4   Prevalence of Infection

The prevalence of infection is the percentage of the population currently infected with a pathogen that being tested at any given time. Prevalence of infection is mainly used to study the infection situation of some infectious diseases or parasitic diseases, evaluate the effect of prevention and control work, and provide reference for the formulation of prevention and control measures.

$$Prevalence\ of\ infection = \frac{The\ number\ of\ people\ who\ tested\ positive\ for\ the\ infection}{The\ number\ of\ people\ tested} \times 100\%$$

19.1.1.5   Mortality Rate

The mortality rate refers to the proportion of the total number of deaths in a certain population in a certain period, and is the most commonly used indicator to measure the risk of death in a population. Mortality rate is used to measure the mortality risk of people in a certain period in a certain area, and can also be used as an indicator of the risk of disease occurrence.

$$Mortality\ rate = \frac{Total\ number\ of\ deaths\ in\ a\ population\ in\ a\ given\ year}{The\ average\ population\ of\ this\ population\ in\ the\ same\ year} \times K$$

K=100%, 1 000‰, 10 000/ten thousand, 1 000 000/ hundred thousand…

19.1.1.6   Case Fatality Rate

Case fatality rate (CFR) refers to the proportion of patients who die of a certain disease in a certain period of time, indicating the risk of death from the disease. Case fatality rate refers to the death probability of patients diagnosed with a certain disease, which can reflect the severity of the disease, as well as the medical level and diagnosis and treatment ability.

$$CFR = \frac{Number\ of\ deaths\ from\ a\ disease\ in\ a\ given\ period}{The\ number\ of\ cases\ of\ a\ disease\ in\ the\ same\ period} \times 100\%$$

19.1.2   Epidemic Intensity and Distribution of Disease

The epidemic intensity of a disease is often expressed as sporadic, outbreak, epidemic and pandemic. It refers to the change in the incidence of a disease in a population in a certain area over a period of time and the degree of association between the cases.

Due to the comprehensive effects of various factors such as the population characteristics, pathogenic factors and natural and social environment, the epidemic intensity and existence status of diseases are different in different populations, different regions and different times. The distribution of diseases reflects not only the biological characteristics of diseases themselves, but also the effects and interactions of various internal and external environmental factors related to diseases. The epidemic characteristics of diseases can be expressed through the distribution of diseases in population, region and time.

19.2   The Descriptive Study

Cross-sectional study, a typical descriptive study, also known as prevalence study, is to collect and describe the data of disease or health status and the distribution of related factors in the population at a specific point in time and within a specific range, so as to provide clues of etiology for further research.

Design of a Descriptive Study

Identify Research Objectives and Research Subjects

The purpose of cross-sectional studies in epidemiology in sanitary inspection is to investigate and analyze the relationship between exposure to food, air, water, environmental factors and health or disease. The research objects of the current study are generally people in a specific range. Appropriate research objects should be selected according to the research purpose.

Determine Sample Size and Sampling Method

There are many factors that determine the sample size of the cross-sectional study, mainly including: the expected prevalence rate (P); the allowable error (d) (the larger the allowable error is, the smaller the required sample size would be); the significance level (α), generally, $\alpha=0.05$.

According to the purpose and object of the study, it is decided whether to use a census or a sample survey. Sampling survey method can be divided into the non-random sampling and random sampling. Since each sample unit is randomly selected, random sampling can not only use sample statistics to estimate the overall parameters, but also calculate the sampling error, which can obtain reliable results.

Collect, Collate and Analyze Data

In a cross-sectional study, the definition of exposure and the criteria of the disease should be clear and uniform. Cases should be defined according to clinical standards. The data obtained either by questionnaire or laboratory measurement need to be checked and entered in database in time, and the integrity and accuracy of the data should be verified.

19.3   Cohort Study

Cohort study is an observational research method that divides the population into different subgroups according to whether they are exposed to suspicious factors, tracks the occurrence of the outcomes of the subjects in each group, and compares the differences in the expected outcomes (such as disease, death) between different groups, so as to determine whether there is a causal relationship between the exposure factors and the outcomes and the degree of correlation. It can be used to test causal hypotheses, evaluate the effect of preventive measures, and observe the natural history of a disease in research.

19.3.1   Design of Cohort Studies

19.3.1.1   Determine Study Exposure Factors and Study Outcomes

On the basis of cross-sectional studies and case-control studies, the suspicious risk factors (exposure factors) usually need to be further identified by cohort study. The outcome is the natural end point of the cohort study, and the expected outcome of the follow-up of the subjects and the outcome include changes at the molecular level, changes at the cellular level and the onset of health or disease. The subjects are divided into the exposure group and the control group according to the exposure situation.

19.3.1.2　Determine Sample Size

The main factors affecting the sample size include: the incidence of diseases studied in the general population (control population) (P_0); the incidence difference between the exposed group and the control group (d); the false positive error a and the false negative error β.

19.3.1.3　Data Collection

The data of cohort study should be collected through follow-up. Baseline data should be collected immediately after the subjects are recruited in the study, and other information should be collected in the follow-up process, and the occurrence of study outcomes should be recorded. Baseline data includes not only personal information such as age, sex, ethnicity, occupation, and education level, but also exposed state to exposure factors.

19.3.2　Calculation of Rates in Cohort Studies

When we calculate incidence rate in cohort studies, the cumulative incidence is generally used in fixed cohorts, that is, the number of people at the starting point of observation is used as the denominator. While in dynamic cohorts, the observation time of every subject is different. Therefore, person-time is used to describe the exposure experience of the subjects, which is the sum of observation time of each subject and used as the denominator. The generally used person-time is person-year.

19.3.2.1　Cumulative Incidence

Cumulative incidence reflects the risk of onset within a specific period of time, and generally vary from 0 to 1. Cumulative incidence must be reported with a description of the length of cumulative time and usually applied to large and stable study populations.

$$Cumulative\ incidence = \frac{Number\ of\ cases\ during\ observation\ period}{The\ number\ of\ people\ at\ the\ starting\ point\ of\ observation}$$

19.3.2.2　Incidence Density

In cohort studies with a long observation period, especially dynamic cohorts, subjects enter the cohort at different times or are lost to follow-up due to death or withdrawal for other reasons. Therefore, it is necessary to calculate the person-time and use it as the denominator to calculate the incidence rate, also known as the incidence density, which theoretically varies from 0 to infinity.

$$Incidence\ density = \frac{Number\ of\ cases\ during\ observation\ period}{Total\ person-time\ in\ the\ study}$$

19.3.2.3　Estimation of Effect

Relative risk (RR) is the ratio of the risk of exposure group (measured as cumulative incidence or incidence density) to the risk of control group.

$$RR = I_1/I_0$$

I_1 and I_0 represent the cumulative incidence or incidence density of disease in the exposure group and the control group, respectively. RR indicates how many times the risk of disease or death is in the exposure group compared to the control group. The higher the *RR* value, the greater effect of exposure, and stronger the correlation between exposure and outcome.

Attributable risk (*AR*), also known as specific risk, is the absolute difference between the incidence of the exposure group and that of the control group. It represents the degree to which the risk of outcome is attributable to exposure factors.

$$AR = I_1 - I_0 = a/n_1 - a/n_0$$

AR refers to the increased number of diseases among exposed people compared with non-exposed people. If the exposure factors are eliminated, the incidence of diseases in this number can be reduced. Therefore, it has the significance of disease prevention and public health.

19.4   Case–Control Study

A case-control study compares the statistical difference in exposure to one or several possible risk factors between patients with a disease and controls without the disease, and analyzes whether these factors are associated with the disease. The control group is divided into matched case-control study and unmatched case-control study. A matched case-control study selects the control group which is consistent with the case group in some factors or characteristics. The purpose is to make matching factors keep the balance between the two groups, and eliminate the interference caused by these factors on the results.

19.4.1   Design of a Case–Control Study

19.4.1.1   Determination of the Purpose and the Type of Research

Refer to relevant domestic and foreign literature to understand the exposure factors that need to be studied in this topic, put forward the etiological hypothesis, and determine the purpose of the study. When testing etiological hypotheses or when it is difficult to compare the control group with the case group in a balanced manner, case-control studies with matched individuals may be used to ensure comparability between the control group and the case group.

19.4.1.2   Identify of Research Subjects

Selection of cases: In case-control studies, the diagnostic criteria of the disease should be clarified before the study is carried out, and the common diagnostic criteria should be used as far as possible. Case can be incident case, prevalent case, or even death case. The investigation of new cases is not prone to recall bias, but it is possible that the expected number of cases may not be obtained within a certain period of time.

Selection of control: The control group should be persons who are diagnosed as free of the studied disease according to international or national diagnostic criteria. Before the case-control study carried out, appropriate control group should be selected according to the research purpose and type.

19.4.1.3   Sample Size

The calculation of sample size of case-control study is mainly influenced by the following factors: exposure rate of exposure factors studied in the control group or population (P); an estimate of the strength of the association between study factors and the disease, the odds ratio (OR); the false positive probability α, generally $\alpha=0.05$; the false negative probability, generally $\beta=0.1$.

19.4.1.4   Collection of Data

Case-control studies can collect information through telephone or letter return visits, online or on-site questionnaires. Exposure information can be obtained through laboratory tests (such as blood samples) or environmental factors measurement (water samples, air samples, etc.) to obtain detailed exposure.

19.4.1.5   Analysis of Data

Association analysis mainly analyzes whether there are differences in exposure factors between the case group and the control group, as well as the association and degree of association between exposure and the disease under study. In case-control studies, the strength of the association between exposure and disease is measured by the ratio of exposure ratios between the case and control groups. This value is called the odds ratio (OR).

In the unmatched case-control study, the data are organized according to Table 19-1 as follows:

Table 19–1   Form of data collation in unmatched case–control studies

Exposure history	Case group	Control group	Total
Yes	a	b	$a+b=m_1$
No	c	d	$c+d=m_0$
Total	$a+c=n_1$	$b+d=n_0$	$N=a+b+c+d$

19.4.2   Correlation Analysis Between Exposure and Disease

The Chi-square test is often used for statistical analysis of differences in exposure ratio between the case group and the control group.

The calculation of the OR: $OR = [a/(a+c) / c/(a + c)]/[b/(b + d)/d/(b + d)] = ad / bc$

In matched case-control studies, the data are organized according to Table 19-2 as follows:

Table 19–2   form of data collation in matched case–control studies

Control group	Case group		Total
	Exposed	No exposed	
Exposed	a	b	$a+b=m_1$
No exposed	c	d	$c+d=m_0$
Total	$a+c=n_1$	$b+d=n_0$	$N=a+b+c+d$

Association analysis between exposure and disease:

Chi-square test formula: $\chi^2 = (b-c)^2/(b+c)$

Calculation of OR: $OR = c/b$ $(b \neq 0)$

OR has the same meaning as RR, which refers to how many times the risk of disease of an exposed person is that of an unexposed person. $OR>1$ means that exposure can increase the risk of disease, and exposure factors are risk factors of disease; $OR<1$ represents exposure can reduce the risk of disease, and exposure is a protective factor. $OR=1$, indicates that there is no statistical association between exposure factors and disease.

Generally, 95% confidence interval of OR needs to be calculated, and Miettinen method and Woolf method are usually used for calculation.

When describing the basic data of case-control studies, T-tests are usually used to compare the differences in age, height, weight between control and case groups. T-test, also known as Student's t test, is used to infer the probability of difference with T-distribution theory, so as to compare whether the difference between two means is significant, and to compare whether factors such as age and height are balanced between the control group and the case group.

If the case-control study studies multiple exposure factors, multiple logistic regression analysis is used to analyze the risk factors and exclude the influence of confounding factors. The response variable Y in the logistic regression model is a dichotomous variable, which is usually coded as 0,1. Y =1 represents the outcome that the researcher focuses on, and Y=0 represents the opposite outcome. Suppose there are P possible influencing factors (i.e., explanatory variables) for the response variable Y, denoted as X_1, X_2... X_P. With P explanatory variables, the probability that Y=1 occurs is denoted as π, and the probability that Y=0 is $1-\pi$. After logit transformation, the following equation can be established.

$$logit(\pi) = \ln\left(\frac{\pi}{1-\pi}\right)$$
$$= \beta_1 X_1 + \beta_2 X_2 + \beta_3 X_3 + \beta_4 X_4 + \dots \beta_P X_P$$

19.5   Experimental Epidemiology

In experimental epidemiology, subjects from the same population are randomly divided into experimental and control groups, artificially adding or subtracting a treatment factor, and then the outcome of each group is prospectively followed up to compare the degree of difference in order to determine the effect of the treatment factor. Experimental epidemiological measures occur before the outcome, and the time sequence of cause and effect is clear. Subjects are randomly divided into the experimental group and the control group, and some factors are artificially imposed or reduced, so the etiology hypothesis can be tested.

Design of an Experimental Epidemiological Study

Definition of Research Objectives and Research Subjects

The study of experimental epidemiology should be designed according to the PICO principle which measures each question in the trial into four sections: patient, intervention, control and outcome. Definition should be clearly made from the four sections of patient or population, intervention, control and outcome. Before a study is carried out, it should be clear whether the effect of a drug or treatment is to be studied or whether the effect of a preventive measure is to be evaluated.

Choose the right research object according to the research question and research purpose. In drug research, patients should be selected as research objects. When evaluating preventive measures such as vaccines, normal people at risk of infection should be selected for the study.

Calculation of Sample Size

In experimental epidemiology, when calculating the sample size, the following factors should be considered: the numerical difference between the experimental group and the control group in the occurrence of outcome events, the smaller the difference, the larger the sample size required; the false positive probability, generally taken as $\alpha=0.05$; the false negative probability, generally $\beta=0.1$; unilateral or bilateral test, the sample size required for unilateral test is smaller than that for bilateral test; the number of the groups of research objects, the more groups, the larger the sample size required.

Randomized Grouping and Application of Blind Method

A key feature of experimental epidemiology is the randomization of subjects into experimental and control groups. Randomization is performed to balance confounding factors known and unknown between the experimental and control groups to improve the comparability of the two groups.

In experimental epidemiological studies, many deviations arise from subjects, from the design stage, or from data collection or analysis. In order to reduce selection bias and information bias in experimental epidemiological studies, blind methods are performed at these stages. Blinding refers to the fact that the subject, the experimenter, and the result measurer are unaware of the participant's group assignment.

Selection of Control Group

When studying the effect of intervention measures, the observed effect is often the comprehensive effect of interaction of various factors. Therefore, selecting reasonable control can successfully expose or identify the real effect of intervention measures objectively and fully, so that researchers can make correct evaluation.

The control group can be divided into standard control and placebo control according to the treatment measures. A standard control is the most common type of control used in clinical trials, using conventional or current best treatments (drugs or surgery) as controls. Standard controls are used for diseases which have therapies with definite effect. Placebo controls are used when there is no effective treatment for the disease being studied or when placebo has no effect on the outcome of the study. A placebo is an object that is indistinguishable from an active drug in appearance, color, taste, smell, and no specific known therapeutic ingredient. Commonly used placebos include sweet pills or injections of saline.

Determination of the Study Observation Period

The study outcome (primary outcome and secondary outcome) is determined, and the measurement method of the study outcome is determined. The duration of prospective observation is determined according to the study purpose, study type and study outcome. The observation period of general chronic diseases is long for cardiovascular diseases such as hypertension, and the observation period of infectious diseases is short, such as influenza.

Collect and Organize Data

Since experimental epidemiological studies are prospective studies, baseline data of the experimental and control groups need to be collected and followed up after the study begins. Follow-up observation mainly includes the following three aspects: implementation of intervention measures; information on relevant influencing factors; outcome variables. The follow-up observation of the experimental group and the control group should be consistent.

Analysis of Data

Experimental epidemiology often uses intention-to-treat to analyze the results of studies. The intention-to-treat is performed on the basis of the original subgroup regardless of which treatment patients are really taken, and comparisons between groups are based on the outcomes of the treatment of initially randomly assigned subjects. The purpose of the intention-to-treat is to avoid selection bias and to maintain comparability between groups.

19.6   Epidemiology of Infectious Diseases

Epidemiology of infectious diseases mainly studies the epidemic process of infectious diseases in the population and the factors affecting the process, and formulates countermeasures and measures for the prevention, control and elimination of infectious diseases. Infectious diseases are diseases caused by various pathogens that can spread between humans and animals. Epidemiology in sanitary inspection examines pathogens in the process of transmission and transmission media, so as to discover and control pathogens that can be transmitted in time and control the spread of infectious diseases.

19.6.1   Pathogen and Host

The infectious process refers to the interaction between pathogens and the host after they enter the host, and it also refers to the whole process of the occurrence, development and outcome of infectious diseases.

Pathogens refer to all kinds of organisms that can cause disease of the host, including viruses, bacteria, rickettsiae, mycoplasma, chlamydia, spirochetes, and many other microorganisms and parasites. Whether a pathogen can cause disease after invading the host is closely related to the characteristics of the pathogen and the immune response of the host. Host refers to the person or animal that can be parasitized by infectious pathogens under natural conditions. The host will be damaged by infectious pathogens, but can resist and neutralize foreign invasion through its own defense mechanisms. The host's own defense mechanism mainly includes skin mucosal barrier, internal barrier and specific immune response.

After a host is exposed to a pathogen, it can generate different outcomes, ranging from asymptomatic to death. Understanding the occurrence, development and outcome of different infectious diseases is helpful to formulate corresponding control strategies and measures.

19.6.2   Epidemic Process

The epidemic process refers to the process in which pathogens are discharged from the source of infection, passing through certain transmission routes, invading the body of susceptible people to form new infections, and interacting with the body of susceptible people, and developing continuously. The epidemic process must have three basic links: source of infection, transmission route and susceptible population. Without any one of these links, the infectious disease cannot spread and prevail in the population. The source of infection refers to those who can produce and discharge pathogens, including patients, pathogen carriers and infected animals.

There are a large number of pathogens in patients with infectious diseases, and at the same time, patients with infectious diseases have certain clinical symptoms conducive to the discharge of pathogens. For example, COVID-19 patients can cough to discharge a large number of pathogens, increasing the chances of infection of susceptible persons. Therefore, the patient is an important source of infection, and the whole period during which the patient excretes the pathogen is called the infectious period. The length of the infectious period can affect the epidemiological characteristics of the disease and is an important basis for determining the duration of isolation of infectious patients. A pathogen carrier is a person who has no clinical symptoms but can expel the pathogen after infection. According to the carrier status and clinical stage, pathogen carriers can be divided into incubative pathogen carriers, convalescent pathogen carriers and healthy pathogen carriers. Infected animals can shed pathogens. Diseases and infections that can spread naturally between vertebrates and humans are called zoonotic diseases, such as plague, rabies and schistosomiasis.

The route of transmission refers to the discharge of the pathogen through the source of infection, the whole process that pathogen experiences in the outside environment before invading a new susceptible person. Infectious diseases can spread by one or more routes.

The level of susceptibility of a population depends on the proportion of susceptible people in the population. The greater the proportion of susceptible people in the population, the higher the population susceptibility, and the higher the incidence and spread of infectious diseases.

19.6.3   Prevention Strategies and Measures for Infectious Diseases

The prevention and control measures for infectious diseases mainly include monitoring of infectious diseases, eliminating or reducing the transmission of infectious sources, cutting off transmission routes and protecting susceptible populations. At present, there are 40 kinds of notifiable infectious diseases in China, including 2 kinds of category A infectious diseases,

27 kinds of category B infectious diseases and 11 kinds of category C infectious diseases.

The measures taken against sources of infection are mainly to eliminate or reduce the role of sources of infection in spreading pathogens and effectively curb the spread of infectious diseases. The measures for patients are mainly early detection, early diagnosis, early reporting, early isolation and early treatment. Pathogen carriers of category A infectious diseases and category B infectious diseases under the management of category A infectious diseases shall be isolated and treated. Those who have been in close contact with the source of infection (patient, carriers, suspected patients) and may be infected should be kept in designated places for check-up, medical observation and other necessary preventive measures. According to the degree of harm and economic value of infected animals, measures such as isolation, treatment, killing, burning and deep burial are taken.

Measures for transmission routes are mainly to eliminate pathogens dispersed by the source of infection in the environment. Infectious diseases with different routes of transmission require different measures. The airborne infectious diseases can be prevented by personal protective measures such as ventilation, air disinfection or wearing masks. For infectious diseases transmitted by the fecal-oral route, the patient's excreta, contaminated objects and the surrounding environment should be disinfected. The insect-borne diseases are mainly controlled by the insecticide.

Vaccination is an effective method to prevent infectious diseases. Before the epidemic of infectious diseases, the susceptibility of the population can be reduced by vaccination, so as to effectively prevent the corresponding infectious diseases. This is an important measure for controlling and eliminating infectious diseases, including active and passive immunization.

Glossary

incidence rate 发病率 the frequency of the occurrence of a new case of a disease in a certain range of people within a certain period

exposure cohort 队列 a group of people with a common exposure or characteristic

attributable risk 归因危险度 also known as risk difference (*RD*) or excess risk, is the absolute value of the difference between the incidence of the exposed group and that of the control group. It indicates the extent to which the risk is specifically attributable to the exposure factor

confounding factors 混杂因素 the external factors that affect the relationship between the studied factor and the studied outcome are called confounding factors. It is an influencing factor of the disease, and is related to the factors studied, and its unbalanced distribution between the groups, would obscure or exaggerate the association between the studied factor and the studied disease

route of transmission 传播途径 the whole process that a pathogen goes through in the external environment after being expelled from an infectious source before invading a new susceptible host. Infectious diseases can spread through one or more routes

source of infection 传染源 people and animals, reproducing, and excreting pathogens, including infectious disease patients, pathogen carriers, and infected animals

（张定梅）

新形态教材网·数字课程学习……

🖥 教学 PPT　　　　📄 自测题　　　　💬 推荐阅读

Chapter 20
Basic Theory of Health Inspection and Quarantine

Learning objectives:

- Know the application of terminology in practical cases.
- Understand the terminology of the public health risk screening process.
- Be familiar with the terminology of public health risk monitoring and control.
- Master the main terms in public health risks and factors.

20.1 Public Health Risk of Health Quarantine Concern

The public health risk of health quarantine concern represents the public health risk that will endanger the life, health and safety of population, and spread across regions, countries and continents, causing serious and direct dangerous events that need to be dealt with by the health and quarantine department. There are four kinds of public health risk of health quarantine concern: infectious disease, nuclear radiation hazard factor, biological hazard factor and chemical hazard factor.

Infectious Disease

Infectious disease is caused by various pathogens and can be transmitted from person to person, from animal to animal or from animal to person. Infectious diseases of health quarantine concern are divided into quarantinable infectious diseases and monitored infectious diseases. Quarantinable infectious diseases specified in the "Frontier Health and Quarantine Law of the People's Republic of China" include plague, cholera, yellow fever and other infectious diseases determined and announced by The State Council the People's Republic of China. Monitored infectious diseases contain malaria, dengue fever, paralytic polio and so on.

Nuclear Radiation Hazard Factor

Radiation sicknesses can be caused by radiation hazard factors. Radiation can be divided into electromagnetic radiation and particle radiation. The body suffering from various types of nuclear radiation will produce various types and degrees of damage or disease, collectively known as radioactive disease. The main sources of nuclear radiation related to human life are medical exposure, occupational exposure, accident exposure, emergency exposure, emission of radioactive substances from nuclear energy production, exposure of radioactive materials, and nuclear weapon explosion.

Biohazard Factor

Biohazard factor refers to those that cause harm to human body by biological means or infectious factors, including bacteria, viruses, fungi, rickettsia, chlamydia and toxins, etc. For example, the anthrax letter attacks happening in the United States in 2001 killed 5 people and infected 17 others.

Chemical Hazard Factor

Chemical hazard factor refers to toxic, corrosive, explosive, combustion and combustion-supporting chemicals that are harmful to the human body, facilities and the environment. The chemical hazard factors focuses on are chemical agents, including nerve agents, erosive agents, systemic toxic agents, asphyxiation agents and incapacitated agents. For example, in 1995, 13 people died and about 5,500 others were poisoned by sarin gas on the Tokyo subway.

The Characteristic of Public Health Risk of Health Quarantine Concern

The public health risk of health quarantine concern has obvious characteristics: relying on the carrier, spreading, causing people group harm and social concern. All public health risks of health quarantine concern must rely on carriers to disseminate. Carriers are generally people, vectors and their hosts, animals, goods and so on. Spreading is the main difference between the risk of quarantine concern and other public health risks. And the public health risk of health quarantine concern not only can cause individual harm, but also cause group harm. Such group harm will cause social panic, and affect normal traffic and trade order.

Factors Influence the Spread of Public Health Risks

The public health risk spreads need three factors: risk sources, transmission route and susceptible population. The influencing factors of risks spread and harm include human factor, natural factor and social factor. The human factor contains the structure of population, the habit of living, the susceptibility to infectious diseases. The structure of population represents age, gender and occupation, etc. The natural factor contains geography, meteorology, ecology, etc. The social factor contains the system of political and social, living conditions, health facilities, medical conditions, educational level and so on. All these factors influence the occurrence and spread of public health risk.

20.2   Public Health Risk Screening Process

Screening of public health risks of health quarantine concern represents the adoption of certain technical means to inspect specific quarantine objects, such as travelers, vehicles, goods, postal parcels, containers and vectors, to discover possible risks of quarantine concern, and to screen and confirm the specific types of risks. The purpose of risk screening is to discover, identify and confirm risks, and provide a technical basis for further treatment, as well as policy making. Therefore, risk screening is the basis of the whole health quarantine's work. The screening of public health risks of health quarantine concern emphasizes promptness and quickness. The technical means of screening mainly include quarantine, medical examination, health declaration, temperature monitoring, medical inspection, document examination, sanitary examination, epidemiological case study and laboratory examination.

Quarantine

Quarantine was first implemented in Italian ports during the plague pandemic of the 14th century. Quarantine is a preventive control measure. It represents the separation of persons, goods or vehicles that may carry health risk factors of quarantine concern from other persons and goods, determining whether they carry risk factors of quarantine concern through quarantine and inspection for a certain period of time, so as to prevent their spread. During the quarantine period, the quarantined people are checked every day to detect patients in a timely manner, and release will not be granted until the incubation period is over and there are no risks.

Medical Examination

The medical examination is the traditional screening method of health quarantine. It is generally aimed at specific infectious diseases, and it can detect infectious disease patients or suspect persons, and distinguish them from the healthy population. For example, when carrying out health quarantine on passenger ships from plague epidemic areas, it is a very important task to have all passengers undergo a health inspection before entering the country. This includes fever, signs of pneumonia, swollen lymph nodes examinations, etc. Taking into account the disruption of medical examinations to travel activities, the rapidness of health quarantine medical examinations is emphasized. The medical examination usually uses the rapid screening method, and the examination results are available within a short time, such as colloidal gold immunochromatographic rapid reagent strip screening for malaria.

Health Declaration

Health declaration refers to the reporting by the responsible person to the health authorities of the possible risks of health quarantine concern, including travelers' reports of infectious diseases related to individuals, as well as the responsible persons' reports on possible risks carried by conveyances, goods, baggage, and postal parcels. According to the classification of declaration, health declaration can be divided into on-site paper declaration and remote electronic declaration.

According to the classification of declaration subjects, health declaration can be divided into personal declaration of travelers, health declaration of ships, health declaration of aircraft and health declaration of other means of transportation. The content of health declaration generally includes whether there are patients with infectious diseases, whether there are suspicious symptoms of infectious diseases, whether they carry medical vectors, whether they carry pathogenic microbial pathogens, and whether there are other risk factors.

Temperature Monitoring

Temperature monitoring is also a traditional method to monitor symptoms of infectious diseases. It refers to the use of certain technical means to take the temperature of the target population to find people with fever symptoms. Fever is the first symptom of most infectious diseases, which always continuous for a long time. Therefore, temperature monitoring can be used to quickly distinguish patients with suspected infectious disease from the general population. At present, infrared temperature measuring tools are commonly used in public places. The surface temperature of the object is related to the size of its infrared radiation energy and the distribution of wavelength. According to this principle, infrared temperature measuring instrument can accurately determine the surface temperature of the object.

Medical Inspection

Medical inspection is an effective supplement to temperature monitoring, usually through the autions of checking, looking, hearing and smelling. Medical inspection is conducted for specific groups of people to detect signs and symptoms of infectious diseases and to detect risk factors carried by travelers. Signs and symptoms to focus on during a medical inspection include dry cough, runny nose, dyspnea, rash, gait changes due to bone, muscle and joint pain, skin flushing, and mental status.

Documents Examination

Documents examination refers to the examination of documents, certificates, records and other materials related to health risks of quarantine concern to find evidence of the existence of risk factors. The documents examination usually include the examination of the traveler's personal information and the relevant records , certification materials of transportation, cargo, luggage and postal parcels. The documents examination on individual travelers generally includes inspecting health declaration forms, identification documents, travel history documents, vaccination certificates, etc. The documents examination on vehicles generally include inspecting employee lists, passenger manifests, medical logbooks for the flight, suspicious cases with a definite diagnosis, sanitary control, manifest, etc.

Sanitary Examination

Sanitary inspection refers to the inspection of transportation vehicles, containers, goods, luggage and postal parcels according to the basic theoretical knowledge of hygiene by means of inquiry, visual inspection, data reference and sampling inspection, so as to find possible risk factors of quarantine concern. Sanitary examination mainly includes inspecting water and food hygiene, solid and liquid wastes, suspicious symptoms and medical vectors.

Epidemiological Case Study

The epidemiological case study is an important means of screening public health risk factors concerned by health quarantine. The epidemiological case investigation targets are persons with positive results through other screening methods, including suspected carriers of infectious diseases, food poisoning, and carriers of other risk factors such as nuclear radiation. The basic information, specific exposure history and health status of individuals are investigated by using specific questionnaire, to provide a basis for the diagnosis of individual cases, tracing of co-contaminated people and close contacts, and timely control of the spread of risks.

Laboratory Examination

Laboratory tests are carried out against risk factors of biological quarantine concern, including infectious agents, toxins, etc. Laboratory tests includes rapid screening and confirmatory monitoring. The samples for laboratory testing are generally from persons suspected of infectious diseases who are discovered by isolation, medical examination, health declaration, medical inspection, epidemiological investigation, document examination, sanitary examination and other methods. There are many types of samples used in laboratory tests, usually including: throat swabs, nasal swabs, serum, whole blood, urine, faeces, vomit, cerebrospinal fluid, etc.

The commonly used methods of laboratory examination include the following four kinds: (a) direct examination (microscope); (b) isolation, cultivation and identification of pathogens; (c) immunological detection; (d) molecular biological detection. Direct examination through microscope usually can directly detect plasmodium, spirochetes, schistosoma, etc. Pathogen isolation, cultivation and identification are using selective media to cultivate and identify different pathogens. Immunological detection usually includes rapid immunochromatographic detection, agglutination test, precipitation test, complement binding test, neutralization test, immunofluorescence detection, radioimmunodetection, enzyme-linked immunosorbent assay. Molecular biological tests are mainly aimed at detecting nucleic acids of pathogens , including ordinary PCR, nested PCR, RT-PCR, nucleic acid molecular hybridization, gene chip technology, DNA sequencing and analysis.

20.3   Public Health Risks Prevention and Control

Public Health Risks Control

Once a public health risk of health quarantine concern occurs, the risk should be controlled as soon as possible to protect the health of the population and prevent the further development and spread of the risk. But how can public health risks be effectively controlled? The control of public health risk of health quarantine concern should focus on the group, and the control methods can be divided into two categories: direct controlling the epidemic; changing the natural and social factors to affect the epidemic. The risk control method should not only have macro management means, but also have specific control measures. There are several specific methods: vaccination, medical observation, sanitary treatment (decontamination, disinfection, deinsectization, deratization), joint prevention and control, etc. Here we introduce the sanitary treatment and joint prevention and control.

Sanitary Treatment

The sanitary treatment concerned in health quarantine refers to disinfection, deinsectization, decontamination and deratization. These sanitary treatment methods are important means to eliminate the source of infection and cut off the way of transmission. Disinfection is one of the most commonly used sanitary procedures. The main purpose of disinfection mentioned in health quarantine is to kill pathogenic microorganisms and prevent their spread. According to the purpose of disinfection, disinfection can be divided into foci disinfection and preventive disinfection. According to the method of classification, it can be divided into physical disinfection and chemical disinfection. According to the disinfection level, it can be divided into high level, medium level and low level disinfection. The foci disinfection refers to the disinfection of the area where is a source of infection so as to prevent the pathogen from infecting other susceptible persons. Preventive disinfection refers to the disinfection of objects, places and human bodies that may be contaminated with pathogens when no source of infection is found. Physical disinfection includes dry heat disinfection and damp heat disinfection, such as incineration disinfection, pasteurization. Chemical disinfection is the use of chemical disinfectant to perform disinfection, such as chlorine disinfectant, and peroxide material disinfectant.

Joint Prevention and Control

Joint prevention and control represent that when dealing with the health risks of quarantine concern, multiple departments related to prevention and control measures are united to establish a unified coordination and command organization, so as to jointly take charge of the risks and prevent their spread. To establish a good joint prevention and control work model, at least three elements should be considered: appropriate components, clear division of responsibilities, and an efficient coordination mechanism.

Public Health Risks Prevention

Risk prevention is based on the theory of public health, technology and method, strengthen the public health capacity building at border, the border traffic hub , such as active implementation of health education, immunization, health cleaning and other environmental health interventions, to prevent the risk development, dissemination and diffusion, and reduce the probability of occurrence of harm and loss . Risk prevention is carried out around three links and three factors of risk transmission: controlling risk sources, cutting off the route of transmission and protecting vulnerable populations. At the same time, attention should be paid to the influence of crowd factors, natural factors and social factors. The risk prevention mainly has four objectives: (a) to prevent the occurrence and development of risks; (b) to prevent the spread and dissemination of helath risks of quarantine concern, (c) to protect the life and health of the population, (d) to ensure the development of traffic and trade order. Risk prevention mainly includes population health prevention, transportation junction public health protection, conveyance operator management.

Population Health Prevention

Population health prevention includes health prevention of whole healthy population and health prevention of key population. Promote public health awareness of the whole population through health education and community activities, and promote preventive intervention measures for key populations through vaccination, health education and travel health security.

Transportation Junction Public Health Protection

Transportation junction is the necessary path for the convergence and spread of risks concerned by health quarantine, and it is the risk prone point, transmission transfer point and key point for controlling the spread. Doing a good job in public health protection of transportation junctions is an important means to cut off the route of risk transmission and protect vulnerable populations. To ensure the public health of the transportation junctions, transportation junctions need to meet the core capacity requirements under the Inernational Health Regulations, including five capacities at all times and seven capacities responding to events that may constitute a public health emergency of international concern. The five capacities are: (a) the availability of medical services at a suitable location and of sufficient medical personnel, equipment and premises for prompt treatment of ill travelers; (b) the ability to mobilize equipment and personnel for the transport of sick travelers to released medical facilities, (c) having trained personnel to inspect vehicles, (d) ensuring a safe environment for facilities at transport hubs through health supervision, (e) developing well-developed operational plans to control vectors and hosts near transport hubs. The seven emergency response capabilities are: (a) emergency plan capability to provide appropriate response measures for public health emergencies; (b) capacity to assess and treat infected travelers and to treat them in isolation; (c) having appropriate places to separate infected travelers from other travelers; (d) ability of assessing suspected travelers; (e) ability of sanitizing multiple traffic cargoes; (f) ability of carrying out entry-exit control measures for travelers; (g) having trained professionals.

Conveyance Operator Management

A conveyance operator represents a natural or legal person in charge of a conveyance or his agent. Management of conveyance operator should include the following contents: (a) establish health management system and ensure the implementation of the system; (b) operators in different positions of transportation and logistics should respect corresponding sanitary requirements; (c) establish corresponding hardware equipment.

20.4   The Cases of Basic Theory of HIQ

Background

At 9:00 PM on August 29, 2011, a group of 33 labors returning from Country C in Africa entered China through a port of entry. Health quarantine officers found a passenger with fever during quarantine. The body temperature was 37.6°C by the infrared thermal imaging system, and 39.7°C by mercury thermometer. Health and quarantine personnel carried out on-site quarantine investigation immediately.

Health Quarantine

The epidemiological case investigation showed that the passenger was male, Chinese, with symptoms such as chills, high fever, joint pain and fatigue, and had worked in Country C for 6 months. He had been treated for malaria and had been bitten by mosquitoes recently. The latest onset was 2 days ago. He was receiving oral and injection of anti-malarial drugs. According to the investigation, on August 28, he and other 32 workers departed from Country C, arrived at Hong Kong Airport in the evening of August 29 and directly took the same bus through a port of entry.

They intended to stay in Shenzhen for one night and return to their original residence on August 30.

The health and quarantine staffs made a preliminarily judgement on the traveler suspected malaria infection based on the epidemiological investigation and medical test results. For further screening, the quarantine staffs collected blood samples and sent them to the Centers for Disease Control and Prevention (CDC) for testing, and transferred him to institutional hospitals for diagnosis and treatment according to the joint prevention and control mechanism. The body temperature of other 32 travelers was measured again one by one, and medical examination was carried out as well, and all of them were normal.

An epidemiological investigation showed that 32 closely contacts had worked in malaria-affected countries in Africa, and 20 of them had suffered from malaria, including 6 persons who had developed malaria one month ago, 9 persons who had developed malaria three months ago, 5 persons who had developed malaria six months ago, and 19 persons who had been treated with drugs. Health quarantine staffs asked the 32 close contacts to fill in health declaration forms, collected their samples, gave them health advice, and issued medical convenience cards before releasing them. The health and quarantine staffs then took mosquito control and final disinfection to the port area that the group passengers passed through, the outstanding quarantine facilities and equipment, the bus they took and the accompanying luggage.

On August 30, CDC conducted a preliminary screening by using colloidal gold method and a nucleic acid test to recheck the samples. This passenger and 5 of his colleagues were tested positive for plasmodium falciparum malaria. Combined with the results of medical examination and epidemiological case study, the 6 persons were confirmed to be malaria patients. The health quarantine staffs immediately contacted the 6 patients, reported their test results, gave them health advice, required them to self-isolation, controlled and eradicated mosquitos, and went to the hospital for treatment. Meanwhile, local health authorities were informed of the situation and asked for assistance in follow-up treatment and supervision.

Case Analysis

Malaria is an important parasitic disease that seriously harms the health and life safety of Chinese people and affects the social and economic development. Clinically, the typical symptoms are periodic chills, fever, headache, sweating, anemia and splenomegaly. It occurs more frequently in summer, and can occur all the year round in tropical and subtropical areas, and is easy to spread. In order to effectively protect the health of the general public and promote coordinated economic and social development, the Chinese government decided in 2010 to carry out the elimination of malaria in a comprehensive manner, to eliminate the disease nationwide by 2020. Quarantine prevention and control of malaria is a key work of health quarantine.

In this case, plasmodium was the risk factor of quarantine, the sick passengers were the risk source, the bus was the route of transmission, and the passengers traveling with the patients and port population were vulnerable groups. Through temperature monitoring, medical investigation, epidemiological investigation, laboratory testing and transferring to designated hospitals for diagnosis and treatment, health quarantine could effectively discover and control the sources of risk concerned by quarantine. Sanitation treatment was carried out on buses and port areas to effectively cut off the transmission routes. Health advice was given to fellow passengers and medical observation was carried out. Subsequently, another 5 passengers were found to be infected with malaria, and relevant departments were notified in time, which effectively protected the vulnerable groups.

Glossary

public health risk 公共卫生风险 the risk that will endanger the life and health safety of people, and will spread across regions, countries and continents, will cause serious and direct dangerous events, requiring the health and quarantine department to deal with it

infectious disease 传染病 the disease caused by various pathogens, which can be transmitted from person to person, from animal to animal or from animal to person. Infectious diseases of health quarantine concern are divided into quarantinable infectious diseases and monitored infectious diseases

carrier *n*. 载体 the substance capable of transmitting infectious pathogens or carrying other substances

susceptible population 易感人群 the population who lack immunity to some infectious diseases and infectious pathogens, who are susceptible to infection

risk screening 风险筛查 adoption of certain technical means to inspect specific quarantine objects, such as travelers, vehicles, goods, postal parcels, containers and vectors, to discover possible risks of quarantine concern, to screen and confirm the specific types of risks

medical examination 医学检查 using the rapid screening method, to detect infectious disease patients or suspect persons, and distinguish them from healthy population

health declaration 健康申报 the reporting by the responsible person to the health authorities of the possible risks of health quarantine concern, including travelers' reports of infectious diseases related to individuals, as well as the responsible persons' reports on possible risks carried by conveyances, goods, baggage, and postal parcels

temperature monitoring 体温监测 using of certain technical means to take the temperature of the target population to find people with fever symptoms

medical inspection 医学巡查 conducting for specific groups of people to detect signs and symptoms of infectious diseases and to detect risk factors carried by travelers

documents examination 文书检查 examination of documents, certificates, records and other materials related to health risks of quarantine concern to find evidence of the existence of risk factors

sanitary examination 卫生检查 inspection of transportation vehicles, containers, goods, luggage and postal parcels according to the basic theoretical knowledge of hygiene by means of inquiry, visual inspection, data reference and sampling inspection

epidemiological case investigation 流行病学个案调查 an investigation in which the basic information, specific exposure history and health status of individuals are investigated by using

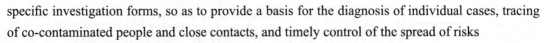

specific investigation forms, so as to provide a basis for the diagnosis of individual cases, tracing of co-contaminated people and close contacts, and timely control of the spread of risks

CDC 疾病预防控制中心 Center for Disease Control and Prevention

（李雪霞）

新形态教材网·数字课程学习……

🖥 教学 PPT   📝 自测题   💬 推荐阅读

Chapter 21
Travel Health

Learning objectives:
- Know travel consultation.
- Understand the relationship between health and climate change.
- Be familiar with the relevant questions in pretravel counseling.

21.1　Introduction

Travel health considers all health maintenance during the whole journey, including both physical and emotional, infectious diseases (ID) and non-infectious diseases (NID), natural environment (extreme weather, temperature, altitude, pressure, solar ultraviolet radiation, etc.), and even the social culture and language. The aims of travel include the following different contents, such as tourism, work, volunteerism, medical care, migration, etc. However, with global climate change and globalization, the challenge of increasing infectious diseases, such as COVID-19, has crept into the field, impacting both the provider and the traveler.

The travel consultation includes three aspects: pretravel consultation, health problems while traveling and post-travel consultation. The pretravel consultation should consider the specific traveler populations with certain purposes in order to offer practical information on the management of pretravel and post-travel related. However, it is not easy to keep up to date in the field of travel medicine because it covers too many fields, for instance, travel medicine, infectious disease and non-infectious disease, general medical journals and national government and international recommendations.

21.2　Travel Consultation

21.2.1　Pretravel Consultation

The pretravel consultation aims to provide evidence-based information that addresses health problems while abroad and upon return home. The pretravel consultation, therefore, covers three main goals:

(1) to assess the travelers' fitness for travel, based on medical history and an understanding of the purpose and type of travel;

(2) to analyze the anticipated and real health risks;

(3) to translate the findings into tailored counseling of prophylactic measures.

Furthermore, travel consultation should include the following suggestions during travel, such as appropriate behavior, self-management, and instruction about seeking medical care when health problems arise. The personal experience of the provider/advisor positively impacts the credibility of suggestions. Informing travelers is a key function of the advisor. Many travelers are overly anxious during travel, possibly due to uncertainty about and fear of infectious diseases or strange circumstances. Thus highlighting the positive influences of travel on health may reassure travelers. International travelers should be vaccinated or take medicine to prevent infectious diseases, such as COVID–19, malaria risk and prevention, safe sex, and even non-infectious diseases (traffic accidents, drowning, altitude sickness, sunburn, mental and psychological problems of travel).

21.2.2　How to Provide the Pretravel Consultation

As a travel health advisor, he/she could provide personalized and relevant tips for a safe journey to travelers, e.g., for malaria, motion sickness, jet lag, extreme weather and accident prevention. The advisors must focus on what they perceive to be the most important health risks and their prevention for every traveler based on the travel destinations, such as considering the epidemiology in the targeted destinations. Any advisor's personal experience is an additional asset during counseling. The assessment of potential exposures should be based on the traveler's detailed itinerary and activity plans. However, travel plans are frequently uncertain before the trip. Travel health providers must recognize potential deviations in itineraries and advise accordingly.

The content of pretravel advice may be defined by the checklists below (Table 21-1). Referral to travel health experts with broad experience is optimal for more complex situations requiring detailed epidemiologic knowledge, special health risks, or advice for immunocompromised travelers. A face-to-face interview by an advisor is an effective method of delivering counseling. However, the expertise and communications skills of the advisor would impact the pretravel consultation.

Key Points of Pretravel Advice Practice

Food　Eat freshly prepared food, try to avoid raw, uncooked food. Check that food is not contaminated by dirty materials or by organisms, e.g., insects or rats.

Water　Drink safe water (such as bottled water) and boiling water. Avoid fresh dairy products without quality.

Mosquitoes　The whole-day prevention of mosquito bites especially relevant in areas endemic for malaria, dengue, chikungunya, zika, and other arthropod-transmitted pathogens. Take

Table 21-1   Relevant questions in pretravel consultation
(modified from Keystone et al., 2019, Travel medicine)

Items	Details
Itinerary/schedule	Where/destination
	Standards of accommodation and food hygiene standards
Duration	How long
Travel style	Independent travel/single or package tour/groups
	Business trip
	Adventure trip
	Pilgrimage
	High risk of infectious disease (malaria, dengue fever) in rural areas with poor hygienic standards
	Refugees
	Expatriates
	Long-term travelers
Time of travel	What season? Epidemic season of infectious diseases, such as mosquito or rats
	How long until departure
Special activities	Hiking
	Diving
	Rafting
	Biking
Healths status	Chronic diseases
	Allergies
	Regular medications
	Mental health issues/problem
Vaccination status	Basic vaccinations
	Special (travel) vaccinations
Travel experience	Tolerated (malaria) medication
	Problems with high altitude
	Accidents
	Animal contacts
Special situations	Pregnancy/breastfeeding
	Disability
	Physical or psychological problems during previous trips

repellents, protective clothing, and mosquito nets, etc.

Hydration/Dehydration   Drink adequate fluid to keep a light yellow color of urine.

Sun   Avoid too much sun exposure, especially for children. Prepare sunscreen, hat, cap, fine-meshed protective clothing, and sunglasses.

Insects Bite/Animals Attack   Do not walk barefoot to avoid the parasites/insects bite; shoes and long trousers are important for preventing attacking of poisonous animals, e.g., bee, wasp, snake, scorpion, and spider.

Sexual Contacts   Avoid casual contacts, and carry condoms at all times, just in case.

Accidents   Accidents include traffic accidents, sports and other leisure injuries, violence and aggression, drowning, drunk and animal bites.

Altitude   Prepare medication to prevent high-altitude sickness for those high-mountain hiking and trekking travelers.

Insurance   Buy the travel insurance prior to departing.

Vaccination is a safe and effective tool to prevent infectious diseases (ID). In travel medicine, vaccines are not only indicated for individual protection of the traveler against destination-specific ID risks but also for public health considerations to prevent the spread of ID. Recommended vaccination schedules and routes of administration should be adhered to, but immune memory is generally sufficiently effective to compensate for delayed immunizations. Some vaccines can be combined to account for a limited time before departure. Special considerations apply to people with an impaired immune system and pregnant women. However, a strict contraindication is relevant only in sporadic cases and thorough risk-benefit considerations should be performed. The availability of efficacious and safe vaccines alone is not sufficient; their adequate use is as important.

21.2.3   Fitness to Travel

Ideally, international travelers should be aware that the stableness of their physical and mental health is necessary for travel. Acute disorders indicate that trip should be canceled. Special risks for small children, pregnant women, older people, or travelers with chronic disorders require careful advice when balancing the benefits and risks of a trip. For example, pretravel consultation should aim to minimize the potential health dangers for a pregnant woman who is obligated to travel to Africa or South America for family reasons. Finally, the travelers need to decide for themselves, but the advisor may also recommend against a journey if the risks are deemed too high (e.g., malaria, Zika virus). Cardiovascular problems (e.g., heart disease) and injuries (e.g., traffic accidents) are the most common causes of death during travel. The destination and the type of travel affect the magnitude of health risks for particular groups. Physical stress accompanies activities such as trekking and diving, and climatic challenges (temperature, humidity, altitude, air pollution).

A priority in the pretravel consultation is to minimize unnecessary exposures, particularly in vulnerable groups. Therefore travel to remote and tropical destinations is typically discouraged for pregnant women and very young children/babies, given the risks ranging from infectious diseases to general stress, dehydration, sunburn, and lack of appropriate medical care in remote areas. Immunocompromised travelers, such as those with chronic diseases, and medical conditions requiring immune modulators, also need special attention and preparation. Additionally, the travel health advisor may need to recommend deferring air travel due to the increased risk for complications for certain travelers, having coronary bypass surgery within two weeks, having stroke within two weeks, diving or having diving accidents within 24 hours, etc.

21.2.4 Health Problems During and After Travel

During the past several decades, travelers who visit remote, extreme, and wilderness adventures have increased obviously. The travelers have more chances to encounter dangerous species (e.g., mosquitoes, flies, fleas, lice, chiggers, scabies) and environments (e.g., sunburn, drowning, flooding and high-altitude sickness, polar area). The dangers travelers may encounter while traveling are classified into 3 sections: nonvenomous injuries (e.g., blood-feeding arthropods and animal attacks); venomous injuries (e.g., arthropods and reptiles); and traumatic or traumatic envenoming injuries (e.g., shark, jellyfish).

For example, two general rules during and after travel to tropical and subtropical countries are to investigate: ① every fever within 24 hours of onset, and ② every diarrheal episode with fever, abdominal cramps, and bloody stool. Medical screening is recommended for long-term travelers in tropical areas, even when asymptomatic, such as exposure history and physical examination, blood chemistry and hematology, stool/urine parasitology. Unless the apparent symptoms exist, some examinations may be performed about 3 months after returning for the incubation periods of possible pathogens. The incubation period must be borne in mind. *Falciparum malaria* usually appears within a few months after returning, but manifestations of malaria after 1 year and longer have been reported. Late-onset or recurrent diarrhea may be a manifestation of giardiasis, amebiasis, or postinfectious irritable bowel syndrome; pruritus with skin swellings can be a result of filariasis. When in doubt, a specialist in tropical diseases should be consulted for such cases. Posttravel screening is an essential process for the diagnosis of latent infection in travelers who return from a region where these diseases are prevalent.

Most travel clinics provide pretravel consultation, posttravel screening, and health care. It is not necessary for every traveler to do a posttravel medical examination. A posttravel medical examination generally aims to rule out a latent (subclinical) disease but is not confirmed. Travelers, who have the following situations, should be advised to have a medical examination on their return if they:

- suffer from a chronic illness;
- are immunocompromised;
- experience illness within 3 months after returning, e.g., fever, vomiting, weight loss, jaundice, urinary disorders;
- expose to a potentially severe ID while traveling;
- have spent more than 3 months in a developing country.

Two general screenings include a medical interview and a physical examination. A medical interview by an experienced physician identifies exposure to specific infectious diseases and estimates the potential risk. Risk assessment in travelers without symptoms should include a basic questionnaire (Table 21-2, and 21-3). The responses will be used for the reference of clinical investigations and counseling. A physical examination has a limited value in asymptomatic travelers. However, unsuspected individuals may manifest skin lesions, splenomegaly, lymphadenopathy, or signs of chronic disease unrelated to travel. The medical interview should guide the extent of the examination.

Table 21–2 Self–administered questionnaire in posttravel screening
(modified from Keystone et al., 2019)

Items	Details
Demographic factors	Age, gender
Travel characteristics	Destination, duration of stay, and date of return
Vaccinations	Document year of last dose, Polio, diphtheria, tetanus, Hepatitis A and B, Yellow fever, Typhoid fever, Meningococcal meningitis type A, C, W, and Y, Japanese encephalitis, Other (rabies, tickborne encephalitis)
Malaria chemoprophylaxis	Drug used and duration of intake

Table 21–3 Interactive posttravel screening questionnaire (modified from Keystone et al., 2019)

Items	Details
Basic medical information	Weight change, tobacco, alcohol and psychotropic drug use, concomitant medication
Travel intentions	Holiday, professional travel, visiting friends and relatives (VFRs), adventure sports, ecotourism, etc.
Physical environment	Destination, duration, transport means, travel route, type of accommodation, altitude
Specific environment	Freshwater contact (rivers, lakes, flooded areas), caves, marine environment, forests, game parks, etc.
Food intake habits	Exposure to raw meat and fish, undercooked food, unusual ingredients, unpurified water, unpasteurized dairy products
Previous disease history	Chronic diseases and allergic conditions (asthma, eczema, urticaria), potentially interfering with screening procedures
Malaria protection	Physical protection, type of antimalaria drugs, dosage, and duration of intake
Sexually transmitted infection (STI risk)	Protective measures, contact with risk groups
Bloodborne risks	Injection drug use, needle-prick accidents, trauma, blood transfusion
Diseases during travel	Febrile, intestinal and skin diseases, STIs

21.2.5 Challenges of Travel Consultation

Much time and effort are needed to stay abreast with the growing body of knowledge in travel medicine (see the **"key points of pretravel advice practice"** above). The regular provision of advice is necessary to obtain and maintain the routine. If such practice is not possible, it may be advisable to work with checklists for standard travel advice, and to refer clients to more experienced colleagues for complex itineraries or special health considerations. Studies on health problems associated with travel have mostly relied on surveys or surveillance networks, and may not be sensitive in capturing injuries that require immediate attention during travel or evaluation by trauma specialists rather than travel medicine, tropical medicine, and infectious disease specialists. Technological advances such as mobile phones and telemedicine platforms may allow improved data capture.

The advisor should be aware of the information sources that their clients use. Some travelers obtain information from travel agencies, which naturally emphasize the positive aspects of travel. Some travelers receive information from friends and relatives; others visit pharmacies for advice. The media publish abundantly about travel destinations as well. A wide range of inadequate or conflicting information from different perspectives often creates confusion rather than clarity. Contradictory information unsettles travelers and raises their skepticism about preventive measures, leading to poor compliance with recommendations. Clear, accurate, and up-to-date information must therefore be conveyed. The organization and order of components in a travel clinic consultation are listed below.

- Ask questions to assess the risk associated with the trip.
- Review and recommend vaccinations (routine, required, itinerary based).
- Discuss vector-borne disease risk and prevention such as malaria chemoprophylaxis and insect precaution.
- Discuss food and water precautions and prevention/treatment of travelers' diarrhea.
- Discuss sexually transmitted infections and bloodborne issues.
- Assess and recommend environmental challenges and preventions (altitude, pollution, etc).
- Determine other risks and their prevention/management based on itinerary and activities (e.g., schistosomiasis, leptospirosis, diving).

The client (traveler) is often overwhelmed with abundant information and is likely to forget most of it. Thus there are five suggestions that may help with all consultations.

- Advise travelers in a personal, individualized conversation that responds to their needs and allows for questions. The assessment should explore details regarding travel itinerary and style, previous travel experience and vaccinations, and existing health problems. Offering concise information is best, but elaborate on areas of concern to the traveler.
- Remind travelers about preventing risks such as sunburn, accidents and injuries, and mental health disturbances during travel.
- Provide written material as additional information. Such information must be consistent with the oral advice given.
- Provide links to reliable Internet sources (WHO, local CDC, and other national recommendations) to guarantee accurate guidance.
- Provide and recommend carrying important documents such as vaccination certificate (or exemption letter), critical medical records, list of allergies, blood type, travel health insurance information, and emergency contacts.

Controversial information must be discussed to avoid confusion and eventual noncompliance. Addressing discrepancies between different sources of information illustrates controversies that travelers may encounter. Many clients will have consulted other information sources or received advice from nonprofessionals, which may vary due to the limited amount of evidence on certain issues. One way to impact health behavior is to combine individualized advice based on scientific evidence with enriched personal experience.

21.3　The Relationship Between Health and Climate Change

The CO_2 concentration in the atmosphere had increased from 280 ppm before the industrial revolution to 417 ppm in 2021. The accumulation of atmospheric CO_2 intensifies the greenhouse effect, which leads to global warming. The global sea surface temperature (SST) has increased by approximately 1℃ over the past century, and it is expected to increase by 2-4℃ by the end of the 21st century compared to the 1870s.

Links between climate change and infectious diseases are complex. However, climate change caused by global warming influences public health significantly. Climate mainly affects the range of infectious diseases, whereas weather affects the timing and intensity of outbreaks. Climate change scenarios include a change in the distribution of infectious diseases with warming and changes in outbreaks associated with weather extremes. Statistical models are used to estimate the global burden of some infectious diseases as a result of climate change. According to the models, by 2030, 10% more diarrheal diseases are expected, affecting primarily young children. If the global temperature increases by 2-3℃, as expected, the population at risk for malaria could increase by 3%-5%. There is now evidence that in some areas, e.g., the Horn of Africa, warm EI Niño Southern Oscillations (ENSO) are associated with a higher risk of emergence of Rift Valley fever, cholera and malaria and during cold La Niña events, dengue fever, chikungunya and yellow fever.

Due to climate change affecting vector biology and disease transmission, Zoonotic tick-borne diseases increase the health burden in Europe. Climate change may also be partly responsible for the change in the distribution of tick (e.g., *Dermacentor reticulatus*). Increased winter activity of tick is probably due to warmer winters. Climate suitability models predict that 8 important tick species are likely to establish more northern permanent populations in a climate-warming scenario. This is a bad phenomenon for public health. However, the models of climate change are required to consider the dynamic biological processes involved in pathogen abundance and pathogen transmission to assess future infectious disease scenarios.

Glossary

pretravel consultation 旅行前咨询 the consultation offers a dedicated time to prepare travelers for the health concerns that might arise during their trips

posttravel consultation 旅行后咨询 the consultation offers a dedicated time to those illness travelers after return from abroad

altitude sickness 高原反应 an altitude sickness if someone travels to a high altitude too quickly. Breathing becomes difficult because you're not able to take in as much oxygen

motion sickness 晕动 sickness occurs when your brain can't make sense of information sent from your eyes, ears and body. Lots of motion — in a car, airplane, boat, or even an amusement park ride — can make you feel queasy, clammy or sick to your stomach

immunocompromised travelers 有免疫缺陷的旅行者 many chronic illnesses, underlying health conditions, and medicines can weaken a person's immune system, this is called being immunocompromised

arthropod-transmitted pathogens 节肢动物传播病原体 a general term used to describe infections caused by a group of viruses spread to people by the bite of infected arthropods (insects) such as mosquitoes and ticks

vaccination *n.* 接种疫苗 the administration of a vaccine to help the immune system develop immunity from a disease. Vaccines contain a microorganism or virus in a weakened, live or killed state, or proteins or toxins from the organism

cardiovascular problems 心血管问题 cardiovascular disease (CVD), a general term for conditions affecting the heart or blood vessels

nonvenomous *adj.* 无毒的 not producing venom

venomous *adj.* 有毒的 producing venom

traumatic *adj.* 创伤性的 deeply disturbing or distressing, relating to or denoting physical injury in medicine

envenom *v.* 使有毒，毒害 to fill or impregnate with venom; make poisonous

asymptomatic *adj.* 无症状的 producing or showing no symptoms

symptomatic *adj.* 有症状的 showing symptoms, or it may concern a specific symptom

falciparum malaria 恶性疟 a unicellular protozoan parasite of humans, and the deadliest species of Plasmodium that causes malaria in humans

lymphadenopathy *n.* 淋巴结病 a term that refers to the swelling of lymph nodes

splenomegaly *n.* 脾肿大 an enlarged spleen

climate change 气候变化 long-term shifts in temperatures and weather patterns. These shifts may be natural, such as through variations in the solar cycle. human activities have been the main driver of climate change, primarily due to burning fossil fuels like coal, oil and gas

EI Niño Southern Oscillations (ENSO) 厄尔尼诺事件 a recurring climate pattern involving changes in the temperature of waters in the central and eastern tropical Pacific Ocean

La Niña event 拉尼娜事件 the periodic cooling of ocean surface temperatures in the central and east-central equatorial Pacific. Typically, La Nina event occurs every 3-5 years or so, but on occasion can occur over successive years

（关万春）

Chapter 22
The Port Inspection and Quarantine

Learning objectives:
- Understand entry and exit health quarantine inspection of China.
- Be familiar with the International Health Regulations.
- Be familiar with the history of frontier health and quarantine in China.

22.1 Overview of International Health Regulations

Founded in 1948, the World Health Organization (WHO) has 194 member states across six regions. One of its central and historical responsibilities is the management of the global regime for controlling the international spread of diseases. The World Health Assembly is authorized by the Constitution of WHO to adopt regulations aimed at preventing the global spread of diseases. In 1969, The World Health Assembly a dopted the International Health Regulations ("the IHR" or "Regulations") to replace the International Sanitary Regulations (ISR) which was adopted by the Fourth World Health Assembly in 1951. Six "quarantinable diseases" were included in the 1969 Regulations and reduced to three (yellow fever, plague, and cholera) after amendments in 1973 and 1981.

In 1995, the Forty-eighth World Health Assembly called for a substantial revision of the 1969 Regulations, in consideration of the growth in international travel and trade, and the emergence or re-emergence of international disease threats and other public health risks. After ten years of endeavor, the IHR (2005) was eventually adopted by the Fifty-eighth World Health Assembly on 23 May 2005, and entered into force on 15 June 2007. The purpose and scope of the IHR (2005) is "to prevent, protect against, control and provide a public health response to the international spread of disease in ways that are commensurate with and restricted to public health risks, and which avoid unnecessary interference with international traffic and trade."

Compared to the 1969 Regulations, the IHR (2005) includes a range of innovations. For example, the scope declared by the revised IHR is not limited to any specific disease or manner of transmission, but includes diseases or medical conditions that cause or are likely to cause significant harm to human, regardless of origin or source. It also sets out the obligations of States Parties. Such as, the State Party is obligated to develop certain minimum core public health capacities, and to notify the WHO of events that may constitute a public health emergency of international concern according to defined criteria. Moreover, many technical and other regulatory functions, including certificates applicable to international travel and transport, and requirements for international ports, airports, and ground crossings, are also updated and revised in the IHR (2005).

22.2   Overview of the Frontier Health and Quarantine in China

As is known to all, the practice of quarantine began to fight against plague epidemics during the fourteenth century. Hundreds of years later, the practice of frontier health and quarantine in China began in 1873 when the deadly epidemic of cholera spread in the vast areas of South east Asia. The imperialist set up institutions of health quarantine at Shanghai and Xiamen ports, and carried out seaport quarantine following some simple health quarantine regulations. Foreign doctors were employed as port sanitary officers to carry out quarantine inspections on ships that came from epidemic areas. This is the beginning of China's entry and exit health quarantine. Unfortunately, throughout the long period of semi-feudal and semi-colonial society, there was little progress in health quarantine. Until the founding of the People's Republic of China, especially since the reform and opening up, progress and contributions have been made for the improvement of disease control and public health.

Since 1950, our country has adopted many health quarantine regulations. The Regulations of the People's Republic of China on Frontier Health and Quarantine was adopted at the 88th meeting of the Standing Committee of the First National People's Congress of the Communist Party of China on December 23,1957. This is the first health and quarantine regulation of the People's Republic of China. It included six quarantinable diseases (plague, cholera, yellow fever, smallpox, epidemic typhus, and relapsing fever). On December 2, 1986, the Frontier Health and Quarantine Law of the People's Republic of China was adopted at the 18th meeting of the Standing Committee of the Sixth National People's Congress of the CPC. The 1986 law was amended in 2007, 2009, and 2018, respectively.

Due to the institutional reform and adjustment of the State Council, the competent authority of health quarantine institution has been changed several times and is now the General Administration of Customs of the People's Republic of China (GACC). The missions of the Department of Health Quarantine under the GACC including ① formulating rules and procedures on entry-exit health quarantine and plans of public health emergency treatment; ② performing entry-exit health quarantine; ③ monitoring infectious diseases and overseas epidemics; ④ conducting health supervision and treatment; ⑤ coping with public health emergencies at ports.

22.3   Entry and Exit Health Quarantine Inspection of China

China is a state party of IHR, and its current laws and regulations of frontier health and quarantine are referred to IHR. What we carry out in frontier health and quarantine should be consistent with the principles stipulated in IHR and international practice. In accordance with the "Frontier Health and Quarantine Law of the People's Republic of China" and its specific rules, all persons, means of transport and transport equipment, luggage, goods and postal parcels that may spread quarantinable diseases must be subject to quarantine inspection when enter or exit the territory. This section mainly introduces quarantinable diseases, and health quarantine of travelers, conveyance and goods.

22.3.1   Quarantinable Diseases

According to the Frontier Health and Quarantine Law of P.R.C, the quarantinable diseases including yellow fever, plague, cholera, and other infectious diseases are determined and announced by the State Council. In line with the prevalence of infectious diseases, the State Council could approve other infectious diseases into the management of quarantinable diseases. For example, ebola haemorrhagic fever and COVID-19 were included in the management of quarantine diseases in 2014 and 2020 respectively. This section mainly introduces plague, cholera, and yellow fever.

22.3.1.1   Plague

Plague is caused by the bacteria *Yersinia pestis*, anaerobic, gram-negative coccobacillus in the family *Enterobacteriaceae*. It is transmitted between animals through fleas. The *Xenopsylla cheopis* flea is the primary vector for transmission, although roughly 80 species of fleas can carry it. The bacteria multiply in infected rodents and block the fleas' alimentary canal, causing the fleas to regurgitate the *Y. pestis* bacteria into its animal host. It is reported that more than 280 mammalian species can serve as carriers, including wild squirrels, rats, prairie dogs, marmots, gophers, and other rodents. Humans can be infected by the bite of infected vector fleas, unprotected direct contact with infectious bodily fluids and tissues or contaminated materials, and inhalation of infected respiratory droplets.

People infected with *Y. pestis* often develop symptoms after an incubation period of one to seven days. There are three major clinical forms of plague infection: bubonic, pneumonic, and septicaemic. Bubonic plague is the most common form and is characterized by painful swollen lymph nodes or "buboes". The bacteria reproduce rapidly in lymph nodes located closest to the flea bites, leading to painful swellings ("buboes") in the groin, cervical, or axillary lymph nodes, which can enlarge to the size of an egg (or up to 10 cm). If left untreated, the case-fatality ratio is estimated at 30% to 60% for the bubonic type. Human-to-human transmission of bubonic plague is rare. However, bubonic plague can advance and spread to the lungs, leading to a more severe type of plague called pneumonic plague. It is especially contagious and can trigger severe epidemics through person-to-person contact via droplets in the air. The septicemic plague is a rarer form (10%-15% of cases). It occurs when the bacteria multiply in the blood, often triggering disseminated intravascular coagulation and gangrene of the extremities, ears, or nose. The latter two clinical subtypes are invariably fatal without treatment.

Historically, the plague was known as the "Black Death" during the fourteenth century, causing more than 50 million deaths in Europe. Currently, plague outbreaks continue to occur and cause occasional deaths throughout the world. The three most prevalent countries are the Democratic Republic of the Congo, Madagascar, and Peru. In fact, between 2010 and 2015, there were 3 248 plague cases and 584 deaths worldwide, with the majority (75%) being in Madagascar.

22.3.1.2   Cholera

Cholera is an acute diarrhoeal infection caused by ingestion of food or water contaminated with the bacterium *Vibrio cholerae* which belongs to the *Vibrionaceae* family. More than 200 serogroups of *V. cholerae* are reported, but only serogroup O1 and O139 cause outbreaks. The O1 serogroup is divided into the classical and El Tor biotypes based on phenotypic and genetic markers. Vibrios secreting cholera toxin usually causes epidemics. The genes for cholera toxins are encoded by filamentous bacteriophages, which differ slightly between classical and El Tor biotypes. Serogroup O1 organisms have caused seven cholera pandemics recorded so far, but only the first six pandemics are caused by the classical biotype, and the seventh by El Tor biotype. *V. cholerae* O139 was first identified in Bangladesh in 1992 and has caused outbreaks in the past, but has recently been identified only in sporadic cases.

There is no difference in the illness caused by the two serogroups. Most people infected with *V. cholerae* do not develop any symptoms, although the bacteria are present in their faces for 1-10 days after infection and are shed back into the environment, potentially infecting others. It takes between 12 hours and 5 days for a person to show symptoms after ingesting contaminated food or water. The majority of people who develop symptoms have mild or moderate symptoms, while a minority develop acute watery diarrhea and vomiting. The stools usually assume the appearance of rice water with flakes of mucus, often with a fishy odor. If left untreated, it can lead to severe dehydration and even death within hours.

V. cholerae spreads through the faecal–oral route, and is closely linked to inadequate access to clean water and sanitation facilities. Cholera outbreak/epidemic can occur in both endemic countries and in countries where cholera does not regularly occur. In a country where cholera outbreaks infrequently occur, an outbreak is defined at least one confirmed case of cholera with evidence of local transmission. Today, cholera remains a global threat to public health and an indicator of inequity and lack of social development. The number of cholera cases reported to WHO has continued to be high over the past years. In 2019, 31 countries notified 923 037 cases, 1911 deaths. Africa seems to be the major locus of this disease burden. A study suggested that approximately 2.9 million cases and 95 000 deaths occur annually in epidemic countries, with 60% of cases and 68% of deaths recorded in Africa.

22.3.1.3 Yellow Fever

Yellow fever is an acute viral haemorrhagic disease transmitted by infected mosquitoes. The yellow fever (YF) virus is an RNA virus of the genus *Flavivirus* and family *Flaviviridae*. It is an arbovirus and transmitted by *Haemagogus*, *Sabethes* or *Aedes aegypti* mosquitoes. Different species of mosquito live in different habitats—some breed around houses (domestic), others in the jungle (wild), and some in both habitats (semi-domestic). There are three types of transmission cycles:

Sylvatic (or jungle) Yellow Fever Monkey are the primary reservoir of yellow fever in tropical rain forests, where they are bitten by wild mosquitoes of the *Aedes* and *Haemogogus* species, which spread the virus on to other monkeys. People who work or travel in the forest occasionally get bitten by infected mosquitoes and develop yellow fever.

Intermediate Yellow Fever In this type of transmission, semi-domestic mosquitoes infect both monkeys and humans. Increased contact between people and infected mosquitoes leads to increased transmission, and outbreaks can occur simultaneously in many separate villages in an area.

Urban Yellow Fever Large epidemics occur when infected people introduce the virus into densely populated areas with a high density of *Aedes aegypti* mosquitoes, and where most people have little or no immunity due to lack of vaccination or previous exposure to yellow fever. In these conditions, infected mosquitoes transmit the virus from person to person.

The incubation period for yellow fever is 3 to 6 days. It is estimated that half of those infected are asymptomatic, but when symptoms do occur, they are most commonly fever, muscle pain with prominent backache, headache, loss of appetite, and nausea or vomiting. These symptoms disappear after 3-4 days in most cases. However, approximately 15% of patients enter a second, more toxic phase, presenting with a high fever, affecting several body systems, usually the liver and the kidneys. In this phase, people are likely to develop jaundice (yellowing of the skin and eyes, hence the term "yellow fever"), dark urine, and abdominal pain with vomiting. Bleeding may occur in the mouth, nose, eyes, or stomach. Half of the patients who enter the toxic phase die within 10-14 days, while the rest recover without significant sequelae.

Currently, the disease is endemic only in the tropical forests of the African continent and Latin America. Forty-seven countries in Africa, Central and South America are either endemic or have some regions endemic to yellow fever. A study based on African data sources estimated the burden of yellow fever during 2013 was 84 000-170 000 severe cases and 29 000-60 000 deaths. Travelers who visit yellow fever endemic countries may occasionally bring the disease to countries free from yellow fever. To prevent the importation of the disease, many countries including China require proof of vaccination against yellow fever before issuing a visa, particularly if travelers come from, or have visited yellow fever endemic areas.

22.3.2 Travelers Quarantine

In China, the travelers quarantine is divided into routine quarantine and temporary quarantine. When a quarantinable infectious disease or a disease suspected to be quarantinable is discovered at a frontier port, or a person dies of an unidentified cause other than accidental injury, the temporary quarantine should be adopted. First, three measures are generally used to screen the public health risks carried by travelers, including health declarations, temperature monitoring and medical inspection. Second, the quarantine department identified risks through epidemiological case study, medical examinations and laboratory examinations. Then, many public health measures would be implemented to control the risks, for example, placing suspected persons under public health observation, implementing isolation and treatment for affected persons.

To better control the infections diseases at points of entry and prevent its spreading across the border, sometimes, the quarantine department may adjust quarantine measures according to the epidemic situation of diseases. For example, during the COVID-19 pandemic, the GACC decided to re-adopt the health declaration measures, requesting all inbound and outbound travelers to fill in the Health Declaration Form on Entry/Exit. This form is not required in the absence of a public health emergency of international concern. The GACC announced to require all inbound and outbound travelers must declare their health conditions to quarantine officers of China Customs, and cooperate with temperature monitoring, medical examination, and observation, as well as other public health measures.

22.3.3   Conveyance Quarantine

22.3.3.1   Ships Quarantine

According to the rules for implementing the Frontier Health and Quarantine Law of the People's Republic of China, entering ships shall undergo quarantine inspection at the port quarantine anchorage or at the specific places approved by institutions of health quarantine. Any ship subject to quarantine at entry points must hang up the quarantine signals and wait for inspection. It is not allowed to lower the quarantine signal before the quarantine certificate is issued by institutions of quarantine.

In the daytime, the quarantine signal is the signal flag of international code hung on the ship. "Q" flag means that the ship is not affected, requesting the entry quarantine certificate; "QQ" flag means that the ship is a suspected or affected ship, requesting quarantine immediately.

At night, the quarantine signal is lamps hung vertically in a conspicuous place on the ship. Three red lamps mean that the ship is not affected, requesting the entry quarantine certificate. Four lamps (red, red, white, and red) mean that the ship is a suspected or affected ship, requesting quarantine immediately.

Based on information received before the ship's arrival, if the quarantine institution considers that the ship's arrival will not cause the introduction or spread of disease, it may authorize the ship free pratique by radio or other means of communication. If a source of infection or contamination is found on board, the quarantine institution shall carry out necessary disinfection, decontamination, disinsection and deratting measures or take other necessary measures to prevent the spread of the infection or contamination.

22.3.3.2   Aircraft Quarantine

Upon the arrival of the aircraft subject to entry quarantine inspection at the airport, the quarantine staff shall board the plane first. The captain or his authorized representative is required to submit the general declaration form, passenger list, cargo manifest, a valid mosquito disinsection certificate, or other relevant certificates. Before the completion of quarantine inspection, no one shall be allowed to get on or off the aircraft, and no baggage, cargo, or parcels shall be loaded or unloaded unless permitted by the quarantine institution. Based on the inspection results, the quarantine staff shall grant a free pratique to a healthy aircraft. If a source of infection or contamination is found on the aircraft, the competent authority shall consider the aircraft as affected and take measures such as disinfection, decontamination, disinsection and deratting. Upon completion of the inspection of the aircraft, the quarantine staff shall sign and issue a quarantine certificate to a healthy aircraft, or issue a quarantine certificate when all sanitary measures required by the competent authority have been completed. If the aircraft is unable to take off as scheduled due to sanitary control, the airport shall be informed in time.

22.3.3.3   Ground Transport Vehicle Quarantine

On arrival of ground transport vehicles that are subject to entry quarantine at the ground crossing, the quarantine staff shall board the vehicle at first. The head of the train or the person in charge of the vehicle is required to report to the health quarantine institution on the sanitary conditions of the vehicle, and the health condition of persons. No one shall be allowed to get on or off the vehicle, load or unload baggage, cargo, or parcels without the quarantine institution's permission before obtaining the quarantine certificate. If the vehicles are considered as affected or suspected of being affected, sanitary measures including disinfection, decontamination, disinsection or deratting should be taken at the designated places. The waste, excreta, vomit, and food in vehicles should be thoroughly disinfected and buried deep or burned.

22.3.3.4   Cargo Quarantine

According to the IHR, cargo means goods carried on a conveyance or in a container. The types of goods are diverse and there are many ways to classify them. The cargo quarantine is to inspect whether a public health risk exists, effectively preventing the possible spread of infectious diseases, medical vectors, and other toxic and harmful substances through goods. When the goods arrive at the port of entry or exit, the carrier, agent, or owner must declare to the health and quarantine institution and accept inspection. Goods having been exposed, or possibly exposed, to a public health risk and that could be a possible source of the spread of disease shall be disinfected, disinsected, deratted, or treated with other necessary sanitary measures. Microorganisms, human tissue, biological products, blood and blood products that are classified as special goods, must be declared and inspected. Without the certificate of approval for special goods, no entry or exit shall be allowed.

Glossary

World Health Assembly 世界卫生大会

International Health Regulations 国际卫生条例

Frontier Health and Quarantine Law of the People's Republic of China 中华人民共和国国境卫生检疫法

General Administration of Customs of the People's Republic of China 中华人民共和国海关总署

quarantinable disease 检疫传染病 infectious diseases that seriously endanger human health and require frontier health and quarantine inspection according to law. For example, yellow fever, plague, cholera

contamination *n.* 污染 the presence of infectious or toxic agents or matter on a human or animal body surface, in or on a product prepared for consumption or on other inanimate objects, including conveyances, that may constitute a public health risk

decontamination *n.* 除污 a procedure whereby health measures are taken to eliminate an infectious or toxic agent or matter on a human or animal body surface, in or on a product prepared for consumption or on other inanimate objects, including conveyances, that may constitute a public health risk

conveyance *n.* 交通工具 an aircraft, ship, train, road vehicle or other means of transport on an international voyage

point of entry 入境口岸 a passage for international entry or exit of travelers, baggage, cargo, containers, conveyances, goods and postal parcels as well as agencies and areas providing services to them on entry or exit

ground crossing 陆路口岸 a point of land entry, including one utilized by road vehicles and trains

a public health emergency of international concern 国际关注的突发公共卫生事件 an extraordinary event which is determined, as provided in IHR, to constitute a public health risk to other States through the international spread of disease, and is to potentially require a coordinated international response

free pratique 无疫通行 permission for a ship to enter a port, embark or disembark, discharge or load cargo or stores; permission for an aircraft, after landing, to embark or disembark, discharge or load cargo or stores; and permission for a ground transport vehicle, upon arrival, to embark or disembark, discharge or load cargo or stores

（柏琴琴）

新形态教材网·数字课程学习……

💻 教学 PPT　　　📝 自测题　　　💬 推荐阅读

PART VI

Lab Management

Chapter 23
Accreditation and Certification of Laboratory

Learning objectives:

- Understand laboratory evaluation system in China.
- Be familiar with the laboratory accreditation system.
- Master the laboratory mandatory approval system.

23.1 Overview of Laboratory Evaluation System

As the economy and technology continue to advance, consumers are demanding higher quality products, which has led to the growth of the inspection and testing industry. To ensure accuracy and reliability, inspection bodies and laboratories must undergo a rigorous assessment process known as laboratory evaluation before issuing data to the public. The first national laboratory accreditation system was established in Australia in 1947, with the creation of the National Association Testing of Australia (NATA). Since then, many developed countries have established their own laboratory accreditation structures, with developing countries following suit. As global trade has increased, the need to eliminate non-tariff barriers has led to the emergence of regional laboratory accreditation cooperation organizations, promoting exchanges and cooperation among national laboratory accreditation systems. In 1975, the Western European Calibration Cooperation Organization (WECC) became the first laboratory accreditation cooperation organization. Later, in 1991, the International Accreditation Forum (IAF) was established with the primary objective of harmonizing certification systems across different countries. The IAF aims to ensure effective international mutual recognition by standardizing auditor qualification requirements, training criteria, and assessment and certification procedures of quality system certification bodies in each member state. As a result, certification bodies accredited by the accreditation bodies that have signed the IAF multilateral recognition agreement can be trusted and recognized globally in areas such as management systems, products, services, personnel, and other conformity assessment projects. In 1992, the Asia-Pacific Regional Laboratory Cooperation Organization (APLAC) was founded. Four years later, the International

Laboratory Accreditation Cooperation (ILAC) was established with the goal of achieving mutual recognition of test reports issued by accredited laboratories. This was accomplished through the signing of mutual recognition agreements (MRA) between laboratory accreditation agencies. Fast forward to 2019, the Asia Pacific Laboratory Accreditation Cooperation (APLAC) and the Pacific Accreditation Cooperation (PAC) merged to form a new regional accreditation cooperation organization, the Asia Pacific Accreditation Cooperation (APAC). APAC's main responsibility is to oversee and enhance a Mutual Recognition Arrangement (MRA) between accreditation bodies in the Asia Pacific area. This MRA allows for conformity assessment outcomes generated by accredited Conformity Assessment Bodies (CABs) from one APAC MRA signatory to be recognized and accepted by all other APAC MRA signatories. This mutual recognition and acceptance of conformity assessment results significantly reduces the need for redundant testing, inspection, or certification, resulting in time and cost savings, improved economic efficiency, and the promotion of international trade.

In China, there are two distinct laboratory evaluation systems: mandatory approval and accreditation. Under the mandatory approval system, both the inspection body and laboratory employ the same set of evaluation methods. Conversely, the accreditation system involves the use of different evaluation methods by the inspection body and laboratory. As such, this article will focus solely on the evaluation method employed by laboratories.

23.2   Mandatory Approval

According to the "44 Administrative Measures for the Mandatory Approval of Inspection Body and Laboratory," an inspection body and laboratory are defined as a legally established entity that uses instruments, equipment, environmental facilities, and professional skills to inspect products or specific objects specified by laws and regulations, in accordance with relevant standards or technical specifications. Mandatory approval is carried out by the Certification and Accreditation Administration of the People's Republic of China (CNCA) and the provincial quality and technical supervision department. This approval process evaluates whether the inspection body and laboratory meet the legal requirements outlined in relevant laws, regulations, standards, and technical specifications. Once the basic conditions and technical capabilities are met, the evaluation licenses are issued. The assessment of mandatory approval involves CNCA and the provincial quality and technical supervision department evaluating whether inspection bodies and laboratories meet the requirements outlined in the "Competence assessment for inspection body and laboratory mandatory approval-general requirements for inspection body and laboratory (RB/T 214-2017) and the supplementary requirements for evaluation." This evaluation is conducted in accordance with the Administrative Licensing Law of the People's Republic of China, either by the departments themselves or by professional technical evaluation institutions. The process involves examining the basic conditions and technical ability of the inspection body and laboratory. Mandatory approval is required for certain bodies and laboratories and is overseen by China Metrology Accreditation (CMA).

23.2.1 History of Mandatory Approval

After the "Measurement Law of the People's Republic of China" was issued in 1986, mandatory evaluation and administrative licensing of inspection bodies and laboratories were implemented in China. The "Detailed Rules for the Implementation of the Metrology Law of the People's Republic of China" was issued in 1987, which named our country's laboratory accreditation system as the "China Metrology Accreditation" system for the first time. In 1990, the State Bureau of Technical Supervision introduced the first laboratory evaluation system in our country, known as the "Technical Assessment Specification for Metrology Accreditation of Product Quality Inspection Organizations" (JJF 1021-1990). Laboratories that passed the assessment of "China Metrology Accreditation" were authorized to use the CMA logo in their inspection reports, as shown in Figure 23-1. Inspection reports with the CMA logo can be used for product quality evaluation, achievement and judicial appraisal, and have legal effect.

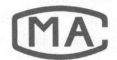

Figure 23–1 CMA logo

Around the same time as the implementation of the Metrology Accreditation system, a laboratory evaluation process was introduced known as the review and accreditation system. This system involves an administrative review and accreditation process that adheres to the regulations outlined in laws such as the Standardization Law, the Implementation Regulations of the Standardization Law, the Product Quality Law, the Management Measures of the National Product Quality Supervision, Inspection and Testing Center, and the Management Measures of Product Quality Supervision and Testing Stations. The review and accreditation system is designed to evaluate the quality inspection institutes of technical supervision departments at all levels, as well as national and provincial quality inspection centers (stations) authorized by quality and technical supervision departments. These institutes are responsible for tasks such as supervision, inspection, and arbitration. Laboratories that have undergone the review and accreditation process are identified by the CAL logo, as shown in Figure 23-2.

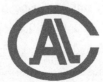

Figure 23–2 CAL logo

The process of review and accreditation, which involves review, acceptance, and legal authorization, bears a striking resemblance to metrology accreditation in terms of implementation and evaluation criteria. However, there are notable differences in the laws, regulations, and application objects. Metrology accreditation is applicable to all laboratories that issue notarized data in society, while review and accreditation are limited to quality inspection centers (stations) established and authorized by the technical supervision bureau in accordance with the law. During this period, the evaluation criteria for metrology accreditation were based on the "Technical Assessment Specification for Metrology Certification of Product Quality Inspection Institutions" (JJF1021-1990).The evaluation criteria for review and accreditation, which includes review and acceptance as well as legal authorization, were established based on the "Detailed Rules for Review and Accreditation of National Product Quality and Technical Supervision and Inspection Center", "Detailed Rules for Acceptance of Product Quality and Technical Supervision and Inspection Institute", and "Detailed Rules for Review and Accreditation of Product Quality and Technical Supervision and Inspection Station". However, in 2000, the former State Bureau of Technical and Quality Supervision decided to streamline the process and avoid repeated on-site assessments by combining the requirements for metrology accreditation and review and accreditation. As a result, the "Evaluation Criteria for Metrological Accreditation/Review and Accreditation (Acceptance) of Product Quality Inspection Institutions (Trial)" ([2000] No. 46) was issued, unifying the evaluation criteria for metrology accreditation and the review and accreditation.

In 2006, CNCA issued the "Laboratory Mandatory Approval Evaluation Criteria" (2006 version) as a replacement for the "Evaluation Criteria for Metrological Accreditation/Review and Accreditation (Acceptance) of Product Quality Inspection Institutions (Trial)." In 2015, the former General Administration of Quality Supervision, Inspection, and Quarantine of the People's Republic of China issued Order No. 163, which introduced the "Administrative Measures for the Qualification Accreditation of Inspection Body and Laboratory." This change shifted the focus of mandatory approval from product quality inspection institutions to inspection bodies and laboratories

23.2.2 Evaluation Basis of Mandatory Approval

The current evaluation basis of mandatory approval is the "Administrative Measures for the Qualification Accreditation of Inspection Body and Laboratory" (Order No.163 of the General Administration) and "Competence Assessment for Inspection Body and Laboratory Mandatory Approval-General Requirements for Inspection Body and Laboratory" (RB/T 214-2017). The "Administrative Measures for the Qualification Accreditation of Inspection Body and Laboratory" includes seven chapters, including general provisions, qualification conditions and procedures, technical review management, inspection and testing institution employed norms, supervision and management, legal responsibility and supplementary provisions, with a total of 50 clauses. The "Competence Assessment for Inspection Body and Laboratory Mandatory Approval, as outlined in RB/T 214-2017", encompasses five key elements: institutions, personnel, site environment, equipment facilities, and management systems. This comprehensive standard comprises a total of 49 clauses and has been issued by CNCA to replace the previous "Criteria for the Evaluation of Qualification Accreditation of Inspection Body and Laboratory." Since its implementation in 2018, RB/T 214-2017 has become mandatory for all inspection and testing fields. However, for inspection bodies and laboratories operating in specialized fields, additional supplementary requirements may apply, and evaluations must be conducted accordingly. For instance, the "Competence Assessment for Inspection Body and Laboratory Mandatory Approval-Requirements for Food Test Body" (RB/T 215-2017), is a set of regulations that must be followed for the mandatory approval of food test bodies. Similarly, the "Competence Assessment for Inspection Body and Laboratory Mandatory Approval - Requirements for Motor Vehicle Test Body" (RB/T 218-2017), is applicable to the mandatory approval of motor vehicle safety technical inspection bodies, motor vehicle emission inspection bodies, and vehicle comprehensive performance inspection bodies. The "Competence Assessment for Inspection Body and Laboratory Mandatory Approval - Requirements for Forensic Identification Body" (RB/T 219-2017), applies to the mandatory approval of forensic identification bodies. "Competence Assessment for Inspection Body and Laboratory Mandatory Approval-Requirements for Medical Device Inspection Body" (RB/T 217-2017), is a set of regulations that must be followed for the mandatory approval of medical device inspection bodies.

The approval for inspection bodies and laboratories is mandatory and remains valid for a period of six years. The accreditation mark for these entities consists of the English abbreviation CMA, which stands for China Inspection Body and Laboratory Mandatory Approval, along with the unique accreditation certificate number.

23.2.3 Levels of Mandatory Approval

There are two levels of mandatory approval in China: national and provincial. National-level mandatory approval pertains to inspection bodies and laboratories that are legally established by relevant departments of the State Council and industry authorities. These institutions fall into four categories: public institutions registered by the State Public Institution Registration Administration, enterprise legal persons registered or approved by the State Administration for Industry and Commerce, institutions directly under the jurisdiction of relevant departments of the State Council and industry authorities, and institutions jointly determined by the relevant departments of the State Council, competent departments of relevant industries, and industry associations, as necessary, in collaboration with the CNCA. Provincial mandatory approval, on the other hand, is the responsibility of the provincial approval department and applies to inspection bodies and laboratories established in accordance with the law within its administrative region. This includes quality inspection institutes (institutions) in provinces, autonomous regions, municipalities directly under the Central Government, sub-provincial cities, cities under deputy provincial level, cities listed in the plan, and provincial fiber inspection institutions.

23.2.4   Procedures for Assessment of Mandatory Approval

According to the "Administrative Measures for the Qualification Recognition of Inspection Body and Laboratory" , the general procedures for assessment of mandatory approval of inspection body and laboratory are as follows.

(1) The applicant, which refers to the inspection body and laboratory applying for mandatory approval, must submit a written application and relevant materials to either the State Administration for Market Regulation or the provincial market supervision and administration department. The applicant is responsible for ensuring the authenticity of the submitted materials.

(2) The department responsible for mandatory approvals is required to conduct a thorough review of the application and accompanying materials submitted by the applicant. Within five working days of receiving the application, the department must make a decision regarding acceptance or rejection and communicate this decision to the applicant in writing.

(3) Within 30 working days of receiving the application, the mandatory approval department will conduct a technical assessment of the applicant in accordance with the basic norms and assessment criteria for mandatory approval of inspection bodies and laboratories. This assessment will include both paper and on-site (or remote) reviews. The technical review time is separate from the qualification accreditation period, and the mandatory approval department will inform the applicant of the review timeline. However, if the applicant is unable to complete the work within the specified time due to rectification or other reasons, the department will make an exception.

(4) The mandatory approval department will make a decision on whether to grant the license within 10 working days of receiving the technical review conclusion. If the license is granted, the applicant will receive a qualification certificate within 7 working days of the decision. If permission is not granted, the applicant will receive a written notification explaining the reasons.

23.2.5   Supervision and Administration

To enhance the supervision and management of inspection bodies and laboratories and standardize their practices, the State Administration for Market Regulation has issued the "Measures for the Supervision and Administration of Inspection Bodies and Laboratories" (Order No.39) in 2021. This ordinance comprises five major parts, including the responsibilities of inspection bodies and their personnel, the norms of inspection and testing practices, the crackdown on false and fraudulent inspection and testing behaviors, the implementation of the new market supervision mechanism, and the legal responsibilities for violations of laws and regulations. With a total of 50 clauses, this ordinance aims to address the main issues in the inspection and testing market and promote the healthy and orderly development of the industry. It is of significant practical importance to reinforce the main responsibility of working institutions, strengthen supervision during and after events, and severely penalize false and fraudulent inspection and testing behaviors.

23.3　Laboratory Accreditation

Accreditation is a process whereby an accreditation body evaluates conformity assessment bodies that are involved in certification, testing, and inspection activities, in accordance with relevant international or national standards. This evaluation confirms that these bodies meet the requirements of the relevant standards, and have the necessary technology, ability, and management skills to engage in certification, testing, and inspection activities. Upon successful completion of the evaluation, the accreditation body issues a certificate of accreditation. Accreditation can be classified into three categories: certification body accreditation, laboratory and related body accreditation, and inspection body accreditation.

Laboratory accreditation means that an accreditation body conducts assessments in accordance with laws and regulations, based on the requirements of GB/T 27011 and different standards in different fields, It formally recognizes conformity assessment bodies that meet the requirements, and issues an accreditation certificate to prove that the organization has the technical and managerial competence to carry out specific conformity assessment activities. These laboratory accreditations include as follows.

(1) The testing or calibration laboratories are reviewed base on GB/T 27025 "General Requirements for Testing and Calibration Laboratory Capacity" (equivalent to adopting the international standard ISO/IEC 17025) to confirm the ability to carry out testing or calibration activities.

(2) Medical laboratories are evaluated according to GB/T 22576 "Specific Requirements for the Quality and Competence of Medical Laboratories" . This standard is equivalent to the internationally recognized ISO 15189. The purpose of this evaluation is to ensure that the laboratory has the necessary skills and resources to conduct medical testing activities with accuracy and precision.

(3) The laboratories that deal with pathogenic microorganisms are subject to a thorough review process based on GB 19489 "General Requirements for Laboratory Bio-safety" . This review is conducted to ensure that the laboratory's bio-safety protection measures meet the corresponding level of safety required for handling such microorganisms.

(4) The proficiency testing plan providers are reviewed base on GB/T 27043 "General Requirements for Conformity Assessment Proficiency Testing" (equivalent to adopting the international standard ISO/IEC 17043) to confirm the ability to provide proficiency testing.

(5) The reference materials producers are evaluated base on GB/T 15000.7 "General Requirements for the Competence of Reference Material/Standard Sample Producers" . This standard is equivalent to the internationally recognized ISO 17034, which confirms that these producers possess the necessary capacity for reference material production.

23.3.1 History of Laboratory Accreditation in China

Laboratory accreditation activities in China have a long history, dating back to 1980 when the former National Bureau of Standards and the former State Administration for Import and Export Commodities Inspection (SACI) jointly organized a group to participate in the International Laboratory Accreditation Cooperation Conference. Since then, several accreditation committees have been established, including the China National Accreditation Committee for Laboratories (CNACL) in 1994 and the China Import and Export Commodity Inspection Laboratory Accreditation Committee (CCIBLAC) in 1996. In 2001, the China National Certification and Accreditation Administration (CNCA) was established to manage national certification and accreditation work. In 2002, CNACL and CCIBLAC merged to form the China National Accreditation Board for Laboratories (CNAL), which is responsible for accrediting laboratories and inspection bodies in China. The unification of the laboratory accreditation system in China has greatly improved the quality and reliability of laboratory testing and inspection services in the country.

In 2002, the Certification and Accreditation Administration of the State Council approved the establishment of the China National Accreditation Board for Certification Agencies (CNAB). This body was formed through the merger of several former accreditation services, including the China National Accreditation Service for Quality System Certification (CNACR), the China National Accreditation Service for Product Certification (CNACP), the China National Accreditation Body for Import and Export Enterprises (CNAB), and the China Accreditation Committee of Environmental Management System Certification Body (CACEB). CNAB's primary responsibility is to accredit certification bodies for a range of management system certifications and product certifications, as well as oversee related work.

In 2006, the China National Accreditation Service for Conformity Assessment (CNAS) was established and approved by CNCA. CNAS is the result of the integration of CNAB and CNAL, and it is responsible for the uniform accreditation of relevant institutions such as certification bodies, laboratories, and inspection agencies. As a full member of IAF, ILAC, and APAC, CNAS plays a crucial role in international recognition activities and is an integral part of the international recognition and mutual recognition system. Therefore, CNAS accreditation is widely recognized as authoritative, independent, impartial, technical, non-native, unified, and international.

23.3.2 The role of Accreditation

The laboratory has voluntarily sought approval to participate in laboratory accreditation. Accreditation organizations offer their services to laboratories of all types, including government, third-party independent, enterprise, and private laboratories. But why is accreditation important for laboratories? Accreditation benefits not only the laboratory but also the country, society, and enterprises. The advantages of accreditation are as follows.

(1) In terms of competency assessment: The purpose of this assessment is to showcase the

conformity assessment body's capability to conduct a specific conformity assessment.

(2) In terms of government supervision: The primary objective of this assessment is to increase the government's trust in the use of conformity assessment results such as certification, testing, and inspection. This assessment helps to reduce the uncertainty associated with decision-making and technical evaluation in administrative licensing. By reducing administrative supervision risks and costs, the government can ensure that the conformity assessment results are accurate and reliable, thereby enhancing public safety and protecting the environment.

(3) In terms of promoting trade: This assessment aim to sign multilateral or bilateral mutual recognition agreements with international organizations, regional organizations, or foreign accreditation agencies. This will facilitate the international mutual recognition of conformity assessment results and ultimately boost foreign trade.

(4) In non-trade areas: The assessment aim to improve normative, quality, and capacity in non-trade areas such as health, safety, and social services.

(5) In terms of market competition: The assessment help to enhance the social visibility and market competitiveness of conformity assessment bodies and their clients.

(6) In terms of continuous improvement: continuous improvement involves implementing systematic and standardized technical evaluations, as well as providing ongoing supervision of conformity assessment bodies.

23.3.3　CNAS Certification Mark

The CNAS certification mark is a graphic symbol that is granted by CNAS. This mark can be used on laboratory test reports and calibration certificates that have been approved by CNAS, including reports on ROHS (Restriction of Hazardous Substance), PAHS (Polycysclic Aromatic Hydrocarbons), safety tests, and calibration. The CNAS certification mark typically includes the CNAS logo, an indication of the approval system, and a registration number. This registration number can be verified on the official CNAS website to confirm that the laboratory's testing and calibration capabilities cover the scope of the report. The CNAS certification mark is depicted in Figure 23-3, with the letter "L" representing laboratory approval and "XXXX" indicating the approved serial number.

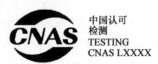　　　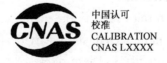

A　　　　　　　　　　　　　　　B

Figure 23-3　CNAS certification marks of testing and calibration laboratory

(A: CNAS certification marks of testing laboratory; B: CNAS certification marks of calibration laboratory)

(Rules for the Use of Accreditation Symbols and Reference to Accreditation, CNAS)

CNAS is proud to be a signatory of the multilateral recognition agreement ILAC. This agreement grants CNAS the right to use the ILAC-MRA international mutual recognition mark, which is used in accordance with relevant regulations. To further enhance our recognition, CNAS typically combines the International Mutual Recognition Mark with our own CNAS Logo, creating the Joint International Mutual Recognition Logo. As shown in Figure 23-4.

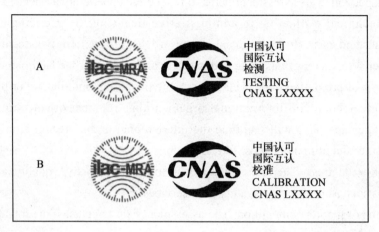

Figure 23–4   International mutual recognition joint recognition identification

A: ILAC-MRA/CNAS of testing laboratory; B: ILAC-MRA/CNAS of calibration laboratory

(Rules for the Use of Accreditation Symbols and Reference to Accreditation, CNAS)

23.3.4   Accreditation Standards

CNAS adheres to international standards, guidelines, and other normative documents issued by renowned organizations such as ISO/IEC, IAF, ILAC, and APAC, as well as the accreditation specifications issued by CNAS. These specifications are normative documents that accredited laboratories must comply with. CNAS conducts compliance assessments on the management and technical capabilities of certification bodies, laboratories, and inspection bodies in accordance with these specifications. Accreditation specifications include accreditation rules, criteria, guidelines, schemes, instructions, and technical reports. While some documents such as accreditation rules, criteria, instructions, and certain schemes are mandatory requirements, accreditation guidelines and technical reports are non-mandatory documents that laboratories can use as a reference.

Accreditation Rules

Accreditation rules refer to the policies and procedures established by CNAS to govern the implementation of accreditation activities in accordance with regulations and international organization requirements. These rules are divided into two categories: general accreditation rules (R) and special accreditation rules (RL). The General Accreditation Rules (R) consist of three documents, namely CNAS-RO1:2020 "Rules for the Use of Accreditation Symbols and Reference to Accreditation", CNAS-R02:2018 "Rules for Impartiality and Confidentiality", and CNAS-R03:2019 "Rules for Dealing with Appeals, Complaints and Disputes" . The dedicated Accreditation Rules (RL) comprise ten documents, including CNAS-RL01:2019 "Rules for the Accreditation of Laboratories", CNAS-RL02:2018 "Rules for the Accreditation of Proficiency

Testing Provider", CNAS-RL05:2016 "Rules for the Accreditation of Laboratory Biosafety", and CNAS-RL10:2020 "Rules for the Accreditation of Biobank".

Accreditation Criteria

Accreditation criteria serve as the fundamental basis for assessing conformity assessment bodies, such as certification bodies, laboratories, and inspection agencies. These criteria outline the basic requirements that these bodies must meet, including both basic and application accreditation criteria. The basic accreditation criteria consist of 10 documents, identified by the CL series code letters, such as CNAS-CL01: 2018 "Accreditation Criteria for the Competence of Testing and Calibration Laboratories". CNAS-CL07:2021 "Accreditation Criteria for the Competence of Reference Measurement Laboratories in Laboratory Medicine". CNAS-CL08:2018 "Accreditation Criteria for the Competence of Forensic Units", CNAS-CL09:2019 "Accreditation Criteria for Research Laboratory", CNAS-CL10:2020 "Accreditation Criteria for the Quality and Competence of Bio-bank". The application accreditation criteria are specific to particular fields or industries and are identified by a criteria name or suffix, such as CNAS-CL01-A001:2018 "Guidance on the Application of Testing and Calibration Laboratory Competence Accreditation Criteria in the Field of Microbiological Testing", CNAS-CL01-A025:2022 "Application of Laboratory Accreditation Criteria in the Field of Calibration", CNAS-CL01-G001: 2018 "Application of CNAS-CL01<Accreditation Criteria for the Competency of Testing and Calibration Laboratories>", CNAS-CL02-A001:2021 "Application Requirements of Accreditation Criteria for the Quality and Competence of Medical Laboratories", CNAS-CL03-A001:2019 "Guidance on the Application of Accreditation Criteria for Proficiency Testing Providers in the Field of Microbiology", CNAS-CL05-A001:2018 "Guidance on the Application of Laboratory Bio-safety Accreditation Criteria: Evaluation of Mobile Laboratories", CNAS-CL08-A007:2018 "Guidance on the Application of Accreditation Criteria for the Competence of Forensic Units in the Field of Forensic Toxicological Analysis and Drugs Testing".

Accreditation Guidelines

Accreditation Guidelines refer to the recommendations and guidance documents provided by CNAS for accreditation rules, criteria, and processes. These guidelines are comprised of a total of 50 files, typically identified by the GL series code. Examples of these files include CNAS-GL001:2018 "Guidance on Laboratory Accreditation," CNAS-GL006:2019 "Guidance on Quantifying Uncertainty in Chemical Analysis," CNAS-GL011:2018 "Guidance on Internal Audit for Laboratories and Inspection Bodies," and CNAS-GL050:2021 "Guidance on Medical Laboratories Accreditation in the Field of Molecular Diagnostics."

Accreditation Scheme

The Accreditation Scheme serves as a complementary framework to the accreditation rules, criteria, and guidelines established by CNAS for various fields and industries, in accordance with legal requirements and the needs of system owners. Typically identified by the S series file code, examples of Accreditation Schemes include CNAS-CL01-SO1:2018 "Accreditation Scheme for NIM," CNAS-CLO1-S02:2018 "Accreditation Scheme for Energy Star® Laboratories," and

CNAS-CL01-S03:2020 "Accreditation Scheme for Anti-Doping Laboratories."

Accreditation Statement

The accreditation statement is a set of specific requirements and clarifications that are necessary for the implementation of accreditation specifications by CNAS. These requirements are outlined in a series of 18 files, generally referred to as the EL series. Each file is assigned a unique code, such as CNAS-EL-03:2016 "Description on the Scope of Accreditation of Testing and Calibration Laboratories", CNAS-EL-06:2013 "Description on the Scope of Accreditation in the Field of Food Testing", CNAS-EL-13:2019 "Accreditation Instructions for Requirements Related to Test Reports and Calibration Certificates".

Technical Report

A technical report is a document issued by CNAS that provides a detailed description of technical procedures and guidelines for relevant conformity assessment bodies. These reports are typically identified by a file code in the TRL series, such as CNAS-TRL-003 "Assessment and Examples of Calibration and Measurement Capability (CMC)", CNAS-TRL-010:2019 "Application of Measurement Uncertainty in Compliance Determination".

Currently, CNAS utilizes CNAS-CL01:2018 "Accreditation Criteria for the Competency of Testing and Calibration Laboratories" as the fundamental standard for laboratory accreditation, which is equivalent to the international standard ISO/IEC17025:2017. In addition, CNAS has developed a series of application notes for laboratory accreditation criteria in specific technical fields. CNAS also requires laboratories to adhere to the relevant application guidelines of APLAC and ILAC. CNAS-CL01:2018 consists of five parts: general requirements, structural requirements, resource requirements, process requirements, and management system requirements. The general requirement includes impartiality and confidentiality. Structural requirements emphasize the laboratory's legal and substantive responsibility. Resource requirements include six elements: general, personnel, facilities and environmental conditions, equipment, metrological traceability, and externally provided products and services. The process requirements include eleven elements: review of requirements, bids and contracts, selection, validation and validation of methods, sampling, handling of testing and calibration items, technical records, evaluation of measurement uncertainty, ensuring the validity of results, reporting results, complaints, nonconforming work, control of data, and information management. Management system requirements include nine elements: options, management system documentation (option A), control of management system documentation (option A), control of records (option A), actions to address risks and opportunities (option A), improvement (option A), corrective actions (option A), internal audits (option A), and management reviews (option A).

23.3.5   Accreditation Process

There are seven stages involved in obtaining initial approval for CNAS accreditation for the first time. These stages include expressing the intention to apply, submitting a formal application and receiving acceptance, undergoing document review, establishing an assessment group, conducting an on-site assessment, undergoing accreditation assessment, and finally, receiving the certificate and having it published.

Intent to Apply

The applicant can express their intention to apply to the CNAS secretariat through various means, including visiting in person, contacting via telephone, fax, or other electronic communication methods. The CNAS secretariat will provide the applicant with the most up-to-date version of the accreditation rules and other pertinent documents.

Formal Application and Acceptance

Once the self-assessment has met the accreditation conditions, the applicant must submit the required application materials to the CNAS secretariat and pay the application fee. The CNAS will then review the submitted materials and determine whether to accept the application, notifying the applicant accordingly. In the event that an initial visit is necessary to determine the application's suitability, the CNAS secretariat will arrange for one. Throughout the data review process, the CNAS secretariat will inform the applicant of any discrepancies found with the accreditation conditions. Generally, the evaluation will be arranged within 3 months of receiving the application.

Document Review

After the CNAS secretariat has accepted the application, an assessment team leader will be assigned to review the application documents. The on-site assessment can only be scheduled if the results of the document review meet the necessary requirements. Any issues discovered during the document review will be communicated to the applicant by the CNAS secretariat. In some cases, a pre-assessment may be necessary to determine whether an on-site assessment can be arranged.

Set up the Assessment Group

To ensure fairness, the CNAS secretariat will establish an assessment group with the appropriate technical expertise based on the applicant's scope of application, including testing, calibration, appraisal, laboratory site, and scale. The applicant's consent will be obtained before proceeding. If an applicant refuses to accept the CNAS assessment group arrangement without valid reasons, the accreditation process may be terminated, and recognition may not be granted by CNAS.

On-site Assessment

On-site assessment is a crucial step in the accreditation process, where the assessment group evaluates the technical capabilities and quality management activities of the applicant's application. The assessment is conducted in accordance with the accreditation criteria, rules, and requirements of CNAS, laboratory management system documents, and relevant technical standards. The assessment should cover all activities and related venues involved in the scope of the application. The on-site assessment time and number of personnel are determined based on the number of testing/calibration/identification sites, items/parameters, methods, standards/norms, etc., within the scope of the application. The on-site review process includes several stages, such as the first meeting, on-site visit (if necessary), on-site evidence collection, communication between the assessment group and the applicant on the review, and the final meeting. During the on-site assessment, if the assessed laboratory is found to have violated relevant national laws and regulations or other circumstances that are detrimental to the reputation and rights and interests of CNAS, the assessment group shall report it to the CNAS secretariat. In serious cases, CNAS has the right to terminate the accreditation process and take corresponding measures. The assessment group leader shall submit the results of the on-site assessment to the assessed laboratory at the final meeting. If non-conformity items are discovered during the on-site assessment, the assessed laboratory shall carry out timely rectification according to the requirements. Corrections/ corrective measures shall usually be completed within two months, and the review group shall verify their effectiveness. If the corrections/corrective actions are effective, the assessment group leader will report the final assessment report and recommendations to the CNAS secretariat.

Accreditation Assessment

The CNAS secretariat is responsible for submitting the evaluation report, relevant information, and recommendations to the evaluation committee. The committee evaluates the applicant's compliance with the accreditation requirements and provides an evaluation conclusion. The evaluation conclusion may fall into one of the following four categories: a) Approved; b) Partially approved; c) Not approved; d) Re-evaluation is required based on additional evidence or information. The secretary-general of CNAS or the authorized personnel makes the accreditation decision based on the assessment conclusion.

Issuance and Publication

The CNAS accreditation cycle typically lasts for 2 years, during which a reassessment is conducted to determine the accreditation status. Accreditation certificates are issued by the CNAS secretariat to accredited laboratories, and these certificates are generally valid for 6 years. To maintain their accreditation status, accredited laboratories must notify the CNAS secretariat of their intention to do so at least one month before the expiration of their accreditation certificate. The CNAS secretariat renews the accreditation certificate based on the laboratory's expressed intention, as well as the results of previous evaluations and accreditation decisions made during the validity period of the certificate. The CNAS secretariat is responsible for publishing and updating information related to the accreditation status, basic information, and accreditation scope of accredited laboratories.

Once a laboratory is approved for accreditation, it is subject to ongoing surveillance assessments by CNAS. These assessments are designed to ensure that the laboratory continues to meet the accreditation requirements throughout the validity period of accreditation. Additionally, they ensure that the laboratory is able to adapt to any changes in accreditation rules, criteria, or technical capabilities. If a laboratory is found to be non-compliant during a surveillance assessment, CNAS will require it to implement corrective measures within a specified timeframe. In severe cases, CNAS may suspend, narrow, or revoke the laboratory's approval immediately. Therefore, it is essential for conformity assessment bodies to operate in accordance with approved requirements to ensure the competence and impartiality of their accredited conformity assessment activities. They must also take responsibility for the authenticity, accuracy, and validity of any certificates or reports issued.

Glossary

mandatory approval 资质认定 Certification and Accreditation Administration of the People's Republic of China (CNCA) and the provincial quality and technical supervision department would implement the evaluation license when the basic conditions and technical capabilities of the inspection body and laboratory meet the legal requirements in accordance with relevant laws, regulations, standards, and technical specifications

inspection body and laboratory 检验机构 a legal establishment, in accordance with relevant standards or technical specifications, using instruments, equipment, environmental facilities and other technical conditions and professional skills to inspect products

accreditation *n.* 认可 an accreditation body conducts assessments of conformity assessment bodies engaged in certification, testing and inspection activities in accordance with relevant international standards or national standards to confirm that they meet the requirements of relevant standards and have the technologies to engage in certification, testing and inspection activities, ability and management ability by issuing a certificate of accreditation

metrology accreditation 计量认证 the first form of madatory approval in China, which performed by national or provincial quality and technical supervision department to confirm the the inspection body and laboratory can meet the legal requirements in accordance with relevant laws, regulations, standards, and technical specifications

CMA 中国计量认证 China Metrology Accreditation

CAL 中国审查认可 China Accreditation of Laboratory

IAF 国际认可论坛 International Accreditation Forum

APAC 亚太地区认证合作组织 Asia Pacific Accreditation Cooperation

ILAC 国际实验室认可合作组织 International Laboratory Accreditation Cooperation

MRA 多边互认协议 Mutual Recognition Agreement

CNCA 中国国家认证认可监督管理委员会 Certification and Accreditation Administration of the People's Republic of China

CNAL 中国实验室国家认可委员会 China National Accreditation Board for Laboratories

CNAS 中国合格评定国家认可委员会 China National Accreditation Service for Conformity Assessment

（黄东萍）

新形态教材网·数字课程学习……

教学 PPT　　　自测题　　　推荐阅读

Chapter 24

Biosafety

Learning objectives:

- Know the concepts related to laboratory biosafety.
- Understand the relevant guidelines and standards of laboratory biosafety.
- Be familiar with the good microbiological practice and procedure in biosafety laboratories.
- Master the classification of biological agents and biosafety laboratories.

There are many biological hazards present in clinical, research, and industrial production laboratories. Work with infectious agents may have the risk of occurrence of laboratory-associated infection (LAI) if there is no proper protection. Laboratory-associated infection means any infection acquired or reasonably assumed as a result of exposure to a biological agent in the course of laboratory-related activities, also known as laboratory-acquired infections. The historical accounts of LAI have raised awareness about the hazards of infectious microorganisms and the health risks to laboratory workers who handle them. Reports of LAI can serve as lessons in the importance of maintaining safe conditions in biological research. Many published accounts have suggested practices and methods that might prevent LAI. In order to reduce LAI and protect the public health and environment, the first edition of the laboratory biosafety manual was published by the World Health Organization (WHO) in 1983. Subsequently, many countries have used the expert guidance provided in the manual to develop national codes of practice for the safe handling of pathogenic microorganisms in laboratories. The fourth edition of the manual was published in 2020. Application of this knowledge and the use of appropriate techniques and equipment will be able to prevent personal, laboratory and environmental exposure to potentially infectious agents or biohazards. Similarly, individual workers who handle pathogenic microorganisms must understand the containment conditions under which infectious agents can be safely manipulated and secured.

24.1　Biological Risk Assessment

The backbone of the practice of biosafety is risk assessment. Risk assessment is a stepwise process used to identify the hazardous characteristics of a known infectious or potentially infectious agent or material, the activities that can result in a person's exposure to an agent, the likelihood that such exposure will cause a LAI, and the probable consequences of such an infection. The purpose of the risk assessment is to gather information, evaluate it and use it to provide a guide for the selection of appropriate biosafety levels and microbiological practices, safety equipment, and facility safeguards that can prevent LAI. The causative incident for most LAI is unknown. Only less obvious exposures such as the inhalation of infectious aerosols or direct contact of the broken skin or mucous membranes with droplets containing an infectious microorganism or surfaces contaminated by droplets may possibly explain the incident responsible for a number of LAI. It is important to note that hazards alone do not pose a risk to humans or animals. The laboratory procedure hazards must be considered when the biological hazard agents are used for laboratory work. Risk assessment requires careful judgment. Adverse consequences are more likely to occur if the risks are underestimated. It is important to note that not all factors will affect risk in the same way, but each should be carefully considered.

24.1.1　Hazardous Characteristics of an Agent

The harm caused by exposure to biological agents can vary in nature and can range from an infection or injury to a disease or outbreak in larger population. The principal hazardous characteristics of an agent are: its capability to infect and cause disease in a susceptible human or animal host, its virulence as measured by the severity of disease, and the availability of preventive measures and effective treatments for the disease. WHO has recommended an agent risk group classification for laboratory describes four general risk groups (WHO Risk Groups 1, 2, 3 and 4) based on these principal characteristics and the route of transmission of the natural disease. The four groups address the risk to both the laboratory worker and the community. The State Council of the People's Republic of China Guidelines established a comparable classification and assigned human etiological agents into four risk groups on the basis of hazard. The descriptions of the WHO risk group classifications are presented in Table 24-1. They correlate with but do not equate to biosafety levels. A risk assessment will determine the degree of correlation between an agent's risk group classification and biosafety level.

24.1.2　Hazardous Characteristics of Laboratory Procedures

Investigations of LAI have identified five principal routes of laboratory transmission. These are parenteral inoculations with syringe needles or other contaminated sharps, spills and splashes onto skin and mucous membranes, ingestion through mouth pipetting, animal bites and scratches, and inhalation exposures to infectious aerosols. The first four routes of laboratory transmission are

Table 24-1 Classification of infective microorganisms by risk group

Risk group classification	Descriptions of risk group	Some common pathogenic microorganism
Risk Group 1 (no or low individual and community risk)	A microorganism that is unlikely to cause human or animal disease	Guinea pig herpes virus, mouse leukemia virus
Risk Group 2 (moderate individual risk, low community risk)	A pathogen that can cause human or animal disease but is unlikely to be a serious hazard to laboratory workers, the community, livestock or the environment. Laboratory exposures may cause serious infection, but effective treatment and preventive measures are available and the risk of spread of infection is limited	Rotavirus, adenovirus, rubella virus, *Streptococcus pneumoniae*, *Enterobacter* spp, *Staphylococcus aureus*
Risk Group 3 (high individual risk, low community risk)	A pathogen that usually causes serious human or animal disease but does not ordinarily spread from one infected individual to another. Effective treatment and preventive measures are available	Human immunodeficiency virus, poliovirus, *Bacillus anthracis*, *Mycobacterium tuberculosis*, *Vibrio cholera*, *Yersinia pestis*
Risk Group 4 (high individual and community risk)	A pathogen that usually causes serious human or animal disease and that can be readily transmitted from one individual to another, directly or indirectly. Effective treatment and preventive measures are not usually available	Ebola virus, smallpox virus

easy to detect, but account for less than 20% of all reported LAI. Most reports of such infections do not include sufficient information to identify the route of transmission of infection. An aerosol generated by procedures and operations is the probable source of many LAI. Aerosols are a serious hazard because they are ubiquitous in laboratory procedures, and are usually undetected. Most manipulations of liquid suspensions of microorganisms produce aerosols and droplets. Small particle aerosols are respirable particles that may contain one or several microorganisms. These small particles stay airborne and are easily dispersed throughout the laboratory. When inhaled, the human lung will retain those particles. Larger particle droplets rapidly fall out of the air, contaminating gloves, the immediate work area, and the mucous membranes of unprotected workers. Procedures and equipment used routinely for handling infectious agents in laboratories, such as pipetting, blenders, centrifuges, sonicators and vortex mixers are proven sources of aerosols. A procedure's potential to release microorganisms into the air as aerosols and droplets are the most important operational risk factor.

Technique can significantly impact aerosol output and dose. The worker who is careful and proficient will minimize the generation of aerosols. A careless and hurried worker will substantially increase the aerosol hazard.

24.1.3   Potential Hazards Associated with Worker Practices, Safety Equipment and Facility Safeguards

Workers are the first line of defense for protecting themselves, others in the laboratory, and the public from exposure to hazardous agents. Protection depends on the conscientious and proficient microbiological practices and the correct use of safety equipment. Carelessness is the most serious concern, because it can compromise any safeguards of the laboratory and increase the risk for coworkers. Training, experience, knowledge of the agent and procedure hazards, good habits, caution, attentiveness, and concern for the health of coworkers are prerequisites for a laboratory staff in order to reduce the inherent risks that attend work with hazardous agents.

Safety equipment such as biological safety cabinets (BSC), centrifuge safety cups, and sealed rotors are used to provide a high degree of protection for the laboratory worker from exposure to microbial aerosols and droplets.

Facility safeguards help prevent the accidental release of an agent from the laboratory. Their use is particularly important for the agents that can transmit disease by the inhalation route or that can cause life-threatening disease.

24.2   An Approach to Assessing Risks and Selecting Appropriate Safeguards

Biological risk assessment is a subjective process requiring consideration of many hazardous characteristics of agents and procedures, with judgments based often on incomplete information. Risk assessments should be conducted in a standardized and systematic way to ensure they are repeatable and comparable. The following describes a five-step approach that gives framework to the risk assessment process.

Identifying Agent Hazards

The principal hazardous characteristics of the agent should be considered, which include its capability to infect and cause disease in a susceptible human host, severity of disease, and the availability of preventive measures and effective treatments.

When new biological agents are being used, or there are specimens for which detailed data are unknown, the information available may be insufficient to be able to make an appropriate assessment of the risk. In such cases, it is sensible to take a cautious approach to specimen manipulation and handle all materials as potentially infectious.

Identifying Laboratory Procedure Hazards

The principal laboratory procedure hazards are high concentration or volume of the biological agent, malfunctioning equipment and laboratory activities associated with aerosolization (for example, sonication, homogenization, centrifugation), and the use of sharps. The complexity of a laboratory procedure can also present a hazard.

Selecting and Implementing Risk Control Measures

A variety of risk control measures including the practices, safety equipment, and facility safeguards will be available depending upon the nature of the risk identified, the available resources, and other local conditions. It should be noted that laboratories worldwide could face unique challenges that will influence the results of a risk assessment and the risk control measures implemented may vary considerably from laboratory to laboratory, institution to institution, region to region and country to country. It must be remembered that even after a risk control measure is selected for your risk strategy, a certain degree of risk will still remain.

Evaluating the Proficiencies of Staff

The protection of laboratory workers, other persons associated with the laboratory, and the public will depend ultimately on the laboratory workers themselves. An evaluation of a person's training, experience in handling infectious agents, proficiency in the use of sterile techniques and BSCs, ability to respond to emergencies, and willingness to assume responsibility for protecting one's self and others is important insurance that a laboratory worker is capable of working safely.

Review Risks and Risk Control Measures

A risk assessments must be reviewed routinely and revised when necessary, taking into consideration new information about the biological agent, changes in laboratory activities or equipment and new risk control measures that may need to be applied.

24.3   Principles of Biosafety

A fundamental objective of any biosafety program is the containment of potentially harmful biological agents. The purpose of containment is to reduce or eliminate exposure of laboratory workers, other persons, and the outside environment to potentially hazardous agents.

24.3.1   Laboratory Practices and Technique

The most important element of containment is strict adherence to standard microbiological practices and techniques. Persons working with infectious agents or potentially infected materials must be aware of potential hazards, and must be trained and be proficient in the practices and techniques required for handling such material safely.

Each laboratory should develop or adopt a biosafety or operations manual that identifies the hazards that will or may be encountered, and that specifies practices and procedures designed to minimize or eliminate exposures to these hazards.

24.3.2   Safety Equipment (Primary Barriers and Personal Protective Equipment)

Safety equipment includes BSC, enclosed containers, and other engineering controls designed to remove or minimize exposures to hazardous biological materials. The BSC is the principal device used to provide containment of infectious droplets or aerosols generated by many microbiological procedures.

Safety equipment may also include items for personal protection, such as gloves, laboratory coats, shoe covers, boots, respirators, face shields, safety glasses, or goggles. Personal protective equipment (PPE) refers to a set of wearable equipment and/or clothing worn by personnel to provide an additional barrier between them and the biological agents being handled, which effectively controls risk by reducing the likelihood of exposure to the agents.

24.3.3 Facility Design and Construction (Secondary Barriers)

The design and construction of the facility contributes to the laboratory workers' protection, provides a barrier to protect persons outside the laboratory, and protects persons or animals in the community from infectious agents that may be accidentally released from the laboratory.

24.4 Biosafety Levels

Four biosafety levels are designated in ascending order as biosafety level 1 (BSL-1), biosafety level 2 (BSL-2), biosafety level 3 (BSL-3) and biosafety level 4 (BSL-4), based on the risk group and protective measures taken for biological agents operated (Table 24-2). The basic practices and equipment are appropriate for protocols common to most research and clinical laboratories. The facility safeguards help protect nonlaboratory occupants of the building and the public health and environment.

Table 24–2 Summary of recommended biosafety levels and practices and equipment

BSL	Laboratory type	Laboratory practices	Safety equipment
1	Basic teaching, research	Good microbiological practice and procedure (GMPP)	Open bench work, autoclave
2	Primary health services; diagnostic services, research	As BSL 1 plus: protective clothing, biohazard warning sign, sharps precautions, limited access, biosafety manual defining any needed waste decontamination or medical surveillance policies	Open bench plus: biological safety cabinet for potential aerosols, autoclave
3	Special diagnostic services, research	As BSL 2 plus: special clothing, controlled access, directional airflow, baseline serum	Biological safety cabinet and/ or other primary devices for all activities
4	Dangerous pathogen units	As BSL 3 plus airlock entry, shower exit, special waste	Class III biological safety cabinet, positive pressure suits, double ended autoclave (through the wall), filtered air

The BSLs should be differentiated from risk groups. Risk groups are the result of a classification of microbiological agents based on their association with, and resulting severity of, disease in humans. The risk group of an agent should be one factor considered in association with mode of transmission, procedural protocols, experience of staff, and other factors in determining the BSL in which the work will be conducted.

Biosafety Level 1

Biosafety level 1 (BSL-1) is the basic level of protection and is suitable for work involving well-characterized agents that are not known to cause disease in normal, healthy humans and present minimal potential hazard to laboratory personnel and the environment. Work is generally conducted on the open bench tops using GMPP.

Biosafety Level 2

Biosafety level 2 (BSL-2) is suitable for work involving agents that pose moderate hazards to personnel and the environment. In addition to meeting all BSL-1 laboratory requirements, the following requirements should be met: access to the laboratory is restricted when work is being conducted, all operations that may create infectious aerosols or splashes are conducted in BSCs or other physical containment equipment, the entrance must be clearly marked with international universal biological hazard signs and the biosafety level, biological agents, information of the person in charge, etc (Figure 24-1).

Biosafety Level 3

Biosafety level 3 (BSL-3) is appropriate for agents with a known potential for aerosol transmission, for agents that may cause serious or potentially lethal infections through the inhalation route of exposure. All operations involving the manipulation of infectious materials must be conducted within BSCs or other physical containment devices. A BSL-3 laboratory has special engineering and design features.

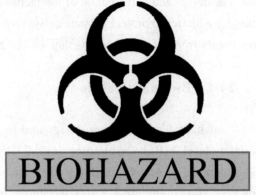

Figure 24-1 Biohazard warning sign for laboratory doors

Biosafety Level 4

Biosafety level 4 is required for work with dangerous and exotic agents that pose a high individual risk of aerosol-transmitted laboratory infections and life-threatening disease that is frequently fatal, for which there are no vaccines or treatments, or a related agent with unknown risk of transmission. The laboratory shall be built in a separate building which shall be far away from the urban area.

24.5 Good Microbiological Practice and Procedure

Good microbiological practice and procedure (GMPP) is a term given to a set of standard operating practices and procedures, or a code of practice, that is applicable to all types of activities with biological agents. It includes general behaviors, best working practice, and technical procedures. The implementation of standardized GMPP serves to protect both the laboratory personnel and the specimens themself from exposure to and/or release of biological agents. It is essential that laboratory personnel are trained and proficient in GMPP to ensure safe working practices. For most laboratory activities, the likelihood of exposure to and/or release of the biological agent is unlikely, GMPP needs to be promoted and laboratory activities needs to be reviewed periodically to ensure that GMPP is effectively implemented.

24.5.1   Best Practice

Best practice describes behaviors that are essential to facilitate safe work practices and control biological risks. For example. (1) Never store food or drink, or personal items such as coats and bags in the laboratory. Activities such as eating, drinking, smoking, and applying cosmetics are only to be performed outside the laboratory. (2) Wash hands thoroughly, preferably with warm running water and soap, after working with potentially hazardous materials and before leaving the laboratory.

24.5.2   Technical Procedures

Technical procedures are a special subset of GMPP which relate directly to controlling risks through safe conduct of laboratory techniques. The following procedures would help avoid certain biosafety incidents occurring.

Avoiding inhalation of biological agents

Use good techniques to minimize the formation of aerosols and droplets when manipulating specimens. For example, it must be done slowly and with care where pipette are used for mixing. Brief centrifuging of mixed tubes before opening can help move any liquid away from the cap.

Avoiding ingestion of biological agents and contact with skin and eyes

Wear disposable gloves at all times when handling specimens known or reasonably expected to contain biological agents. Shield or otherwise protect the mouth, eyes and face during any operation where splashes may occur, such as during the mixing of disinfectant solutions.

Avoiding injection of biological agents

Wherever possible, replace any glassware with plastic-ware. If glassware must be used, check it on a regular basis for integrity Never re-cap, clip or remove needles from disposable syringes. Dispose of any sharps materials in puncture-proof or puncture-resistant containers fitted with sealed covers.

Preventing dispersal of biological agents

Place waste containers, preferably unbreakable (such as plastic, metal), at every workstation. Ensure all waste is properly conducted. Decontaminate work surfaces with a suitable disinfectant at the end of the work procedures and if any material is spilled.

24.6 Biosafety and Biosecurity

Biosafety and biosecurity are related, but not identical, concepts. Laboratory biosafety is the term used to describe the containment principles,technologies and practices that are implemented to prevent unintentional exposure to pathogens and toxins, or their accidental release.

Laboratory biosecurity refers to institutional and personnel security measures designed to prevent the loss, theft, misuse, diversion or intentional release of biological agents, and research-related information. This is accomplished by limiting access to facilities, research materials and information.

While the objectives are different, biosafety and biosecurity measures are usually complementary. Effective biosafety practices are the foundation of laboratory biosecurity and biosecurity risk control measures must be performed as an integral part of an institution's biosafety programme management.

24.7 Transportation of Infectious Substances

It is often necessary to transport specimens, biological materials or waste that are known or expected to contain biological agents between rooms, laboratories, regions or even countries for further testing, treatment or storage. The materials from the laboratory that may contain biological agents are known as infectious substances, which may exist as cultures, patient or animal specimens, infected body parts or organs, and biological products such as live attenuated vaccines or similar therapeutic products, infectious genetically modified organisms or medical/clinical wastes. For transport purposes, these infectious substances may be further subdivided into Category A, Category B and Exempt human/animal specimens. Category A infectious substances are defined as any material(s) known or reasonably expected to contain, biological agents capable of causing permanent disability, or lifethreatening or fatal disease in otherwise healthy humans or animals. Any material(s) containing biological agents capable of causing infection in humans or animals, but which do not meet the criteria for inclusion in Category A are defined as Category B. Exempt human or exempt animal specimens are defined as s substances or materials derived from human or animal patients (that are clinical specimens) for which there is a minimal likelihood that infectious biological agents are present.

Transportation of infectious substances and materials is subject to regulatory controls. Most of the regulations for the transport of infectious substances are based upon the United Nations Model Recommendations on the Transport of Dangerous Goods. International and domestic transport regulations for infectious substances are designed in order to reduce the likelihood of an exposure to a release of the infectious substance during transit to protect the public, workers, and the surrounding environment. Protection is achieved through rigorous packaging requirements and hazard communication. In addition, shippers and carriers must be trained on these regulations so they can properly prepare shipments and recognize and respond to the risks posed by these materials.

Glossary

biosafety *n.* 生物安全 the safety from exposure to infectious agents

biohazard *n.* 生物危害 the hazard to humans or the environment resulting from biological agents or conditions

droplet *n.* 小滴，微滴 a very small drop of liquid

aseptic technique无菌技术 the conditions and procedural measures designed to effectively prevent contamination

inhalation *n.* 吸入 the act of inhaling; the drawing in of air (or other gases) as in breathing

aeration *n.* 通风，充气 the process of exposing to air

prerequisite *n.* 先决条件 something that is required in advance

containment *n.* 控制 the act of containing; the act of keeping something from spreading

gauze *n.* 纱布，薄纱 bleached cotton cloth of plain weave used for bandages and dressings

respirator *n.* 口罩 a protective mask with a filter; to protect the face and lungs against poisonous gases

（李迎丽）

新形态教材网·数字课程学习……

🖥️ 教学 PPT　　　📝 自测题　　　💬 推荐阅读

References

[1] 涂建成，梁纯子. 医学检验专业英语. 北京：人民卫生出版社，2022.

[2] 吕斌，张际文. 卫生检疫学. 北京：人民卫生出版社，2015.

[3] 曲章义. 卫生微生物学. 6 版. 北京：人民卫生出版社，2017.

[4] 黎源倩，叶蔚云. 食品理化检验. 2 版. 北京：人民卫生出版社，2015.

[5] 康维钧，张翼翔. 水质理化检验. 2 版. 北京：人民卫生出版社，2015.

[6] 吕志平. 口岸公共卫生与传染病检疫核心能力. 北京：人民卫生出版社，2013.

[7] 袁长祥. 口岸检验检疫实务. 北京：中国质检出版社，2014.

[8] 葛志荣. 质检专业英语检验检疫部分（上）. 北京：中国标准出版社，2004.

郑重声明

高等教育出版社依法对本书享有专有出版权。任何未经许可的复制、销售行为均违反《中华人民共和国著作权法》，其行为人将承担相应的民事责任和行政责任；构成犯罪的，将被依法追究刑事责任。为了维护市场秩序，保护读者的合法权益，避免读者误用盗版书造成不良后果，我社将配合行政执法部门和司法机关对违法犯罪的单位和个人进行严厉打击。社会各界人士如发现上述侵权行为，希望及时举报，我社将奖励举报有功人员。

反盗版举报电话　（010）58581999　58582371

反盗版举报邮箱　dd@hep.com.cn

通信地址　北京市西城区德外大街4号　高等教育出版社法律事务部

邮政编码　100120

读者意见反馈

为收集对教材的意见建议，进一步完善教材编写并做好服务工作，读者可将对本教材的意见建议通过如下渠道反馈至我社。

咨询电话　400-810-0598

反馈邮箱　gjdzfwb@pub.hep.cn

通信地址　北京市朝阳区惠新东街4号富盛大厦1座　高等教育出版社总编辑办公室

邮政编码　100029

防伪查询说明

用户购书后刮开封底防伪涂层，使用手机微信等软件扫描二维码，会跳转至防伪查询网页，获得所购图书详细信息。

防伪客服电话　（010）58582300